A CLINICIAN'S GUIDE TO

RHEUMATIC DISEASES IN CHILDREN

A CLINICIAN'S GUIDE TO

RHEUMATIC DISEASES IN CHILDREN

Thomas J. A. Lehman

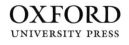

OXFORD

UNIVERSITY PRESS

2009

OXFORD

UNIVERSITY PRESS

Oxford University Press, Inc., publishes works that further
Oxford University's objective of excellence
in research, scholarship, and education.

Oxford   New York
Auckland   Cape Town   Dar es Salaam   Hong Kong   Karachi
Kuala Lumpur   Madrid   Melbourne   Mexico City   Nairobi
New Delhi   Shanghai   Taipei   Toronto

With offices in
Argentina   Austria   Brazil   Chile   Czech Republic   France   Greece
Guatemala   Hungary   Italy   Japan   Poland   Portugal   Singapore
South Korea   Switzerland   Thailand   Turkey   Ukraine   Vietnam

Published by Oxford University Press, Inc.
198 Madison Avenue, New York, New York 10016

www.oup.com

Oxford is a registered trademark of Oxford University Press

Library of Congress Cataloging-in-Publication Data

Lehman, Thomas J. A.
A clinician's guide to rheumatic diseases in children / Thomas J.A. Lehman.
p. ; cm.
Includes bibliographical references and index.
ISBN: 978-0-19-534190-4
1. Rheumatism in children. 2. Pediatric rheumatology. I. Title.
[DNLM: 1. Rheumatic Diseases—diagnosis. 2. Rheumatic
Diseases—therapy. 3. Adolescent. 4. Child. WE 544 L523c 2009]
RJ482.R48L447 2009
618.92′723—dc22
2008021621

1   3   5   7   9   8   6   4   2

Printed in the United States of America
on acid-free paper

This book is dedicated to the many physicians and other professionals who care for children around the world with muscle, bone, joint pain, or arthritis.

On a more personal note, I would like to dedicate this book to the memory of five physicians who greatly inspired me but are no longer with us:

Dr. Harry O. Zamkin, a pediatrician who loved his patients;

Dr. Virgil Hanson, a pediatric rheumatologist who taught me that pediatric rheumatology was not learned from textbooks—it is learned by listening and carefully evaluating the children you treat every time you see them;

Dr. Barbara Ansell, a pediatric rheumatologist who taught me that an "atypical case of A" was most likely a "typical case of B" that I had not thought of, and so much more;

Dr. Arthur D. Schwabe, a gastroenterologist who taught me to never stop asking questions of the children, their families, and myself until all the answers fit together and made sense;

Dr. John Decker, for many years the "Dean" of rheumatology at the National Institutes of Health in Bethesda, Maryland, who inspired so many by his quiet confidence combined with a willingness to endorse any idea that seemed sensible, no matter that it had "never been done before"; and last, to

Dr. Jack Klippel (who is very much still with us!), for continuing to say, "If not you, who? It's your idea—do it."

Contents

PART III: LIVING WITH A CHILD WHO HAS A CHRONIC CONDITION

Introduction

This is not a textbook. It is a guidebook. Like a traveler's guidebook, it will help you find your way in unfamiliar territory. This book provides the information physicians need to make sure that children with muscle, bone, or joint pain or arthritis in their care, and the families of these children, are getting the best care and the information they need.

This book will give pediatricians and other primary care providers the information necessary to ask meaningful questions of both the parents and the specialists to whom they refer children so that they can properly evaluate the alternative choices available and help families determine the best course for the child's care.

This book is designed to help physicians recognize the children who need to be referred to a specialist and care for those who do not. More importantly, parents will seek help from their primary physician or other health professionals when they have questions about the specialist's recommendations. This book provides the information needed to explain these recommendations and help parents understand their choices.

This is not a traditional textbook of pediatric rheumatology or pediatric orthopedics. It is a guide to the chronic rheumatic and orthopedic conditions of childhood. Like every guidebook, it does not cover everything. I have empha-sized the more common conditions and the more important problems where early recognition and treatment can make a lifelong difference in the outcome. Not everyone will agree with all that I have written—just as travelers' guidebooks may disagree on which are the best restaurants and hotels in a given city. If you are looking for long lists of detailed references, put this book down. This book will provide you with the insights I have gained from over thirty years of expe-rience in caring for children with muscle, bone, and joint pain and rheumatic diseases. Very few of the key insights concerning how to take a history of joint pains or even how to properly examine a child with joint pains are reflected in the literature. Pediatric rheumatology remains a young specialty with relatively few patients and fewer practitioners.

Today, millions of dollars are spent annually on research on causes of disease and newer medications, but few of the children I see do poorly because doctors lack the necessary tools to treat them. The majority of children with rheumatic disease do well. Most who do poorly do so because too much time elapsed before they came to proper medical attention or because their parents and caregivers had too little understanding of the many treatments available and the importance of proper treatment. It is vital that primary care providers recognize children with significant conditions and refer them promptly to appropriate specialists. Most forms of arthritis are not life-threatening, but the damage done by chronic pain and disability in childhood will have a lifelong effect. This is especially true for the child who was repeatedly told, "There's nothing really wrong with you. It's just growing pains."

I am writing this book in the hope that it will speed the proper diagnosis and referral of many children with unrecognized or improperly treated problems. Much of the information is not in textbooks, and in many cases it has not been rigorously proven. This is the type of information for which you go out of your way to find an experienced specialist. Often when parents discuss treatment options with their physicians, reference will be made to "controlled clinical trials." It is important to understand that there are far too few children with rheumatic disease for large-scale controlled trials of any but the simplest questions, and even then the results are sometimes contradictory.

When physicians, trained in the field, cannot all agree on the right answers, how can parents make the proper choices? They will be forced to rely on the experience of the specialist they have chosen; for most parents, that will be the specialist they were referred to by their primary care provider. When parents have questions about what the specialist recommended, it will be the primary care provider they return to for guidance. This book reflects my experience. The care of children with muscle, bone, and joint pain and arthritis is still more an art than a science. As in cooking, the best results depend far more on experience, careful monitoring, and minor adjustments than on strict adherence to the written recipe. Not every physician will share my opinions. Not every physician is willing to go beyond the "proven" in reaching for the best possible outcome. The final decisions will always be in the hands of the parents. They will need not just their specialist's guidance, but yours as well.

A NOTE ON THE CASE HISTORIES

I have included many illustrative stories throughout the text. The names, ages, and other identifying details have been changed to protect patient confidentiality, but the examples are all real ones from my experience.

How to Use This Book

The purpose of this book is to guide health care providers through the process of determining and responding to whatever is causing the children they care for to have muscle, bone, or joint pain or arthritis. Everyone reading this book will have different needs and a different background. I have tried to make the writing clear and the science easily understood, with as little jargon as possible.

If you are the physician of a child who has been given a specific diagnosis, you should begin by reading about that diagnosis to see whether it describes the child in your care. When the child's diagnosis is known, this book has useful chapters on medications, the meaning of laboratory test results, family issues, getting the best care, and reconstructive surgery. You will find a lot of information that will allow you to make informed choices and help get the best possible results.

If you are caring for a child with many complaints who does not have a diagnosis, begin with Chapter 2, "Figuring Out What's Wrong." It is my goal to help you think about what the correct answer might be. This book will help you to consider what questions to ask. Make sure that children and families with chronic complaints are getting the time and attention needed. Often there is a significant underlying reason for these complaints that might be medical, psychosocial, or both. Whatever it is, it needs to be addressed.

This book will give pediatricians and other primary care providers the information they need to properly evaluate children with musculoskeletal pain before deciding to refer them. It will help you know what tests to do and help you to decide whether and to which specialist to refer the child. This book will also help you evaluate the advice your patients are being given. Specialists need your help in explaining to families what they are doing to take care of the children and why. If the situation doesn't make sense to you, call the specialist yourself. If you don't get the answers you need to make things clear to the family, there's a problem. Knowing when to recommend that your patient seek an additional opinion is one of the most important services you can provide. No specialist should ever be afraid of listening to a different viewpoint.

PART I

A CHILD COMPLAINS OF PAIN

1

Growing Pains?

Little Jennifer S. was fourteen months old when her mother noticed that she did not want to put her left foot firmly on the floor when she was taken out of her crib one morning. She did not walk correctly for a few minutes, but an hour later she seemed fine. This did not happen again until a couple of weeks later. After six weeks, Jennifer's mother noticed that it was happening more frequently. She mentioned this to the pediatrician when she brought in Jennifer for her immunizations one afternoon. The pediatrician wiggled Jennifer's leg around, watched her walk a few feet, and reassured Jennifer's mother that she was fine. When Mrs. S. called the pediatrician a month later to discuss bringing her in, she was told that the problem was probably just "growing pains." By the time Jennifer was seen in the pediatric rheumatology clinic at the age of two years, her left knee was markedly swollen, she could not straighten her left leg all the way, and the muscles of her left leg were much weaker than those of her right leg. Jennifer had obvious arthritis. Reassured by what the pediatrician had told her, her mother had continued to believe that Jennifer just had growing pains until Jennifer screamed when the nurse tried to straighten her leg at her two-year-old checkup.

Quick Summary

- Growing pains never occur during the daytime.
- No matter how severe the pain is at night, children with growing pains are always fine the next morning.
- Any child with pain or a limp on awakening in the morning or recurring during the day requires a full medical evaluation.

EVALUATING REPORTS OF PAIN

Whenever a child limps or complains that an arm or leg hurts, the first thought is that he or she must have injured it. Even if a child is old enough to deny it, we often assume an injury. The family is likely to seek medical advice only if the pain is very severe or persists for more than a day or two. Even when the pain or limp continues beyond a few days, parents and many physicians often dismiss the problem as growing pains. Children do have growing pains; in fact, they are fairly common. But unfortunately, many children with serious problems are misdiagnosed with growing pains for weeks or even months. Children with arthritis are often first noticed because they walk abnormally when they wake up in the morning, but since the problem often comes on gradually and "they get better in a few minutes," no one is concerned.

Growing pains typically occur in young children between the ages of three and eight years. The child will wake up suddenly complaining that his or her legs hurt. Parents become aware of the problem because the child is crying in bed. Most often the episodes occur a few hours after the child has gone to sleep, but they may occur in the middle of the night. Typically, the child will point to the front or back of the knee or the muscles just above the knee. The pain usually disappears with ten or fifteen minutes of gentle massage and is completely gone in the morning. The pain is always in a large joint such as the knee, not in a finger or toe. Sometimes the pains will wake up the child two or three nights in a row, but more often they occur episodically. Growing pains often occur after days of extra activity. They may disappear for months or years, only to start again during another period of rapid growth.

The key finding in evaluating a child for growing pains is that the child is absolutely fine when he or she wakes up in the morning. There is no pain, limp, or any other abnormality. If any pain is still present when the child wakes up in the morning or occurs while the child is awake, this must not be dismissed as growing pains. Minor aches and pains during the day have many possible explanations, but they are not growing pains.

For a child with typical growing pains, laboratory and radiologic testing is not usually necessary. If a child has absolutely classic pains and is always fine in the morning, the family can usually treat the child with gentle reassurance. However, if the pains are persistent or unusually severe, a complete medical evaluation is warranted. Any child with recurrent pain during the day should be evaluated.

If blood tests or X-rays are done at the time of medical evaluation, a child with growing pains should have absolutely normal results. Bone scans, magnetic resonance imaging (MRI), and other special tests are not necessary for a child with growing pains. But they may be necessary to exclude other causes of pain in children who have atypical findings, persistent severe pain, or pain during the day as well. Bone tumors and osteoid osteomas are uncommon, but they may initially present with pain at night.

WHAT ARE GROWING PAINS?

There are a variety of possible explanations for growing pains. The best explanation is that growing pains result from tendons and muscles being stretched as the bones of the legs become longer. The fact that they only occur at night is related to the gate control theory of pain. This is easy to explain. As you read these words, you will suddenly become aware of feeling the shoes on your feet (if you're wearing shoes). A minute ago, you probably were not aware of the feeling. The nerves in your feet did not suddenly turn on. They were always sending their message to your brain. However, the posterolateral thalamic nucleus filters these inputs and suppresses those that can be ignored.

During the day when children are active, any message to the brain from tendons and muscles being stretched by growth is lost in all the other things going on. But when a child is falling asleep at night and there are no distractions, the pain impulses from stretching of the muscles and tendons may be passed on to cortical centers, causing the child to wake up. As a result, growing pains occur most often during periods of rapid growth and after days with extra physical activity.

Growing pains can be disturbing to both parents and children, particularly when they occur several days in a row. Most often, gentle massage and reassurance are enough to help the child go back to sleep. Children with more severe pain usually will respond to a dose of acetaminophen or ibuprofen. It may be helpful to give children who wake up with pain several nights in a row a dose of medication at bedtime. This will decrease the perception of pain and may prevent the child from waking up. After two or three nights without episodes, the medication should be stopped.

Growing pains will go away. They may come back when the child goes through another period of rapid growth, but they never stay. While inconvenient, they have no long-term significance. They do not interfere with proper growth or development. If the child complains of pain during the day, a more complete investigation should be done. If the pains persist despite medication use or return as soon as the medication is stopped, a full medical evaluation should be done.

2

Figuring Out What's Wrong

Before going to medical school, I had to take all the required classes in college. Many of the classes required for medical school satisfied the requirements for majoring in zoology in college. I enjoy the outdoors and was happy to sign up for field zoology as one of the required courses. Armed with guidebooks, we walked around the local hills in small groups with an instructor looking for and identifying birds. Sometimes the instructor would hear a noise or see a bird vaguely in the distance and tell us what it was. Frequently, it was too far away to see the identifying characteristics noted in the guidebook, but when we got closer, we saw that his identification was correct. At other times, one of us would become very excited and announce that we had just seen a bird we had never seen before and we were sure it was, for example, a Mexican jay. The instructor would just shake his head. No matter how sure we were that it matched the picture in the book, he would point out that we were not in (or even close to) Mexico and that a common bird in our area looked a little bit like the Mexican jay. A few minutes' investigation would invariably prove that he was right and we were wrong. He had been teaching this course in the same hills for many years. Each bird had a typical behavior, a typical place where it was likely to be seen, and a typical time of year when it was likely to be there. These things were not in our guidebooks, but the instructor knew them from experience. With years of experience, it was easy for him to recognize birds from much farther away than we could and to know when we could not have seen what we thought we saw. He knew that there were rare exceptions, but they were always unlikely.

Quick Summary

- Know the typical age when certain diseases tend to occur.
- Always give the child a chance to talk; even young children can explain more about what's happening to their bodies than you think. The parents may not be aware of many of the symptoms.
- Look at the entire child, not just the part that you know hurts.
- Question the diagnosis when symptoms stray from the expected.

When evaluating a child with muscle, bone, or joint pain, it is important to understand that each of the conditions that may be responsible has a typical set of symptoms, a typical age group in which it occurs, and other typical findings that make it easy for an experienced physician to diagnose. At the same time, if a child does not have the typical problems or is not the typical age, it's much less likely that the suspected condition is the proper explanation. Throughout this book, I have clearly indicated the typical presentation for each of the conditions discussed.

TAKING THE HISTORY

Imagine, if you will, that a fourteen-year-old boy is brought to the doctor because his knee hurts. "Most of the time I'm fine, but when I put my foot down and turn to the left, I get a sudden sharp pain on the side of my knee. After five or ten minutes the pain gets better, but then it happens again if I put my foot down and turn left again." (This story clearly suggests a mechanical problem in the knee and probably a torn meniscus.) If the boy says, "My knee hurts all the time," we have much less information. "It hurts when I walk on it" does not tell us very much. We need to know if it is stiff when he wakes up in the morning or hurts only with activity. Sometimes the child and parents are not sure. You may have to ask the same question several different ways. "Are you stiff when you wake up in the morning? Do you have trouble getting out of the car after a long car ride? Do you have trouble getting out of your seat in the theater after a long movie? Suppose you and I are walking in a shopping center; how far can you walk without stopping? If we stop and sit, does your knee immediately get better or does it take five or ten minutes to get better? If we get up to go again after your knee has improved, does it start to hurt immediately and get worse? Does it seem stiff, but then get better after a few steps? Is it fine until we've been walking for ten or fifteen minutes again?" The answers to these questions will help determine the correct diagnosis.

If the child is old enough to explain, let him or her answer some initial questions. You'd be shocked to realize how often parents are surprised by meaningful findings that they were unaware of that their child tells the doctor. Sometimes even four- or five-year-olds add valuable information. For teenagers, it is very important to let them explain their own problems. The parents may have to help out, but let the child go first. If the parents and child argue about what the problem is, that itself is significant information.

The key pieces of information about a problem often can be captured with just a few questions.

- **The quality**. Is it a sharp pain or a dull ache?
- **The exact location**. Some problems cause the front of the knee to hurt; some affect the side. Sometimes the pain is above the knee; sometimes it's below. Each suggests a different diagnosis.
- **The length of time**. How long has the pain been going on, and how did it start?
- **Development over time**. Is it getting better over time or worse?
- **Factors that affect symptom severity**. What lessens the pain, and what makes it worse?

The answers to these questions can rapidly lead to the diagnosis.

Nuances of the Diagnosis

Joints with mechanical problems often hurt after a period of use. They get better with rest. Then they start to hurt after a period of use again. Arthritic joints may begin to hurt after a period of use and then get better with rest as well. However, children with arthritis will feel stiff when they get up to walk again but will improve after a few steps (see Part II). That's not what happens with injuries. The child with arthritis will often describe trouble with long car rides or sitting in a movie theater. Children with injuries are much less likely to do so.

There is a lot of important information to be gained by asking detailed questions. A child with chondromalacia patella may have a chief complaint of knee pain. There is no suggestion of stiffness, but it hurts when he or she walks long distances. If you ask whether it hurts more going up- or downstairs, children with chondromalacia patella characteristically complain of more pain going downstairs. In contrast, children with unrecognized dermatomyositis may also complain of leg or knee pains (see Chapter 16). They will have much more trouble going upstairs. Children with mechanical problems or arthritis may complain of pain going both up- and downstairs. Children with these different problems may be the same age and the same sex. They all complain of leg pains and point to their knees, but these are very different conditions with different causes and treatments.

Another important variable is how the pain began. If the child says, "My knee hurt immediately after I was tackled from the left crossing the forty-yard line with the football," the differential diagnosis is very different from that of the child who cannot explain how the pain began. At the same time, you need to be very careful about unclear histories of trauma. In small children and even in teenagers I have often seen swollen fingers or toes with the explanation "We did not see anything, but we assumed she must have jammed it." Someone in the family should remember if a child has injured a finger or toe badly enough for it to be markedly swollen. Children who exhibit an unexplained "sausage digit" often have psoriasis-associated arthritis (see Chapter 9). I see many children with spondyloarthropathies who complain of repeatedly spraining their ankles or wrists. They cannot really tell you when they sprained it; it just happens "all the time." These are not sprains at all. The condition is spondyloarthropathy— a type of arthritis that commonly causes tendons to be inflamed where they insert into the bone, mimicking a sprain.

The Challenges of Taking a History

Typically, children with injuries know exactly what happened. But children with arthritis or other diseases cannot tell you exactly how or when it started. They just assume they must have twisted it or otherwise somehow injured the joint. Parents of children with pauciarticular-onset arthritis are rarely able to tell you when it began. This is a subtle arthritis that most often sneaks up on people. If the parents can tell me that the child was fine until Tuesday, I know that the diagnosis is not pauciarticular-onset arthritis. Many other diseases also start gradually, and the parents and children cannot tell you when they began. Conversely, you won't always get a history of trauma. You may fail to get this history because the child is ashamed and did not admit the accident to the parents (jumping on the bed or doing something else he or she wasn't supposed to be doing) or because the trauma was caused by a sibling, parent, or other person.

Children with a History of Injury

Most children with a definite history of injury have an orthopedic problem. These problems are usually easily diagnosed by the appropriate history, physical examination, X-rays, or MRIs. Sometimes there is a definite history of injury that leads everyone in the wrong direction. A child may be brought to the emergency room limping because he or she fell a few days earlier and is not getting better. The X-ray evaluation may show arthritis or a bone infection, not an injury. In this situation, it was formerly taught that the child probably fell because of the infection or arthritis and that the fall brought attention to the problem. However, we now know that an initial injury can alter the dynamics of the bone and joint, making the child more vulnerable to the onset of an infection or arthritis.

Children without a History of Injury

I was once working as a general pediatrician in the farm country of California. A mother called me and asked whether I had any experience with malaria. Knowing that malaria does not occur in California, I asked, "Why?" She explained that she and her family had been living in a malarial region of Southeast Asia until two months previously. She was working there as a teacher. She and her family had returned to California, but now one of her own children was "showing the same symptoms the children in my classes in Southeast Asia showed when they had malaria. I must have stopped the medicine we were taking to prevent malaria too soon." This was easy. But imagine how long it would have taken for a physician to suspect malaria and do the right tests if the parent had simply brought the child to the doctor and said, "He has a fever and looks sick."

Often when I'm evaluating a child with pain that started on a certain day, I ask what happened in the days or weeks "just before that." Infection-associated arthritis often begins ten to fourteen days after an episode of sore throat or flu. The travel history may be important as well. Palm frond synovitis is an arthritis that results from a palm frond breaking off inside the child's knee at the time of a fall. The fall usually took place six or eight weeks before the child developed symptoms. The family has no reason to think that their trip to Florida in February has anything to do with the child's knee pain in April. As a result, they will not mention it unless you ask about their travel. There are many similar situations. You cannot rely on the parents to recognize the importance of travel, unusual pets, or other unusual exposures that might be important.

We cannot know all about the lives of the children we are taking care of. Parents do not know what is important and what is not. The key is an open exchange of information. Often at the very end of a long history, one parent will say, "I do not know if this is important, but . . . " Surprisingly often, that may be the key piece of information. To get this information, we have to ask families a lot of questions that seem unrelated and unimportant. I ask all families these questions because I have no way of knowing, in advance, when the answers will make a difference.

- Is the child growing well?
- Has there been any fever or rash?
- Has the child had frequent infections?
- Has there been any recent travel?

Children with chronic or severe problems often have been losing weight. Have they been having fevers or night sweats? These types of problems often suggest a long-standing problem and perhaps a more severe one. Has the child had many infections? Children with a history of frequent ear or upper respiratory infections may have immunoglobulin A (IgA) deficiency or other immune deficiencies that are associated with an increased frequency of arthritis and other rheumatic diseases (see Chapter 9).All these questions may seem a silly waste of time when the answer is no, but they are very important when the answer is yes.

Medications

It is important to ask about all of the medications a child is taking, including vitamins, herbal supplements, and medications obtained without a prescription. ("I gave Johnny one of Grandma's pills that she had left over from when she had a cold" can turn out to be the explanation for the problem if it was an allergic reaction to Grandma's medicine.) You need to know what has been done to treat the problem in the past. It's also important to know what other medical problems the child is being treated for and how.

Past Medical History

> Not long ago, a child was sent to me because of blood in the urine and joint pains. The referring physician was worried about lupus. After I'd gotten all the relevant information from the mother and was asking about past medical problems, she told me that the child had frequently been treated for an infected parotid gland. Then I asked the child whether he had trouble making tears or eating certain foods. When I got the right answers, I knew it was necessary to evaluate him for Sjögren's syndrome. Even though the child had been treated for various symptoms for several years, the correct diagnosis had not been considered because no one had obtained the pieces of information necessary to see how everything fit together to suggest this diagnosis.

You need to know whether the child has other illnesses that may be related to the joint pains or the treatment—even though the family may think that they can't possibly be related. A child might be ten or eleven years old, but the strange problem he or she is having may be the result of something that happened in the neonatal intensive care unit shortly after birth (children who have short bowel syndromes secondary to necrotizing enterocolitis [NEC] have an increased incidence of arthritis; children transfused years ago with hepatitis C–contaminated blood also have frequent joint complaints). You cannot even begin to suspect these problems if you do not know that the child was in the neonatal intensive care unit or received several units of blood in Africa after an automobile accident six years ago.

Family History

This is one of the most important parts of evaluating children with chronic disease. Often I request extra tests for a disease that I would not initially have suspected because there is a strong family history of the disease. I have discovered children with inflammatory bowel disease (IBD) long before abdominal symptoms developed because I requested the appropriate tests when I realized that they had joint pains and a family history of bowel disease. Celiac disease, rheumatic fever, psoriatic arthritis, spondyloarthropathies, and many other diseases tend to run in families.

Social History

Many people think that the social history consists simply of asking where a child goes to school, what grade he is in, and what he wants to be when he grows up. But it also includes asking about smoking or ethanol and other drug use in teenagers. It means that I know whether a child lives at home or in a boarding school. Does the child come home to mom or a babysitter or go to an after-school club? All these pieces of information may provide the answer to the problem. It's easy to consider psittacosis (pigeon fancier's disease) if you know that a child raises birds as a hobby or helps someone who does. But you have to ask about hobbies to know the answer. As physicians, we have to recognize that the social history may not always be accurate, especially with regard to sexual activity and drug use by teenagers, but you have to ask to have any chance of obtaining the information.

Review of Systems

The review of systems is your last attempt to find out anything the family forgot to mention. Is the child allergic to any drugs? Does the child have any bleeding problems? Are there any problems with the hair, eyes, or ears? I ask about everything from the top of the head to the bottom of the feet. Neither the physician, the child, nor the family knows for sure whether the answer to the problem is going to become obvious from these questions. Often it does not, but no one knows until one asks.

THE COMPLETE PHYSICAL EXAMINATION

Sam was a fourteen-year-old boy brought to my office by his mother because his ankle hurt. Sam was a good athlete and loved to play baseball and basketball. Over the last year he had suffered from repeated ankle sprains. He'd been evaluated by several orthopedists and sports medicine doctors and was given a diagnosis of tendonitis. When his problems did not go away despite casting and physical therapy, he was referred to me for "chronic pain syndrome." Sam's ankle had been X-rayed, and computed axial tomography

(CAT) and an MRI had been done. Sam and his family were very frustrated. He could not play, and the doctors seemed to be implying that he did not want to get better. After taking the history from Sam and his family, I sat down next to him and begin to examine his fingers and wrists. Sam immediately said, "It's my ankle that hurts, not my hands." A moment later, he jumped when I flexed his wrist fully. Careful examination revealed that Sam had inflammation in many tendons and obvious limitation of motion in his back and hips. After completing my examination, I told Sam and his family that he had mild arthritis and prescribed medication. They were dubious at first, but two weeks later, Sam was again playing basketball without problems. The key was in examining all of Sam's joints, not focusing only on the one he complained about. Even Sam had not realized that he had other problems. A complete examination was the key to the proper diagnosis.

There are several key aspects to the physical examination of a child. If the child has an obvious injury to an arm or leg, you should examine it carefully. However, if the child is having recurrent injuries or has complaints without an obvious explanation, you must examine the child completely.

Margie was the twelve-year-old daughter of a doctor. She had not been feeling well for several weeks. One morning she woke up with severe pain in her left knee. The pediatrician could not find anything wrong with the knee and sent her to an orthopedist. The X-rays were normal and the orthopedist was stumped. When I saw Margie the next day, she was tense and anxious. Lying on the examination table, she was holding her knee bent and complaining of pain. I sat down next to her and had her relax as best she could, then carefully moved her knee. It was easy to move and was not swollen. However, when I squeezed her thigh above the knee, she was tender. Then I put my hand on her abdomen and immediately noticed an enlarged, hard spleen. Margie had leukemia. Since she was complaining about her knee pain, her leg had been carefully evaluated, but no one had done blood work or examined her fully. When I did this, the diagnosis was immediately evident.

The key to the proper diagnosis is a careful and complete physical examination. We need to look everywhere for the answer, not just where the child points. Diagnosing illness is like solving puzzles. You'll never do a good job if you do not collect all the clues.

George was a sixteen-year-old boy whose family moved to the Southwest because he had severe problems with numb fingers in cold weather. He had been diagnosed with Raynaud's phenomenon (see Chapter 14) and was given medicine. Moving to the Southwest had mostly corrected the condition, but he was having ankle pain. When George walked in to be examined, he had noticeable round red spots on his face and hands. He had seen a dermatologist, who told him he had telangiectasia. This is a common finding and is nothing to be worried about. In talking to George, I also learned that he had seen a gastroenterologist because food sometimes got stuck when he swallowed. He had been told that his esophagus was weak. When I examined him, his fingers were long and thin, and there were little sores on the fingertips. Careful examination also revealed dilated blood vessels in his nail folds (you need a magnifying glass to see this—see Fig. 14–1 in Chapter 14). George also had a lump on his left elbow. An orthopedist had seen this and told him it was calcium buildup, "probably from an old injury." CREST syndrome is a variant of scleroderma (see Chapter 15). The key findings are calcinosis (the bump on his arm), Raynaud's phenomenon, esophageal problems (the difficulty swallowing certain foods), sclerodactyly (long, thin fingers), and telangiectasia (the red spots on his face and hands). Different physicians had seen George for each of the findings, and when asked, he knew about all of them. But no one had put them all together to make the proper diagnosis.

When examining a child with pain in the muscles, bone, or joints, there are several important steps. The first is to determine carefully where the pain is located:

- Is the pain in the joint (where the bones come together)?
- Is the pain just above or below the joint?
- Is the pain in the middle of the arm or leg—far away from a joint?
- Is the child in pain without being touched, or does it hurt only if you squeeze?
- Is this the only joint that hurts, or do other joints hurt if you squeeze them?
- Is the area that hurts hot or warm to the touch?
- Is it red? Is it obviously swollen?
- Does the child have other findings (a rash, bumps, etc.)?

Children should be much more flexible than forty-year-olds. If you are worried about a joint, can the child bend it without pain? Can he or she bend it all the way? Normal children under age ten can put their heels on their buttocks without difficulty. Young children should also be able to bend their hips so that their heels can reach their abdomen. Often I see children who were told that they were normal because they could do everything a forty-year-old can do.

If a child presents with fever and ear pain and has an ear infection, it is highly unlikely that you will check the child's knees. However, if a child has chronic problems that aren't getting better, you want to be sure that he or she has been properly evaluated.

LABORATORY TESTS AND OTHER EVALUATIONS

Proper diagnostic testing may include blood tests, radiographs (X-rays), bone scans, MRI, ultrasound (sonograms), and even biopsies of affected joints and tissues. Chapter 24 provides an extensive discussion of the laboratory and diagnostic tests commonly used in the evaluation and monitoring of children with muscle, bone, or joint pain or arthritis. Diagnostic tests are not a substitute for knowledge and judgment. I often have children referred to me with thousands of dollars of wasted tests and the wrong diagnosis. The key to proper diagnosis and treatment is a careful history and a thorough physical examination. After those have been done, appropriate diagnostic tests can help to pinpoint the cause of the problem and aid in planning treatment.

Simply performing a large battery of poorly thought-out tests not only wastes time and money, but also exposes the patient to unwarranted risks associated with both the testing procedures and the pursuit of false leads. I am often asked to evaluate children who had a positive blood test that suggested a rheumatic disease when no one can tell me why the test was done. The child never had any of the symptoms associated with the disease the test suggests, but somehow it was ordered and now no one knows what to do with the result.

A careful history and a complete physical exam are often sufficient to establish the diagnosis. Further tests should be ordered only to confirm the diagnosis and ensure that nothing else is wrong. Only if physicians are having difficulty finding the cause of a child's problems is a much more extensive evaluation warranted (see Chapter 4).

I have seen several children who complained to their parents of knee pain. When their physicians noted that the knee appeared swollen and there was no history of injury, the children were sent for MRIs. The results were interpreted as showing "synovial tissue proliferation," and the children were operated on for possible tumors. A careful history and a physical examination made it clear that they had typical juvenile arthritis. In many cases, it was obvious that the problem was not a tumor because there were other swollen and tender joints when a full examination was done. Thousands of dollars were wasted, and the children were put through unnecessary hospitalizations and operations. Even the initial MRI that suggested a "possible tumor" would not have been needed if the child had been carefully examined.

Even when appropriate tests are done, it is important to be sure that they are properly interpreted.

A ten-year-old boy was sent to me because of hip pain. Although the pain was severe, he could walk. The family brought an X-ray of the hip that had been interpreted by the radiologist and showed "no hip damage." A bone scan of the hip was also done and showed "no abnormal uptake in the hip," that is, no damage. When I examined the child, it was clear that his pain was not in the hip but adjacent to it. The X-ray and the bone scan were indeed negative for hip damage, but both showed a fracture of the pubic ramus (a bone near the hip). Looking at just the hip, the radiologist had overlooked the fracture nearby. The child pointed right to the location of the fracture when he was asked where it hurt.

3

Common Causes of Pain

KNEE PAIN

When evaluating a child with knee pain, it is important to separate mechanical problems from problems resulting from infections or inflammation. Children with mechanical problems typically hurt with activity. Stop the activity and the pain goes away. Resume the activity and the pain comes back. If there is a fracture or an infection, the pain is there all the time. If there is a torn ligament or meniscus, the pain may be intermittent. It will come on with activities and clear more slowly.

Most knee pain is initially thought to be the result of an injury. If we do not remember having seen a fall, we assume the child must have twisted it. If a child is complaining of knee pain, there are several important questions to answer:

- Did the pain begin immediately after an injury? Or did the parents notice that the child was in pain and then have to "remember" the injury?
- Does the knee hurt all the time?
  - Does it hurt only in the middle of the night?
  - Does it hurt only when the child is running on the soccer field?
  - Does it hurt only in the evening?
- Can the child play but then have to come off the field?
  - If the child comes off the field, is he or she better in five minutes and back in the game?
  - Or is the child out for the rest of the day?
- When the child wakes up the next morning, does he or she feel better or worse?
- Is the knee stiff the next morning? Does it loosen up in the morning after the child gets up and starts moving?
- Has the knee ever been swollen?

- Are any other joints ever stiff or swollen?
- Has there been any fever?
- Has there been any recent diarrhea or viral illness?

The answers to these questions will suggest a variety of explanations for the pain.

Box 3-1 Common causes of knee pain in childhood

Mechanical conditions
Osgood-Schlatter disease

Osteoid osteoma

Blount's disease

Growing pains

Meniscal injuries

Torn ligaments

Overuse syndromes (see Chapter 5 for a discussion of these problems)

    Iliotibial band

    Chondromalacia patella

    Osteochondritis dissicans

Other orthopedic conditions

Common infections
Staphylococcal infections

Tuberculosis

Lyme disease

Rheumatic diseases
Juvenile arthritis

Spondyloarthropathies (enthesitis-associated arthritis)

Systemic lupus erythematosus

Dermatomyositis (weakness in the thighs may be described as "knee pain")

Psoriatic arthritis

Miscellaneous conditions
Pigmented villonodular synovitis

Plant thorn synovitis

Metabolic diseases
Hemophilia
Sickle-cell anemia

Proper Evaluation

The key elements in evaluating a child with knee pain are the presence or absence of stiffness and the description of the pain. X-rays are important if the pain seems to be coming from the bone. If the joint is swollen, then withdrawing fluid from the knee may provide useful answers. Bacteria in the fluid indicates an infection, while a large amount of blood suggests an injury (see the synovial fluid analysis in Chapter 24).

If the knee appears to be absolutely normal, it is important to examine the child and make sure that the pain is not coming from the shaft of the bone or even the hip. Blood tests may be helpful in detecting an infection or arthritis. A sonogram and bone scan can also help. Magnetic resonance imaging can be very useful in diagnosing injuries to the soft tissues around the knee. See Chapter 25 for a more complete discussion of these tests.

Pain After a Fall

If a child is in severe pain after a fall, he or she should immediately be appropriately evaluated. In these cases, X-rays are usually done. Most often, fractures are immediately obvious on the X-ray. However, some fractures may be very small and will be seen only on a follow-up X-ray. This is because callus formation is easily seen on the follow-up X-ray even though the original small fracture was not evident on the first X-ray. Sometimes children with pain who do not have an obvious fracture are presumed to have a growth plate injury that is hard to see on the X-ray. If a fracture is seen or suspected, the child will be put in a cast for an appropriate period. Following cast removal, the child should recover quickly. Repeated injuries in which the fractures are hard to see should be regarded with suspicion. Many children with arthritis are originally diagnosed incorrectly with "small fractures."

If the X-rays are negative, a sprain is often diagnosed. If there is no obvious swelling, such children are often treated with an Ace wrap and crutches or a "walking boot." Often the problem disappears quickly and there is no need for concern. However, children with recurrent injuries of this type need careful medical evaluation. Injuries to the supporting ligaments of the knee or the menisci will require further attention. These injuries are most often associated with swelling. If the knee is aspirated, the fluid will often be bloody. Careful orthopedic evaluation is mandatory, as bloody synovial fluid (fluid from the joint) suggests a significant injury. Children with hemophilia may have recurrent bleeding in their knees. A rare type of synovial disease called **pigmented villonodular synovitis** is also associated with bleeding into the knee joint. Typical childhood arthritis is not associated with bloody synovial fluid unless the needle hits a vein (which does happen). However, this will produce fresh blood, which can be differentiated from old blood in the knee fluid when it is examined under the microscope.

If a child continues to have knee pain after the initial treatment, a repeat and thorough examination should be done. Repeat X-rays of the knees may be needed. It is also important to be sure that the hips have been carefully evaluated. Some children with hip problems complain about pain in their knees. Everyone is misled because the knees are normal. The most common example of this is a child with a slipped capital femoral epiphysis (SCFE) of the hip (see the next section in this chapter on common causes of hip pain). The child should also have blood work that includes a complete blood count, a metabolic profile, and muscle enzymes.

Continuing knee pain during the day should not be dismissed as growing pains or Osgood-Schlatter disease without thorough evaluation. Some children with muscle disease will initially complain of knee pain (in fact, it is probably thigh pain). There are also children with infections or tumors of the bones and joints and children with arthritis who are first brought to the doctor because of pain after falling. Most of these conditions are evident on X-rays, sonograms, or MRI if the appropriate area is examined.

Pain That Comes and Goes

Pain that comes and goes may have many different explanations. If this happens with changing levels of activity, it may have a mechanical explanation. On the other hand, if it occurs with changing barometric pressure (rapidly rising or falling air pressure, as when a storm is coming), it may be the beginning of arthritis or the result of an old injury or a chronic infection. Pain that is much worse with activity but disappears when the activity stops suggests a mechanical problem.

Pain that begins with activity but does not disappear when the activity stops and often results in stiffness the next morning suggests arthritis.Physicians are often fooled when examining children because they believe that arthritis in childhood must be associated with either a positive test for rheumatoid factor or an elevated sedimentation rate. Neither is required for a child to have arthritis (see Chapter 7). Children who are stiff when they wake up in the morning, or have difficulty getting out of the car after a long ride or out of their seat after a long movie, need to be carefully evaluated for arthritis. Small children may have obviously swollen knees and difficulty walking when they first wake up but never seem to be in pain. Again, this is often a sign of arthritis.

When evaluating children with knee pain, it is important to be sure that the pain is in the knee joint and not in the shaft of the bone. At the beginning, children with tumors or infections in the bone may complain of intermittent pain. Most often these conditions are diagnosed by X-ray, ultrasound, MRI or bone scan (see Chapter 25). Typically, these children have pain in the bone itself rather than in the joint. The child will say only that the knee hurts, but the distinction between bone pain and joint pain can be made easily if the child is carefully examined. However, some children have both. Children with growing pains may have intermittent complaints of pain in and around the knee. Normal test results and the occurrence of pain only at night help to differentiate these pains from more serious conditions (see Chapter 1).

Specific Conditions

Osgood-Schlatter Disease

Overview

This condition is the result of inflammation of the insertion of the patellar tendon where it attaches to the anterior tibial tubercle. The role of the patellar tendon is to transmit the force from the muscles in the thigh to forward motion of the lower leg. In children who are developing rapidly (the nine- to fifteen-year-old age group), the muscles often strengthen more rapidly than the bones. Running and kicking, such as while playing sports, leads to repeated pulling on the tendon where it attaches to the bone. With repeated pulling, children develop inflammation at the tendon insertion. As a result, the anterior tibial tubercle becomes swollen and tender (Fig. 3-1).

Diagnosis

The pain in Osgood-Schlatter disease is brought on by activity and relieved by rest. It is never associated with stiffness or swelling of the knee itself, although the anterior tibial tubercle may become tender and swollen. It does not cause pain when children wake up in the morning, and it does not wake children up from sleep. The key to diagnosing Osgood-Schlatter disease is to realize that the pain is not in the knee (although that is how the children usually describe it). On careful examination, the knee is entirely normal. The pain is reproduced by pressing on the anterior tibial tubercle (the prominent bump just below the knee). Most often the tenderness is present on both sides,

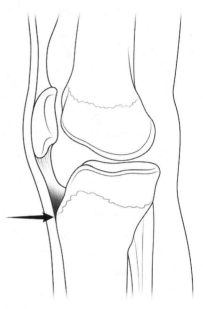

Figure 3-1 *Inflammation of the tendon insertion in Osgood-Schlatter disease producing pain just below the knee. The arrow indicates the anterior tibial tubercle.*

but it may be only on the dominant side (e.g., the right side if the child is right-handed).

Treatment

The key to treatment is to enforce relative rest so that the inflamed tendon and bone can heal and the bone can become stronger and withstand the pulling by the muscles.

Osteoid Osteoma

Overview

Osteoid osteomas are benign tumors of the bone, much like knots in wood. Often they never cause difficulty. They are most common in the region of the hip (see below) but may occur either above or below the knee. However, in some children they cause pain. Most often the pain occurs in the middle of the night and is sufficiently severe to wake the child. Osteoid osteomas occur in boys more often than girls and frequently become symptomatic during the teenage years.

Diagnosis

Osteoid osteomas around the knee are usually diagnosed easily on routine X-rays, but sometimes a CAT scan is required to recognize them.

Treatment

The pain from an osteoid osteoma is usually relieved easily by acetaminophen or ibuprofen. All children in whom it is possible that the lesion may be a serious bone tumor and all children whose pain is not easily relieved by these medications require careful evaluation by an orthopedist with extensive experience in these lesions.

Plant Thorn Synoviti

Overview

Plant thorn synovitis is an arthritis that occurs in children who have fallen on a palm frond, cactus thorn, or similar piece of sharp plant material and part of the plant has broken off inside the knee.

Diagnosis

The typical story involves a four- to six-year-old child who is brought to the doctor with a single swollen knee. The knee is usually red and hot, with no history of injury. The family doctor sends the child to an orthopedist, who removes fluid from the knee. The fluid looks infected. The orthopedist sends the child to the hospital for intravenous antibiotic therapy. When the cultures of the knee fluid reveal no bacteria and the knee fails to improve after four or five days of antibiotic therapy, it may be thought that the condition is Lyme disease that is not responding to the antibiotics. When the knee still does not get better after the antibiotics are changed, a diagnosis of juvenile arthritis is considered.

The key to recognizing plant thorn synovitis is a proper travel history. Usually the child traveled to a warm place (e.g., Florida, the Caribbean, Southern California) several weeks before the problem started. Typically, the child is just old enough to get out of sight and fall down. There is a small cut on the knee that heals quickly. No one remembers this cut when the knee is hot and swollen weeks later.

Treatment

It is important to recognize plant thorn synovitis because it will not respond to antibiotics or nonsteroidal anti-inflammatory drugs (NSAIDs; see Chapter 23). Proper treatment requires a synovectomy (cleaning out all of the inflamed tissue lining the knee). When this is done, the diagnosis of plant thorn synovitis can be confirmed by looking at the tissue under polarized light. This will show starch granules from the plant material that broke off inside the knee.

Orthopedic Conditions

Blount's Disease

Overview

Blount's disease involves bowing of the legs (genu varum). There are two major groups of children with the disease. Young children may develop it with no apparent explanation. There is a sudden shift in growth of the tibia so that the inner edge does not grow as well as the outer edge. With progressive growth of the outer edge, the legs are forced to bow. In small children, this is most often painless and it affects both sides. In teenagers, Blount's disease is often associated with obesity. In these children, it is suspected that the excessive weight puts too much stress on the medial side of the tibia and the growth plate is damaged. Under these circumstances, only one side may be affected. Blount's disease in teenagers may be associated with progressive pain.

Treatment

At first, the pain may be intermittent and relieved by acetaminophen or other pain relievers, but over time it may steadily worsen. If it is left untreated, the pain will continue and the damage to the joint may result in the premature development of mechanical arthritis. An orthopedic surgeon should monitor children of all ages with Blount's disease. Bracing and surgical intervention are sometimes necessary.

Overuse Syndromes

Chondromalacia Patella, Osteochondritis Dissicans, and Iliotibial Bands

These are all mechanical conditions that result primarily from excessive wear and tear on the knee and surrounding tissues. Because these diagnoses are frequently given to explain pain with athletic activities, I have chosen to discuss these conditions in detail in Chapter 5, which deals with injuries.

Infections

Overview

There are two types of infection that must be considered in a child with joint pain. Septic arthritis is an infection in the joint itself. But in the region of the knee, osteomyelitis, an infection in the bone, is more common than septic arthritis.

Diagnosis

Often osteomyelitis occurs near the ends of the bones and produces pain in the joint near the infected bone. The pain of osteomyelitis may wax and wane, but the child is never free of it. In children with osteomyelitis, the pain usually worsens steadily over a few days at most. These children often have fevers and look ill, but occasionally they look well and are only limping. If the infection has been present for a period of time, it should be easy to see on X-rays. However, during the first few days after an infection begins, the X-ray may not show changes. Bone scans and MRIs will demonstrate infections in the bone even at the earliest stages when pain is present.

One problem that requires attention is the possibility of a *sympathetic effusion*. In this situation, there may be an infection or a tumor (even leukemia) in the bone. At the same time, the child will complain of pain and have an obviously swollen knee. Aspiration of the knee will show fluid that suggests arthritis rather than an infection. The key factor is that these children are in more pain than would be expected. In addition, careful examination will indicate great tenderness in the shaft of the bone, not just in the joint itself.

Bone Cysts

Overview

Unicameral bone cysts are large cystic malformations of the bone that may occur in the femur or the humerus. Aneurysmal bone cysts are expansile osteolytic lesions containing blood-filled cystic cavities.

Diagnosis

Unicameral bone cysts usually are entirely asymptomatic unless there is a fracture, in which case the child should be cared for by an experienced orthopedist. Aneurysmal bone cysts differ in having a significant blood vessel component in the cyst. They tend to grow more rapidly than unicameral bone cysts and are more likely to be discovered because they are causing pain. Like unicameral bone cysts, they are easily discovered by routine X-ray. The majority of bone cysts are minor and found by accident.

Treatment

Fractures that occur have to be treated appropriately. Following healing of the fracture, the orthopedist may choose to treat the lesion by direct injections of corticosteroids or curettage. However, because bone cysts can be associated with more serious problems, these children should all be referred to an experienced orthopedist for evaluation.

Bone Tumors

Overview

While many bone tumors are benign, some are malignant and life-threatening.

Diagnosis

The key to recognizing bone tumors is appropriate evaluation of the child with pain. Like tumors elsewhere, bone tumors begin very small and grow relatively slowly. Often they are easily visible on routine X-ray by the time they are producing pain. Children with pain during the day should never be dismissed as simply having growing pains without further evaluation (see Chapter 1). It is true that growing pains and tumors may both wake up children during the night. However, the child with growing pains is fine during the day, while the child with a tumor will most often have pain during the day if carefully examined.

A full discussion of the types of bone tumors and their treatment is far beyond the scope of this book. If you desire further information on this subject, you should contact your local office of the American College of Orthopedic Surgeons or a similar organization.

HIP PAIN

Hip pain is a particularly disturbing finding in children. Most often, children with hip pain walk with a very abnormal gait. If the pain is sudden and severe, the child may not be able to walk at all. A child who is suddenly unable to walk after trauma or a fall needs immediate medical evaluation to exclude fractures and other orthopedic injuries. A child who, without warning, wakes up in the morning with hip pain and has difficulty walking may be suffering from a variety of conditions. If the pain does not disappear after a few minutes, the child should be brought in for immediate medical attention to exclude the possibility of an infection. All children with hip pain should receive a careful and thorough medical evaluation, including children with pain that disappears after a few minutes but keeps coming back.

Box 3-2 lists the common causes of hip pain in childhood, along with the ages at which they occur.

Box 3-2 Common causes of hip pain in childhood

Small children (under age ten)

Toxic synovitis

Observation hip

Bacterial infection

Legg-Calve-Perthes disease

Tumors

Osteoid osteoma

Sickle-cell anemia

Teenagers

Slipped capital femoral
   epiphysis

Sports injuries

Stress fractures

Apophysitis

Labrial tears

Meralgia paresthetica

Osteoid osteoma

Tumors

Iliotibial band syndrome

Spondyloarthropathies

Often pain in the hip is in fact pain in various parts of the pelvis. With excessive physical activity, it is common to develop pain at muscle insertions around the pelvis. These are often referred to as *pointers*. Children with chronic hip injuries typically report pain with certain movements and activities. The pain is relieved by rest. The hip is a deep-seated joint, and injuries such as ligamentous tears are infrequent in childhood.

Chronic and recurrent hip pain in younger children may be the result of Legg-Calve-Perthes (LCP) disease, arthritis, an infection, or tumor in the bone. In older children, SCFE and spondyloarthropathies (enthesitis-associated arthritis; see Chapter 9) are more common. These conditions often begin with vague complaints of hip pain that become progressively worse over time. Children with all of these conditions may initially describe knee or thigh pain. None of these conditions is difficult to diagnose if the child is properly evaluated with X-rays, blood tests, and, if necessary, a bone scan or MRI.

Specific Conditions

Toxic Synovitis

Overview

Toxic synovitis is an inflammation of the hip that typically occurs in children in the four- to six-year-old age group. Although it often occurs in children with evidence of a viral respiratory infection, its cause is unknown.

Diagnosis

Children with toxic synovitis have a very characteristic story. Most often the child went to bed well or with "a slight sniffle" the night before. In the morning, the child has severe hip pain and is unable to walk. Because the symptoms are so dramatic, the child is immediately brought to the doctor. Often there is a low-grade fever, and blood tests may show an elevated white blood cell (WBC) count and slight elevation of the erythrocyte sedimentation rate (ESR). The immediate concern is to exclude a bacterial infection of the hip. Frequently, these children are referred to an orthopedist, who may aspirate the hip to look for a bacterial infection. Bacterial infections of the hip rapidly worsen over a period of hours. In contrast, I have often seen children with toxic synovitis who are already improving by the time they reach my office. If there is doubt, aspiration of the hip, hospitalization, and antibiotic therapy are appropriate until the possibility of an infection has been excluded. Musculoskeletal ultrasound is now being used in an increasing number of institutions. An experienced sonographer is often able to differentiate infection from toxic synovitis. However, the joint should be aspirated if there is uncertainty.

Treatment

Once the diagnosis of toxic synovitis has been made, children may be treated with NSAIDs and rest. They usually recover completely within a few days. However, careful examination may reveal residual irritability of the hip for several weeks. The prognosis for these children is very good. It was long thought that the incidence of LCP was increased in children who had recovered from toxic synovitis, but recent reports suggest that the two conditions are unrelated.

Children with "recurrent" toxic synovitis should be regarded with suspicion. Some have LCP that has not been recognized. In other children, recurrent episodes of synovitis in the hip may be the first manifestation of what will ultimately become an obvious spondyloarthropathy. Any child with recurrent toxic synovitis should have a thorough evaluation by a pediatric rheumatologist if possible. True toxic synovitis is not a recurrent condition, and the correct explanation for the recurrent hip pain should be vigorously sought.

Legg-Calve-Perthes Disease

Overview

Legg-Calve-Perthes disease results from softening of the head of the femur, which gradually becomes distorted and may flatten or crumble (see Fig. 3-2). This is thought to result from problems with the blood supply to the head of the femur. These problems may be the result of an injury or a congenital abnormality. One report has suggested that LCP occurs far more frequently in the children of parents who smoke. However, problems with the environment or the blood supply cannot be the whole answer, since LCP occurs four times more often in boys than in girls.

Diagnosis

Legg-Calve-Perthes disease usually begins in young children (four to six years of age most commonly),

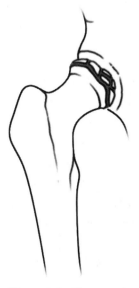

Figure 3-2 *Changes in the head of the femur resulting from LCP.*

who usually limp before there is any complaint of pain. Over time, the limp becomes more noticeable and the child may begin to complain of pain. At the earliest stages, MRI may be required to diagnose LCP. However, if the symptoms have been present for more than several weeks, it should be possible to make the diagnosis with a regular X-ray of the hip. This will show flattening of the head of the femur. Most cases of LCP involve only one hip, but in a few children both hips are affected. Premature birth and problems during the newborn period increase the risk of LCP, as does a family history of the disease.

Treatment

Children diagnosed with LCP should be under the care of an orthopedist. Treatment often consists initially of traction followed by casting. Once the cast is removed, physical therapy is important to restore strength and range of motion. The purpose of the traction and casting is to keep the femur properly seated in the hip while decreasing the pressure on the femoral head. Often this allows the bone to reestablish its blood supply and begin to repair itself. The precise treatment details will depend on the age of the child and the degree of damage to the bone at the time the problem is discovered.

Monitoring

Children with bilateral LCP should be thoroughly evaluated. In some instances, this is a sign of an underlying condition such as hyperthyroidism or sickle-cell disease. In others, the deformed head of the femur may be the result of more widespread conditions, such as multiple epiphyseal dysplasia or spondyloepiphyseal dysplasia tarda. These conditions are recognized by the presence of abnormal epiphyses in multiple joints when a skeletal survey is done. These orthopedic conditions are beyond the scope of this book.

The long-term prognosis for children with LCP who are diagnosed early is good. If the disease has been present for a long time, the bone may already have begun to heal by the time the disease is recognized. In many children, this healing is adequate and things go well. However, in some children, there may be permanent damage to the bone. There is also concern that children with residual damage from LCP may have persisting mechanical problems that will cause mechanical arthritis of the hip, leading to problems when they become adults.

Sickle-Cell Anemia

Overview

Sickle-cell anemia may cause pain in the bones because blood vessels are blocked by the abnormally shaped blood cells. This may occur in the blood vessels that supply the hip and result in damage to the femur. When it does, it looks exactly like—and essentially is—LCP. In children with severe sickle-cell anemia, other bones may be damaged and there may be widespread joint problems. Usually a child with these problems will have been diagnosed with sickle-cell disease long before the bone problems begin.

Infections

Overview

There are two basic types of infection that must be considered in children with hip pain. **Septic arthritis** is an infection in the joint itself, where foreign organisms are growing in the space between the bones. Osteomyelitis is an infection in the bone. In the hip, septic arthritis is more common than osteomyelitis. **Hemophilus influenzae** was the most common bacterial infection of the hip for many years. Now most children are vaccinated against this infection (with the HIB vaccine), and it has become rare. Staphylococcal and streptococcal infections of the hip still occur. It is also possible to have a tuberculosis infection in the hip. At present, Lyme disease may be the most common cause of infectious arthritis involving the hip for people living in endemic areas of the United States (see Chapter 10).

Diagnosis

Most infections in the hip are sudden in onset and associated with rapidly worsening symptoms of pain, fever, and difficulty in walking. A child with these symptoms should be seen by an orthopedist or rheumatologist as soon as possible. Tuberculosis may cause slowly worsening hip pain. A child with an acutely painful hip should be seen by an orthopedist. Although there may be some initial confusion between children with infections and children with toxic synovitis, children with toxic synovitis usually improve rapidly without treatment. If there is a strong suspicion that the joint may be infected, it should be aspirated for appropriate studies, including bacterial cultures. Chronic hip pain associated with stiffness is more likely to be the result of enthesitis-associated arthritis involving the hip (see Chapter 9), but the possibility of an infection should always be given careful consideration.

Osteomyelitis

Overview

Osteomyelitis is an infection in the bone. Often it occurs near the ends of the bones and produces pain in the joint near the infection. The pain of osteomyelitis may wax and wane, but it never disappears and usually gets steadily worse over a period of a few days.

Diagnosis

The children with osteomyelitis often has fever and appears ill, but occasionally the child looks well and is only limping. If the infection has been present for more than a few days, it should be easy to detect on X-rays. However, during the first few days after an infection begins, the X-ray may not show changes. Bone scans and MRIs will demonstrate infections in the bone at the earliest stages when pain is present.

Pain in the lower abdomen near the hip may cause confusion. When dealing with younger children, it can be difficult to know exactly where the pain is located. Children with severe lower abdominal pain may walk with an abnormal gait, suggesting arthritis or an infected hip. As a result, I have seen children brought for evaluation of hip pain and limp who turned out to have an abscess resulting from a ruptured appendix. This possibility should always be considered in children with pain in the right side of the pelvis with no obvious explanation. It can be easily detected by appropriate CAT scan or ultrasound examination of the hip and abdomen.

Osteoid Osteoma

Overview

Osteoid osteomas are benign tumors of the bone, much like knots in wood. Often they never cause difficulty. However, in some children they cause pain.

Diagnosis

Most often the pain is low-grade but constant. Typically it is worse during the night and often is sufficiently severe to wake the child. Careful evaluation is required because malignant bone tumors can also cause chronic bone pain that may awaken a child at night. All children in whom a serious bone tumor is suspected, as well as all children whose pain is not easily relieved, require careful evaluation by an orthopedist with extensive experience with these lesions.

Osteoid osteomas occur more often in boys than girls. Most frequently, they become symptomatic during the teenage years. However, they may cause pain and become troublesome earlier. They are most common in the region of the hip but may also occur around the knee. Osteoid osteomas in the hip area are easily diagnosed on routine X-rays or bone scans.

Treatment

In most cases, no therapy is necessary once the diagnosis has been established. The pain from an osteoid osteoma is usually easily relieved by acetaminophen or ibuprofen. However, in some children the pain is more severe. Surgical removal of the lesion is possible in most of the troublesome cases.

Slipped Capital Femoral Epiphysis

Overview

Slipped capital femoral epiphysis (SCFE) is an injury to the growth plate of the femur that results in the growing end of the bone slipping off the shaft (see Fig. 3-3). This injury occurs most often in boys between the ages of ten and fifteen years but may occur in girls and occasionally in older children. It occurs more often in African Americans and in children who are overweight.

Diagnosis

The most dramatic cases of SCFE occur as an injury with sudden slipping of the epiphysis. This produces acute hip pain and inability to walk. These children are promptly evaluated with X-rays to established the correct diagnosis. The X-rays should include both standard views and "frog leg" views in which the child is

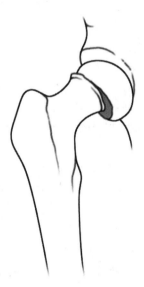

Figure 3-3 *This is the characteristic appearance of an SCFE. The epiphysis is the rounded portion of the bone in the hip joint. It has literally slipped off the end of the long bone (femur). Compare this with Figure 3-2, where the epiphysis has crumbled but remains in the proper position.*

instructed to bend the knees and spread them apart. Slipped capital femoral epiphysis may be missed on standard views of the hips, but the slippage is usually obvious on the frog leg views.

Some children develop SCFE more gradually. No one is sure why this happens. These children have progressive pain and stiffness in the involved hip. Because deep pain may be difficult to localize, the child may describe the pain as coming from the groin, the thigh, or the knee instead of the hip. Children with a chronic slip usually have an obvious limp. The changes in the bone may force the hip on the affected side to rotate outward. The abnormal alignment of the bones that results triggers muscle spasm. This muscle spasm causes children with chronic SCFE to report stiffness with rest and increased pain with activity, symptoms that suggest arthritis. The chronic slip should be evident on X-ray. In uncertain or difficult cases, an MRI may be useful to confirm the diagnosis.

Slipped capital femoral epiphysis may occur in children with hypothyroidism and other growth problems. In about one-third of children, the disease is bilateral. The slip on the opposite side may be present when the first SCFE is noted or it may occur later.

Treatment
Slipped capital femoral epiphysis is treated by orthopedists. They will put a pin in the bone to hold the epiphysis in place while the bone heals. If the condition is detected and treated early, children with SCFE usually do well. Chronic SCFE that is not promptly treated may damage the head of the femur. This can result in a permanent limp, a difference in the length of the two legs, and early onset of arthritis due to mechanical damage.

Iliotibial Band Syndrome
Overview
Iliotibial band syndrome is a common injury of the knee.

Diagnosis
Iliotibial band syndrome may produce pain at the hip or knee. When it produces pain at the hip, children typically complain of a snapping sensation with certain movements. Often this is associated with trochanteric bursitis (see Fig. 3-4), which may be the result of excessive activity. Iliotibial band syndrome may also occur in children with a spondyloarthropathy (see Chapter 9).

Treatment and monitoring

Iliotibial band syndrome itself is a benign condition that does not normally require therapy. However, if the snapping is associated with a sensation of pain, further evaluation is warranted.

Trochanteric Bursitis

Overview

The greater trochanter is the large bump that protrudes on the side of the femur where it turns toward the knee. Because this protrusion is just under the skin at the side of the hip, it is protected by a bursa. The bursa is a small sac of fluid that allows easy movement of the tissues over the

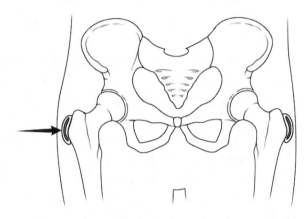

Figure 3-4 *Trochanteric bursitis results from irritation in the fluid-filled sacks (bursas) that are located just under the skin and over the greater trochanter.*

bone (see Fig. 3-4). With excessive running or other activities, this bursa may become inflamed.

Diagnosis

Typically, this is a problem of teenagers or adults rather than younger children. The classic complaint is pain along the side of the leg that can be reproduced by pressure over the greater trochanter. The pain often is described as moving both up and down the side of the leg.

Treatment

Trochanteric bursitis is treated with ice, stretching exercises, and, in more severe cases, NSAIDs. In rare cases, children require injection of steroids into the bursa for relief.

Congenital Hip Dislocation

Overview

Congenital hip dislocation results from improper formation of the sockets into which the heads of the hip bones insert on the pelvis (improper development of the acetabulum, which covers the femoral head).

Diagnosis

This condition should be diagnosed in early childhood. Often it is first suspected when the pediatrician notices a "hip click" in the nursery. This is a sensation of clicking when the hip is moved in what is called the *Ortolani maneuver.* In most children, the hip click will disappear after a period of observation and perhaps "double diapering." However, if it persists, an orthopedic evaluation is needed.

Children with congenital hip dislocation walk with a waddling gait that is obvious to a trained observer but may be overlooked by parents. If the hip dislocation is present on only one side, it may be suspected when the parents or physician notice that the line under the curve of the buttock is not in the same position on both sides (asymmetric gluteal folds). The children will have decreased range of motion of the hips, if carefully examined, and X-ray findings will be abnormal. Congenital hip dislocation is easily diagnosed if appropriate X-rays are done. However, because the condition has always existed, the children may never have complained of pain.

Treatment

Congenital hip dislocation is treated by orthopedists. Cases detected in early life can often be managed without surgery. However, in severe cases, surgical correction is necessary. If the dislocation is not detected and corrected, the hips may become severely damaged because of mechanical damage leading to degenerative arthritis. It is important that any child who walks with a waddling gait be appropriately evaluated and not simply dismissed because "she's always walked like that."

Arthritis Involving the Hip Joint

Overview

The hip joint is rarely the first joint involved in children with juvenile arthritis (Chapter 7), but it may become involved over time. In contrast, the hip is commonly the first joint involved in children with spondyloarthropathies (Chapter 9).

Diagnosis

Children with arthritis involving the hip joint often begin to complain of stiffness in the hip or lower back when they wake up in the morning. Over time, they develop symptoms in other joints. However, they often have to be asked and examined carefully for evidence of pain or limitation in the back, wrists, knees, or ankles, as they will not associate the problems in other joints with their hip pain. This often results in a delay in proper treatment while the cause of their repeated injuries is investigated (see Chapter 9 for more detail). Since spondyloarthropathies rarely begin before the age of ten, younger children with hip pain must be carefully evaluated to exclude other causes.

Mechanical arthritis may occur in children with damage to the bones of the hip resulting from SCFE, congenital hip dislocation, or previous infection. These conditions and the mechanical cause of the arthritis are often evident on routine X-rays. If these X-rays do not provide an explanation for the pain, an MRI may be necessary to exclude less common causes of hip pain.

Muscle and Systemic Diseases

Overview

Some children with muscle or systemic diseases experience significant pain in the muscles in the front of the thigh. This pain may be mistakenly reported as coming from the hip or the knee (and in fact, hip and knee problems may cause pain in the same muscles).

Diagnosis

Whenever a child complains of chronic pain and disability without obvious findings in the bones or joints, a careful evaluation for muscle or systemic diseases should be performed. I have seen children with hypothyroidism, hyperthyroidism, dermatomyositis, leukemia, lymphoma, and rhabdomyosarcoma who were referred with "hip" problems. Proper evaluation for these conditions includes blood tests with muscle enzymes, thyroid function studies, a complete blood count, and appropriate MRIs and X-rays.

Bone Cysts and Bone Tumors

Overview

Unicameral bone cysts are large cystic malformations of the bone that may occur in the femur or the humerus.

Diagnosis

Unicameral bone cysts usually do not produce any symptoms unless there is a fracture. The common bone tumors of childhood are briefly discussed in the section earlier in this chapter on knee pain. They should be considered in the evaluation of children who initially have pain in the hip as well.

Treatment

Like bone cysts near the knee, unicameral bone cysts should be cared for by an experienced orthopedist.

BACK PAIN

A friend's daughter carefully loaded up her book bag for her first day in seventh grade, sat down on a bench, and promptly went over backward with the weight. In this age of larger and larger book bags and backpacks, backache is becoming an increasingly common complaint among adolescents. However, despite the muscle strains associated with heavy book bags and other activities, serious back problems fortunately remain uncommon. As is true for other regions of the body, the key to properly diagnosing the cause of a child's back pain is a careful history and physical examination. It is important to know the answers to the following questions:

- When the pain began, did it come on suddenly, following an injury or a fall, or did it come on slowly over a period of days without an injury?
- Does the pain wake the child up at night?
- Is the pain associated with stiffness, and is it worse when the child gets up in the morning, or does the pain begin only with activities?
- Is the pain relieved by rest or does the child stiffen up if he or she sits for a long period?
- What position or activity reduces the pain? What position or activity makes the pain worse?
- Is the pain confined to a single location or does it move up and down the back?
- Does the pain extend down into one leg or out into one shoulder?

The answers to all of these questions are important in providing a clear understanding of the cause of the child's pain. Common causes of back pain are listed in Box 3-3.

Box 3-3   Common causes of back pain in childhood

Scheuermann's disease

Spondylolisthesis

Spondylolysis

Disc disease

Spondyloarthropathies

Scoliosis

Benign tumors

Infections

Disciitis

Osteoid osteomas

Serious back injuries are typically associated with severe trauma, such as accidents, falls, and sports activities. Trauma and serious injuries will not be covered here.

True backaches not associated with injuries are rare in childhood and are particularly unusual in children less than ten years old. Structural abnormalities are the most common cause. Any young child complaining of back pain requires careful evaluation, since infections and tumors are serious causes of back pain that may be present in this age group. These problems must not be ignored.

Scoliosis and spondylolisthesis rarely come to medical attention before the age of ten years, but in older children they are the most common structural abnormalities that cause back pain. Usually scoliosis and spondylolisthesis begin without symptoms, but over time compensatory changes occur that often cause mechanical pain.

Specific conditions

Scoliosis

Overview

Scoliosis is an abnormal curvature of the spine with rotation of the vertebrae. This curvature often results in one shoulder appearing higher than the other or the hips appearing uneven.

Diagnosis

Since the curvature occurs with growth, it is rare for scoliosis to become evident before the age of ten years. Children are routinely screened for scoliosis at school, but the expertise and thoroughness of the examiners vary widely. Most scoliosis is idiopathic (unexplained). In rare cases, it may be the result of tumors, infections, or damage to the spinal cord. These cases may appear at an earlier age than idiopathic scoliosis and be more severe. Any child whose spine appears crooked or who has an abnormality on the scoliosis screening should have a careful orthopedic evaluation.

It is easy to examine a child for scoliosis. Have the child stand in front of you with the feet together and the heels aligned. Then have the child bend forward to touch the toes. Two findings suggest a scoliosis. The most common finding is a "rib hump," in which the ribs on one side appear higher than the ribs on the other (Fig. 3-5). In some children, there is a prominent low back (lumbar) component that is easily felt by putting your hand on the lower part of the back. If one side of the back is lower than the other, further evaluation by an orthopedist is necessary.

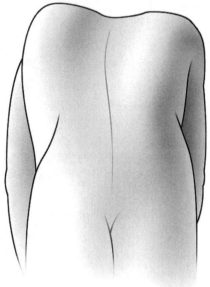

Figure 3-5 *A positive scoliosis screen with the ribs on the left side appearing higher than those on the right when the child bends over. The shoulders may also appear uneven when the child stands up, but this is more difficult to notice.*

Treatment and monitoring

Once detected, scoliosis should be carefully evaluated and followed. Many children have only mild curvatures and require no treatment, but others have progressive disease requiring bracing and, less frequently, surgery. Scoliosis is usually painless and is detected only on examination (see Fig. 3-5). Pain suggests that the scoliosis has been present for a prolonged period with secondary mechanical problems.

Spondylolisthesis

Overview

Spondylolisthesis is an anterior slippage of one vertebra over another. Most often this occurs at the junction of the lumbar and sacral spines (L5–S1 level). Some cases may be due to a congenital weakness and others to poor healing after an injury. Either cause results in weakness of the posterior elements. Spondylolis-thesis results when this weakness allows one bone segment to slide forward over another.

Diagnosis

Although mild spondylolisthesis may be asymptomatic, more severe involve-ment characteristically leads to low back pain that may radiate down the back of the thighs.

Treatment and monitoring

Most children with this condition can be followed conservatively, but some require orthopedic intervention. Because the symptoms can worsen over time, all children with chronic back pain should be monitored by an experienced orthopedist.

Kyphosis

Overview

Kyphosis is an excessive curvature of the spine in which the spine is bent forward.

Diagnosis

Looking at the child from behind, you will not see a curvature, but if you look at the child from the side when he or she is bending over, you will see that the upper part of the back angles forward sharply instead of assuming the normal C shape (see Fig. 3-6). This abnormal forward curvature may be the result of abnor-malities in the bone resulting from fractures or infections. However, most often it occurs with-out explanation. In severe cases, the child may appear to have a hunchback.

Some children have a **postural kyphosis**. This is usually a mild increase in the forward bend of the spine, leading to the appearance that they are always slumping over. In these children, there are often no abnormal findings on X-ray. They can lie face down with their

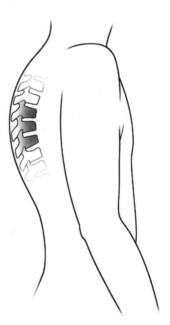

Figure 3-6 *Appearance of the spine with wedge-shaped vertebrae in a child with kyphosis due to Scheuermann's disease.*

backs perfectly flat. Children with more significant abnormalities usually have changes in the bones. As a result, they cannot lie perfectly flat on their stomachs.

Kyphosis may also be the result of damage to the vertebrae by an infection, tumor, or poor bone formation. These conditions are all rare. Children with conditions that are known to damage the spine should be carefully monitored. Parents of children with poor bone formation or of children who are taking medications that can damage the bones need to be reminded that their children should be watched carefully for spine problems. If a child has been diagnosed with an infection or a tumor in or around the spine, the parents should be aware of the need to monitor the spine as the child grows.

Treatment

All children with kyphosis need to be investigated by an orthopedist with appropriate X-rays to find out why they have this condition. For children without significant abnormality, a program of exercises is often adequate.

Scheuermann's Disease

Overview

Scheuermann's disease is a common cause of kyphosis in teenagers. It is thought to result from abnormalities in the growth of the vertebrae, which results in the front being compressed relative to the back (see Fig. 3-6).

Diagnosis

The diagnosis is easily made when abnormal bone structure is seen on appropriate X-rays. Children with this condition may need to wear a brace to relieve their pain and prevent worsening of the condition. More severe or worsening cases may require orthopedic surgery.

Infections

Overview

There are a variety of infections that may damage the spine. Fortunately, none of them is common in childhood. Staphylococcal bacteria are common causes of infections that may affect the vertebrae. Tuberculosis can also affect the vertebrae. In the old literature, tuberculosis that affects the spine is called **Potts' disease**. Bacterial infections of the spine are usually very painful.

Diagnosis

Bacterial infections are easily diagnosed by either X-rays or bone scans (see Chapter 25). Despite many claims to the contrary, back pain in children is not a result of Lyme disease. The last child I saw with "back pain from chronic Lyme disease" had cancer that had gone undetected and untreated through six months of chiropractic and antibiotic treatment.

Disciitis

Overview

Disciitis is a confusing cause of back pain in younger children. Typically, it affects children under the age of ten. The etiology of disciitis remains unclear, but in some cases a bacterium such as staphylococcus is identified. In many cases, no causative bacterium is identified.

Diagnosis

Children with disciitis may have initial symptoms of a cold or flu-like illness. They then develop severe back pain, but in this age group they may not be able to describe it. **The key to recognizing this illness in very young children is that they suddenly refuse to sit up or walk.** This illness is usually diagnosed on the basis of the typical clinical picture with a bone scan and MRI or X-rays to be sure that no other problem is present.

Treatment

When a bacterium is identified, the infection can be treated with antibiotics.

Osteoid Osteomas

Overview

Osteoid osteomas are a cause of chronic low-grade bone pain that may occur in many different locations. While many osteoid osteomas never cause sufficient discomfort to attract attention, some are problematic.

Diagnosis

Osteoid osteomas in the spine typically come to parents' attention when a child complains of chronic back pain that comes and goes without explanation. Larger osteoid osteomas are easily seen on X-rays. Smaller lesions may be found on bone scans. A typical child with an osteoid osteoma reports a sense of deep aching pain, which is often worse at night.

Treatment

Pain is usually relieved by NSAIDs but continues to recur until the osteoid osteoma is removed. Untreated painful osteoid osteomas may cause major problems because the pain results in muscle spasms.

Herniated Discs

Overview

Herniated discs are a common complaint among adults and a frequent explanation for back pain that starts in adulthood. Disc herniation is usually the result of excessive stress put on the spine, with resultant rupture of the cushioning material in one of the intervertebral discs. This condition is quite rare in children because they have more flexible bones and are less likely to do the work-related heavy lifting that often causes disc problems.

Diagnosis

Although an MRI of the spine is very accurate in identifying disc problems, the minor disc problems it reveals are not a reliable explanation for back pain. Many individuals who deny ever having back pain show minor disc herniation on an MRI. Although it is not impossible for a teenager to have a damaged disc, pediatricians should be extremely skeptical about this diagnosis as the cause of back pain. Gradual onset of back pain with stiffness on awakening is more likely to be associated with a spondyloarthropathy or another illness.

Low back pain and morning stiffness are commonly due to spondyloarthropathies in teenagers. However, adolescents rarely come to the doctor complaining of low back pain when they wake up in the morning. Since the onset is very gradual, most of them accept this stiffness as normal. The diagnosis of a spondyloarthropathy as the cause of an adolescent's back pain is based on carefully examining the teenager and finding evidence of arthritis or tendon insertion pain (enthesitis) elsewhere. A strong family history of back pain also should suggest this diagnosis even though the other family members with back pain will all have "good excuses" for this condition. A key indication is that children with spondyloarthropathies almost never have the ability to bend over and touch their toes. See Chapter 9 for a full discussion of spondyloarthropathy.

NECK PAIN

Neck pain in children is rare. Most often it is due to irritation involving the muscles that hold the head and shoulders in the proper position. Muscle irritation that the child describes as neck pain may be the result of an improperly carried backpack, especially if a heavy backpack is slung over just one shoulder.

Carrying an excessive weight on one side places unnecessary strain on the back, the shoulder itself, and the neck muscles.

Box 3-4   Common causes of neck pain in childhood

Muscular irritation
Wryneck
Sprains and strains (e.g., whiplash)
Severe sore throat
Jaw pain
Uncorrected visual problems causing the child to hold the head tilted
Bone problems
Congenital abnormalities
Osteoid osteoma
Herniated disc (rare without known injury)
Infection
Spondyloarthropathies (enthesitis-associated arthritis)
Juvenile arthritis

When evaluating a child's complaints of neck pain, think about the answers to the questions at the beginning of the section on back pain. Since the neck is simply the top portion of the back, the same questions need to be asked about complaints here. Several additional questions should also be asked:

- Is the child having headaches? Do they occur at the same time as the neck pain?
- Is the child having jaw pain? (Spasm in the muscles around the jaw may be reported as neck pain.)
- Is the child having problems seeing?
- What type of pillow does the child use?

Muscular Irritation

Wryneck (torticollis) is a condition in which the child holds the head to one side because of problems with the sternocleidomastoid muscle. This muscle at the front of the neck is sometimes injured at birth and becomes shortened as a result of the injury. Children with this problem do not usually report pain, since it has been present since birth. However, they may develop neck pain as their muscles try to compensate for the injury if the problem is not corrected as they get older. Wryneck in older children is due to muscle irritation (see below).

Sprains and strains are the most common cause of neck pain in children. The muscles of the neck must simultaneously support the head and protect the spinal cord while allowing maximum flexibility for looking up, down, and to both sides. This combination of strength and flexibility can be provided only by using several overlapping sets of muscles. Injury to any one of these muscles will be reported as neck pain. If the pain is severe, there may be muscle spasm, forcing the child to hold the head tilted to one side for comfort. Pain due to irritation of the sternocleidomastoid muscle radiates into the front of the chest. In contrast, pain due to irritation of the trapezius muscle radiates down into the middle of the back and out toward the shoulder on the affected side.

Older children may injure the sternocleidomastoid muscle or the trapezius muscle, causing pain and a tilted head position. They also may suffer an overuse injury when they carry a heavy backpack on just one side. Constant contraction of the muscles necessary to keep the head level when the shoulders are slanted by a heavy load will fatigue the muscles, leading to spasm. The child may go to bed without a complaint but wake up stiff and sore, unable to straighten the neck. The muscles of the neck may also become inflamed by a severe sore throat resulting from infections in the tonsils and infections or other causes of irritation elsewhere in the nose and throat. Similar problems may result from irritation of the jaw, producing spasm of the muscles where the neck and jaw meet. Any child in whom this is a persistent problem without explanation should be evaluated by an ear, nose, and throat specialist (otolaryngologist).

There are congenital bone problems that affect the neck, such as the **Klippel-Feil syndrome**. These are easily diagnosed on X-ray. Other bone problems such as **osteoid osteoma** may occur in the neck, with findings identical to those occurring lower in the back. **Herniated discs** and **infections** may also occur in the neck as elsewhere. **It is important to recognize that these problems may initially be reported as headaches and not recognized as coming from the neck.**

Spondyloarthropathies predominantly affect the low back. However, there are children with neck pain due to irritation of the muscle insertions. In most but not all cases, involvement of multiple joints was previously found. Certain forms of juvenile arthritis commonly lead to problems with the bones in the neck. These children have limited neck motion (often they cannot look up or down or turn their head from side to side without moving their back). In some cases this loss of motion is associated with pain, but more often it occurs gradually and the patient is not immediately aware of the problem.

Any child with prolonged, severe, or unexplained neck pain should be thoroughly investigated with a complete physical examination. If the problem is persistent and the answer has not been found, consideration should be given to evaluation by a neurologist, an ear, nose, and throat specialist, a neurosurgeon or orthopedist who deals with neck problems, and a rheumatologist.

FOOT, ANKLE, HEEL, AND TOE PAIN

It takes a moment to realize that when a child says, "My feet hurt," he or she could be referring to the heels, the toes, the ankles, or anywhere in the middle of the foot. Each area of the foot has a different set of common problems and solutions. Often parents initially assume that foot pain in childhood is the result of shoes that do not fit properly. It is only when the pain continues despite a new pair of shoes that medical care is sought.

When evaluating a child who is complaining of foot pain, it is important to determine whether the pain is in the toes, the ball of the foot (the area just behind the toes), the middle of the foot, the heel, or the ankle. You can both ask the child to point and examine the child's foot yourself to see whether any part of it is red, swollen, or tender. As with most other complaints of muscle, bone, and joint pain in childhood, the first response is likely to be "Maybe he or she banged or sprained it." If the pain has been present for more than a few days, a more thorough evaluation should be done.

There are some very knowledgeable podiatrists, but children should be thoroughly evaluated by an orthopedist and, if appropriate, a rheumatologist before being referred to a podiatrist. Do not forget that heel pain is a common early manifestation of a spondyloarthropathy. Putting cushions in the shoes may alleviate the heel pain, but it will do nothing to correct the associated problems in children with arthritis. X-rays will exclude major fractures, but beware of the diagnosis of hairline fractures or growth plate fractures. These are real conditions, but they are also often convenient explanations when the child hurts and nothing is evident on the X-rays. The care with which the child is evaluated is the key to finding the correct diagnosis. Common conditions causing pain in the toe, heel, and mid-foot are listed in Boxes 3-5, 3-6, and 3-7. Rare conditions such as Fabry disease may initially present with complaints of severe burning foot pain for which there is no obvious explanation.

Box 3-5   Common causes of toe pain

Trauma

Tennis toe

Ingrown toenails

Dactylitis with arthritis

Freiberg's infarct

Box 3-6   Common causes of heel pain

Trauma

Sever's disease

Plantar fasciitis

Achilles tendonitis

Spondyloarthropathies

Box 3-7   Common causes of mid-foot pain

Flat feet

    Tarsal coalition

    Accessory tarsal navicular

Bunions

Kohler's disease

Pes cavus

Arthritis of the subtalar joint

Toe Pain

In young children, toe pain is often a source of confusion because small children cannot reliably tell you what happened. When a child points to one toe and says that it hurts, we all start by thinking that it was banged, was stepped on, or was pinched in the shoe. Real trauma to the toe is usually obvious. A fractured toe is not subtle. The toe is very painful and there is often bleeding under the skin, so that a large area of the toe appears bruised. Whenever this occurs, the foot should be X-rayed to make sure that nothing is broken. With the exception of fractures, minor trauma to the toe should improve in a day or two.

When the toe has been injured, there is often discoloration under the toenail. If there is no discoloration and the pain persists, you should look carefully to see whether the toe is red or swollen. Compare it to the same toe on the other foot. If it is very red and swollen, it may be infected. This should be evaluated immediately. Any child with red marks spreading up the foot that are warm and tender should be assumed to have a serious infection. If a toe looks bigger than the one on the other side but the child is not complaining, squeeze it gently. Often the toe is tender, and the child will pull the foot away. If that happens, gently take the foot in your hand and squeeze just behind the place where the toe attaches to the foot. If that area is also tender, it suggests arthritis. Certain forms of arthritis commonly start with tender swelling involving the entire toe that is often mistaken for an infection or a tumor.

Tennis Toe

Overview

Tennis toe is pain due to bleeding under the toenail. It is most commonly an injury in older children but may occur in younger children whose shoes are too small. It is the result of the toes forcibly colliding with the front of the shoe during activities.

Treatment

The acute pain can be relieved by allowing the blood to escape from under the toenail, which releases the pressure. It is important to recognize that the pain is an indication of improper footwear and that the shoes should be changed.

Ingrown Toenails

Overview

Ingrown toenails may result from a variety of conditions. Although a number of possible explanations have been put forward, the most common cause of ingrown toenails in children is that the nails were cut too short. This results in the nail growing under the skin in front of it.

Treatment

Most often, ingrown toenails can be treated with warm soaks and local antibiotic creams. But this can be an extremely painful condition and may be associated with serious infections. Severe cases may require antibiotics and surgical removal of the offending toenail. Prevention is important. Encourage parents not to cut the child's toenails too short.

In older children, toe pain may be due to a variety of injuries. **Freiberg's infarct** is a degeneration of the end of the metatarsal bone. The metatarsals are the long bones in the foot that extend to the base of the toes. Freiberg's infarct most often occurs in girls and usually at the base of the second toe. It is easily diagnosed if the appropriate X-rays are taken. It is treated with casting and use of an orthotic device to relieve the pressure placed on that portion of the foot. This condition may occur in other toes, but it rarely if ever involves the small toe.

Children complaining of pain at the base of the toes should be carefully examined for problems in other joints. A number of children have come to me after being treated with casting and orthotics for months. The orthopedists were considering surgery. However, the children were not getting better because the toe pain was due to arthritis. This was not obvious from examination of the toe, but when the whole child was examined, obvious arthritis was found in other joints. The toes got better when the arthritis was treated.

Heel Pain

Direct trauma to the heel is rare. It may occur if the foot is stepped on or if something falls on it. These injuries are obvious. Injuries to the heel may also occur with landing wrong after jumping, but again, the injury is immediately evident. Chronic heel pain associated with activities may be thought to be **Sever's disease**. This is a common condition of preteenagers that is associated with increased physical activity. In this condition, the bone of the heel is often tender to pressure and the heel cords may be tight. Sometimes this diagnosis is based on X-rays showing irregularity and sclerosis of the calcaneal apophysis. This is incorrect, as identical changes are commonly found on X-rays of children without foot pain. **Sever's disease is not associated with pain in the tendons above or below the**

heel. Heel pain accompanied by pain in these tendons is often a sign of a spondyloarthropathy (Chapter 9).

Children may develop recurrent injuries and irritations of the tendons in the foot. In small children, these are thought to be cysts, sprains, and strains. In older children, they are often thought to be recurrent athletic injuries. Isolated **plantar fasciitis** and **Achilles tendonitis** occur as overuse injuries in runners and other athletes. Since these findings may also be part of a spondyloarthropathy, the key to proper diagnosis is a careful history and a physical examination. Often a child with recurrent ankle sprains turns out to have back stiffness and hip limitation, too, all of which are indicative of a spondyloarthropathy. Once the entire history has been obtained and a careful examination done, it is clear that the ankle pains are part of a larger diagnostic picture.

Midfoot Pain

A number of conditions may cause pain in the middle of the foot. Again, acute injuries are obvious and easily recognized with appropriate X-rays. Chronic pain in the middle of the foot is often the result of a variety of bony abnormalities. The most common of these is **flat feet**. Painless flat feet are most often a variation of normal and require no treatment. However, if a child with flat feet has foot pain, it requires evaluation. Often no significant abnormality is found, and the pain is relieved with the use of an orthotic.

Some children have a "rigid" flat foot. This is easy to recognize because it is difficult to move the different parts of the foot in relation to each other. (You should be able to simply hold the child's foot in your hand and turn the front part in different directions while holding the heel steady [see Fig. 3-7]. If the child has normal feet, this is easy to do and causes no pain.) In children with a rigid flat foot, it is necessary to determine whether the rigidity is caused by **tarsal coalition** or another correctible abnormality. Every child with a rigid flat foot should be evaluated by an orthopedist.

Tarsal coalition is the formation of fibrous bands between two or more of the tarsal bones. These fibrous bands restrict motion and thus reduce the flexibility of the foot itself. This fibrous banding is thought to be present at birth, but it becomes symptomatic over time. It can be diagnosed with routine X-rays or CAT scans. Casting may provide relief, but surgery is necessary for more difficult cases.

An **accessory tarsal navicular bone** is an extra little piece of bone that forms at the base of the navicular bone in the midfoot. This is easily seen on X-ray. This extra piece of bone protrudes on the inside of the foot and may be painful and tender where it rubs against the inside of the shoe. Many people have this bone and never realize it. If there is pain where the shoe rubs

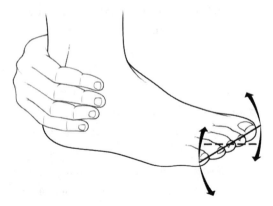

Figure 3-7 *Twisting the front of the foot while holding the heel steady. This is the way to evaluate for the possibility of a rigid flat foot. The front of the foot should twist easily.*

against the inside of the foot, stretching the shoe or wearing wider shoes often will eliminate the problem. Rare cases may require surgery. Occasionally, this leads to a mistaken diagnosis of a fracture.

Bunions are commonly thought of as a disease of adults. However, they may occur in teenagers, girls more often than boys. With activity these bunions may cause pain. Treatment usually centers on finding properly fitting shoes and other conservative measures. Surgery is generally unnecessary.

Kohler's disease is an irregularity of the navicular bone located in the middle of the foot, behind the metatarsal of the big toe. A typical patient with Kohler's disease is a child under the age of ten who complains of pain when walking and tenderness when the bone is pressed. Kohler's disease usually resolves without treatment. Severe or persistent cases are often treated by casting. This condition can be diagnosed by appropriate X-rays or a CAT scan.

Pes cavus is a condition in which the arch of the foot is unusually high. Children with this condition often complain of foot pain when running or pursuing other activities. Pes cavus is not a common condition. Usually both feet are affected equally. If only one side is affected, there is often a neurologic problem. Even when both sides are affected, there may be an underlying neuromuscular condition. All children with pes cavus should be carefully examined by an orthopedic specialist. Surgery to correct the deformity may be necessary.

Arthritis involving the subtalar joint may occur as a complication of many different forms of childhood arthritis. Because the subtalar joint is responsible for twisting movements of the foot, children with arthritis of this joint experience pain and difficulty when walking on uneven surfaces. Subtalar joint involvement is just one part of a much larger picture in children with arthritis. Careful and complete examination of the child makes it easy to recognize that the subtalar arthritis is not an isolated finding. This arthritis is easily diagnosed by careful examination of the foot. It may be treated with NSAIDs or local injection. Some children with persistent pain benefit from the use of orthotics that prevent motion in the subtalar joint by holding the foot in a rigid position inside the shoe.

Diffuse foot pain is infrequent. One of the most common causes is **reflex sympathetic dystrophy** that may begin after an injury to the foot. Children with reflex sympathetic dystrophy often experience color changes in the foot accompanied by profound hypersensitivity. Many of these children cannot put on a shoe or even a sock. This is a complex condition requiring specialized treatment. See Chapter 20 for more details on reflex sympathetic dystrophy.

ELBOW, SHOULDER, WRIST, AND FINGER PAIN

Pain in the fingers, wrists, elbows, and shoulders is common in older adults. But in young children, complaints are infrequent. Most complaints of pain in children under the age of ten are associated with minor injuries. Over the age of ten, overuse with athletic competition becomes more of an issue.

Elbow Pain

"Nursemaid's elbow" is one of the more common causes of distress in young children. Parents usually notice that a young child (two to three years is the peak age group) is holding the arm bent and not using it. It is most often the left arm, but either arm may be involved. Typically, the injury occurs when a parent or sibling who is anxious to go tugs hard on the arm. It might happen when crossing the street, arguing over whether or not it is time to leave the playground, or any other time the child is leaning away from a parent, guardian, or sibling who is pulling him or her by the arm. It can also happen if someone picks the child up by the arm (this should be avoided). The excessive stress on the elbow causes the bones to shift out of position, or dislocate. As a result, the child has pain and cannot straighten the arm.

Commonly, the dislocated nursemaid's elbow will snap back into place by itself. If not, an experienced physician can usually snap the elbow back into place by holding it steady and rotating the thumb toward the middle of the body. The bones often shift back into place with a pronounced clunk. An orthopedist should evaluate children complaining of continuing elbow pain because there may be an associated fracture or other problems requiring correction. Elbow fractures are not always easily seen on X-rays. Although isolated episodes of nursemaid's elbow happen to almost everyone, parents should be instructed to be more careful in handling their children. Repeated or prolonged dislocations of the elbow may lead to permanent damage. The most common causes of hand, wrist, elbow, and shoulder pain are listed in Box 3-8.

Box 3-8   Common causes of pain in the elbow, shoulder, hand, and wrist

---

Elbow

Nursemaid's elbow

Green stick or buckle fractures

Little Leaguer's elbow

Osteochondritis dissicans

Tennis or golfer's elbow

Shoulder

Little Leaguer's shoulder

Rotator cuff injuries

Wrist and fingers

Trauma

   Mallet finger

   Boutonniere deformity

   Navicular fractures

   Dactylitis

Trips and falls are the major causes of pain in the hand or wrist. Serious fractures are unusual without major trauma, but **green stick** or **buckle fractures** may occur. In these situations, a child falls on an outstretched arm and immediately experiences pain. The arm may seem undamaged, but if it remains very tender at a specific point, the child should be taken for X-rays. In these fractures, one side of the bone breaks but the break does not go all the way through. They should be cared for by an orthopedist, as improper treatment could result in unbalanced growth of the bone, causing the arm to curve. All fractures require immediate orthopedic care.

Chronic elbow pain in childhood is most often the result of overuse. The bones and ligaments of young children lack the strength to endure the repeated stress associated with throwing hard and other sports-related activities. While the number of innings pitched during games is strictly limited in organized Little League baseball, many parents fail to recognize that too many hard pitches in practice can also cause damage. **Parents concerned about their child's possible future career in professional sports must recognize that excessive hard practice at an early age will most likely result in injuries that make a professional career impossible.** Symptoms of "**Little Leaguer's elbow**" include pain or swelling along the inner aspect of the elbow and difficulty straightening the arm fully. Although X-rays may be normal, children with these complaints should be forced to rest and not be allowed to throw until the symptoms have entirely disappeared. Continuing to throw despite having elbow pain most likely will lead to long-term disability.

Older children in throwing sports such as football and baseball may develop **osteochondritis dissicans** of the elbow. In this condition, a small fragment of the humerus may drop off the end of the bone. This is the result of repeated stress on the bone from overuse. It can be extremely painful. If the fragment falls into the joint space, it may block normal motion of the joint and cause locking. This can be detected by X-ray, ultrasound, or MRI. If the fragment is blocking normal motion, surgical removal may be necessary.

Tennis elbow is a degenerative change at the origin of the muscle that is used to flex the wrist for activities such as backhanding a tennis shot. This muscle (the extensor carpi radialis brevis) is anchored to the arm just below the elbow. Excessive jerking of the muscle with strong contractions causes pain and irritation where it attaches to the bone. This is rarely seen in young children but may occur in adolescents who are overusing the arm. **Golfer's elbow** is a similar injury occurring on the inside of the elbow with excessive tugging on a different group of muscles. Like all such overuse injuries, these problems are best treated with rest and modification of the activity to prevent further injury.

Juvenile arthritis infrequently begins in the elbow joint without findings of pain, swelling, or limitation of motion elsewhere. However, any child who exhibits swelling of the elbow and difficulty straightening the arm fully should be carefully evaluated for other conditions. Children with arthritis beginning in the elbow may be labeled as having pauciarticular-onset arthritis, but such children most often go on to have more widespread joint disease over time (see Chapter 7).

Shoulder Pain

Fractures in the area of the shoulder are usually the obvious result of direct trauma. All require orthopedic intervention. The most common chronic conditions producing pain in the shoulder are overuse injuries associated with sports. **"Little Leaguer's shoulder"** is an inflammation of the growth plate in the shoulder. It results in pain when the shoulder is pressed and, in more severe cases, weakness. Advanced cases are easily diagnosed on X-ray, but any child experiencing pain should be prevented from further throwing and other stressful shoulder activities until the pain has resolved. Excessive use of the shoulder can occur with tennis, gymnastics, swimming, baseball, basketball, football, and many other sports. As with overuse injuries in other joints, continuing the activity despite having pain is more likely to produce chronic disability than an athlete of superior ability.

The great range of movement possible at the shoulder is due to the fact that unlike the hip, the shoulder is not limited by a deep bone socket. As a result, the shoulder is much more dependent on strong ligaments to maintain proper alignment. Young athletes with relatively loose ligaments are therefore uniquely susceptible to recurrent shoulder injury and dislocation. Any child with recurrent shoulder dislocations without an obvious explanation should be carefully evaluated for ligamentous laxity and associated conditions (see Chapter 18).

Rotator cuff injuries are typically caused by irritation of the muscles in the rotator cuff because they are being compressed between the humerus and the scapula (see Fig. 3-8). This compression is thought to result from imbalances in the strength of the muscles and ligaments that normally keep the bones properly aligned. Most often the children report pain with throwing and other overhand activities. Children with these problems should be carefully evaluated, required to rest, and started on a careful program of rehabilitation. Allowed to rest and rehabilitate appropriately, most children can resume full activity. X-rays are rarely helpful in this condition. Magnetic resonance imaging may be warranted if the problems persist. Surgical intervention is usually unnecessary unless the rotator cuff has been torn by continued overuse.

Children with chronic shoulder pain and repeated injuries should be carefully evaluated for the presence of underlying conditions. Some adolescents with chronic shoulder problems

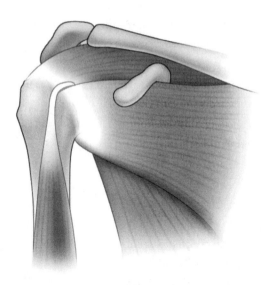

Figure 3-8 *The muscles of the shoulder and the rotator cuff. Injuries often result from enlargement of the muscles with athletic activity to the point where they are irritated as they pass between the bones.*

have underlying conditions such as spondyloarthropathies or ligamentous laxity, which require further investigation and specialized treatment (see Chapters 9 and 18).

Hand, Wrist, and Finger Pain

Finger injuries are extremely common in children of all ages. Obvious fractures are easily recognized and quickly diagnosed by appropriate X-ray examination. Children with persistent finger injuries require careful evaluation. Children with blunt trauma to the ends of the fingers may suffer damage to the tendons resulting in mallet finger or boutonniere deformity. A **mallet finger** is one in which the tip of the finger is pointed downward. It cannot be raised because of damage to the tendon. Whenever a child suffers a blunt injury to the end of the finger, you should check that he or she can move all parts of the finger appropriately. If a tendon is ruptured, so that the child cannot move the tip of the finger up or down, the injury should be corrected surgically. **Boutonniere deformity** results from trauma to the finger tendons as they pass over the middle knuckle of the finger. As a result, the damaged tendon may slip down while the tip of the finger is pulled up (see Fig. 3-9). These are common sports-related injuries. However, boutonniere deformity may also be the result of arthritis.

Young children with swollen fingers or toes without explanation are often thought to have banged or stubbed them. But if the pain or swelling persists, the child should be carefully examined for evidence of arthritis. Persistent swollen

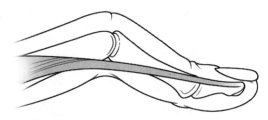

Figure 3-9 *Boutonniere deformity resulting from tendon slippage.*

fingers (**dactylitis**, or a sausage digit) may be the first manifestation of serious arthritis. See Chapter 9.

Wrist injuries are common in normal athletic activity. Younger children rarely experience wrist fractures, but they commonly occur in adolescents engaged in vigorous sports activities. Like fractures in other parts of the body, most wrist fractures are immediately apparent and easily diagnosed with appropriate X-rays. One exception is fractures of the scaphoid bone, located at the center of the wrist. Fractures usually occur when a

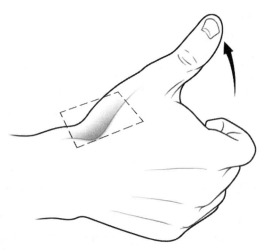

Figure 3-10 *Pain in the anatomic snuff box, the base of the thumb, is an important finding suggesting a fracture of the scaphoid bone in the wrist.*

child falls hard on the outstretched hand. Although the child may complain of pain in the wrist, there is often no obvious problem. However, the pain will persist and the wrist will be tender if it is moved in the direction of the thumb or pressure is applied to the space at the base of the thumb (see Fig. 3-10). Fractures of the scaphoid often are not seen on regular X-rays unless special views are taken. Children with persistent wrist pain after a fall should be evaluated by an orthopedist.

Tendon irritation, sprains, and strains are uncommon in children under the age of ten except as the result of trauma. In older children, overuse injuries are common, especially with tennis and gymnastics. Children experiencing wrist pain in association with sports activities should be allowed to rest and recuperate to avoid worsening the inflammation.

Several forms of arthritis commonly begin in the wrist. Although long-standing arthritis is obvious on X-rays, the key to recognizing arthritis early is a careful examination. In most children with arthritis, several joints are involved. This will be noted on careful examination of the whole child. Children with a chronic injury usually have only one involved joint.

Several genetic conditions may initially present with complaints of hand and wrist pain without an obvious explanation. Metabolic storage diseases may cause a buildup of abnormal materials that first cause pain in the hands because the wrist is a narrow space where nerves can be compressed. Although Fabry disease and mucopolysaccharidosis type I are very rare conditions, children with these diseases often complain of unexplained hand pains for years before the other manifestations of the disease became obvious. Appropriate screening tests can be done on blood and urine. Because these are storage diseases that can be treated, early diagnosis and institution of therapy is very important.

4

The Child Who Hurts All Over and the Child Who Is Failing to Thrive

There are many possible explanations when a child is not doing well, ranging from serious illnesses to problems adjusting at home or in school. Children who aren't thriving or who complain of constant pain are of great concern for both parents and physicians. Some parents worry that their child is not able to keep up with the other children when playing. Others are concerned about repeated athletic injuries, wondering why their child has so many sprains and strains. Still others notice that the child seems withdrawn or irritable or has lost interest in activities.

Most physicians who care for adolescents are aware that a dramatic change in behavior without obvious findings on examination may be a sign of drug use or depression, but it may also be the first indication of rheumatic or other serious diseases. Inability to keep up with other children may simply be an indication that the child in question is not athletic, but it can also be the first sign of many serious illnesses, including muscle weakness from dermatomyositis or arthritis due to any of its many causes. Repeated athletic injuries and recurrent tendonitis may be due to poor stretching techniques, but they may also be the first signs of a spondyloarthropathy that can be easily treated.

Without an obvious explanation for the child's complaint, parents can become frustrated. This frustration can be minimized if physicians take a systematic approach. **When parents are concerned that their child is not doing well, an appointment should be made for a full and unhurried physical examination. Don't let parents catch you with this in the middle of a school or camp physical exam, where the temptation is to quickly dismiss anything that is not obvious. If you don't have time to sit and talk carefully with the parents when they first bring up the problem, encourage them to schedule a detailed examination in the near future. You want to be able to take your time and think about the problem.**

One of the greatest difficulties for families and physicians is that some children with widespread complaints do not look ill. A routine physical examination of the heart, lungs, and abdomen will not reveal muscle pain, weakness, or tender joints. Some conditions, such as celiac disease or mild variants of genetic diseases (e.g., Scheie syndrome or Fabry disease), present with chronic complaints of pain in children who otherwise may look well. These conditions will be diagnosed in their early stages only if they are thought of and tested for. While these diseases are rare, the usual delay between initial complaints and diagnosis is several years. Since treatment can prevent further damage, but cannot always reverse the damage that has been done, early diagnosis is desirable. The routine tests will all be normal. You need to carefully evaluate the child for joint pain or weakness and consider the rare diseases that cause chronic pain. If you don't have time for that in your office, consider a specialist referral. Diagnosing rare diseases is like diagnosing meningitis. If every time you think of it you are right, you are missing most of the cases.

For young children, there are well-established algorithms to evaluate the child who is failing to thrive. Unfortunately, there are no similar algorithms for older children who are not doing well. As a rheumatologist, I have developed my own standardized list of tests to evaluate these children (see Box 4-1).

Box 4-1   Tests for the evaluation of children who are not doing well

Purified protein derivative (PPD; skin test for tuberculosis)

Complete blood count (CBC)

Erythrocyte sedimentation rate (ESR)

Triiodothyronine (T3), thyroxine (T4), thyroid-stimulating hormone (TSH) anti-thyroid antibodies, anti-thyroid peroxidase (thyroid function studies)

IgA tissue transglutaminase (anti-endomyseal antibodies, associated with celiac disease)

Creatine kinase (CK), a muscle enzyme

Aldolase (another muscle enzyme)

Complete metabolic profile (a broad panel of general tests, including liver and kidney function tests)

Glucose, calcium, albumin, and total protein

Electrolytes including sodium, potassium, carbon dioxide, bicarbonate, and chloride

Kidney tests including blood urea nitrogen (BUN) and creatinine

Box 4-1   Continued

Liver tests including alkaline phosphatase (ALP), alanine aminotransferase (ALT; also called serum glutamate pyruvate transaminase [SGPT]), aspartate amino-transferase (AST; also called serum glutamic-oxaloacetic transaminase [SGOT]), lactic acid dehydrogenase (LDH), and bilirubin

Urine analysis (UA)

Serologic markers including antinuclear antibody (ANA), rheumatoid factor (RF), and Lyme titer

Amylase and lipase if there is abdominal pain, dry eyes, or dry mouth

Total immunoglobulin levels including IgG, IgA, and IgM

Clotting studies: prothrombin time (PT) and partial thromboplastin time (PTT)

HLA B27

Urine for glycosaminoglycans

Blood testing for Fabry disease in children with chronic burning hand or foot pain without explanation

Note: I do not routinely screen for drug use in my rheumatology practice. However, in the setting of a general pediatric practice this may be necessary. Testing for human immunodeficiency virus (HIV) and other sexually transmitted diseases may also be needed in the appropriate situations.

It is not practical to recommend that a physician do all of these tests on every child who does not feel well and complains of pain. Most children whom I evaluate with these complaints have previously seen a number of physicians or have been complaining for a long time. I do all tests in the first portion of the list on every child I evaluate who is reported to not be doing well. I reserve the amylase and lipase tests for children with complaints of abdominal pain, the IgG, IgA, and IgM level tests for children with complaints of frequent infections, and the HLA B27 test for children with joint pains. The clotting studies are reserved for children with easy bruising or bleeding, heavy menses, or chest pain. The genetic studies are done on children who have an appropriate family history or persistent unexplained pain suggestive of these conditions. Every physician has a sense of how far it is appropriate to go in the office and when to refer the child to a specialist.

The majority of children with a significant illness of the musculoskeletal system have specific findings on physical examination or abnormalities on at least some of these laboratory tests. Sometimes the abnormalities seem minor, but they must be viewed as part of a pattern of findings that may indicate the diagnosis. In isolation, **normal values on these laboratory tests are not**

enough to eliminate a significant medical condition. Many children with spondyloarthropathies and other conditions have no laboratory test abnormalities. Nonetheless, these children can be easily diagnosed by careful physical examination. Sometimes children have vague complaints during the earliest stages of a disease, even before obvious abnormalities occur. It may not be possible to make a definite diagnosis in these children, and they may not require treatment. However, it is one thing to reassure the family that you are taking their concerns seriously and will follow up on the problem and another to say, "There's nothing wrong with your child." Many rare conditions, such as Fabry disease and Scheie syndrome, will be diagnosed only if they are specifically thought of and tested for.

In many cases, the family history is the key.

I recently saw a five-year-old boy whose mother was concerned because he repeatedly woke up at night complaining of pain in his knees. At first, the story sounded like a typical case of growing pains. However, as I continued to take the history, the mother described episodes of pain in the back and ankles that occurred during the day as well. The pains were usually short-lived (minutes to hours). A careful evaluation had been done by the referring physician, including an MRI of the spine because of concern about a possible tumor. All of the laboratory tests and X-rays were entirely normal. But the pains had been occurring for several months.

When I completed the history and physical examination of the child, there were only two key points. On examination the child was certainly normal, but he was not limber. There was some tightness in his hips and at his ankles. However, it was not enough to be considered abnormal. In addition, when taking the family history, I learned that the father had significant ulcerative colitis. This form of inflammatory bowel disease (IBD) is associated with arthritis (see Chapter 9), and the arthritis may precede the abdominal manifestations. I did not tell the mother that the child had arthritis. Nor did I tell her that the child had IBD. What I did tell her was (1) that her child's complaints were not normal, (2) that there was a possibility that the child's complaints were an early indication of IBD, and (3) that no treatment was necessary at present, but routine follow-up was important so that we could monitor for the possible development of IBD or increased symptoms that did require therapy.

I do not know whether this child will ever develop IBD. I do know that he is at increased risk based on the family history alone. Knowing that there was a possible explanation for the child's complaints and that he would be followed gave his mother reassurance that she had not gotten from being told that "Everything is normal." Some persons may argue that I have unnecessarily made this mother worry about her child developing IBD. However, she was already concerned and knew that IBD could be inherited. What she did not know was that it could produce joint pains. Knowing she was being listened to and her child followed did not make her more worried. It made her more comfortable that her child was being watched carefully and would be treated appropriately if more problems developed.

Box 4-2 Diseases that hurt all over

Fibromyalgia

Systemic lupus erythematosus (SLE)

Mixed connective tissue disease (MCTD)

Scleroderma

Dermatomyositis

Spondyloarthropathies

Leukemia

Lymphoma

Neuroblastoma

Tuberculosis

Epstein-Barr virus (infectious mononucleosis)

Parvovirus B19 infections

Lyme disease

Scheie syndrome (mucopolysaccharidosis I)

Fabry disease

HIV and other sexually transmitted diseases

LABORATORY FINDINGS

There are two key elements that must be considered when evaluating the laboratory results of a child who is failing to thrive:

1. **Entirely normal tests do not ensure the absence of disease.** Many children with chronic diseases begin to lose energy and feel unwell long before their routine laboratory test results become abnormal. It is important to make sure that all appropriate tests have been done.

2. **Things change over time.** On a number of occasions, I have evaluated children who have been followed for months with unexplained chronic complaints. Blood tests done when the child first presented were all normal. However, six months later, this was no longer the case. In the search for an explanation for a child's chronic illness, it is important to reevaluate everything periodically. Even though most children with a low-titer positive ANA but otherwise normal laboratory tests do not have a rheumatic disease, studies have shown that as many as ten years can elapse between the initial finding of a positive ANA and the development of clinical SLE. Periodically repeating the tests is important.

Often the earliest abnormalities in children with rheumatic diseases include a mild elevation of the ESR, a mild anemia, or mild hypoalbuminemia (see Chapter 25). Each of these findings is nonspecific, but an increasing number or gradual worsening of these nonspecific findings should prompt concern.

Many children with normal laboratory test results but continuing complaints are diagnosed as having fibromyalgia or a similar condition. However, it is important to be sure that other significant illnesses have been excluded. Extra steps should be taken if the child has any abnormal laboratory findings including a positive ANA, elevated ESR, or anemia. Even without such abnormalities, consideration must be given to uncommon conditions such as storage diseases. Careful evaluation of such children may include a bone scan and a gallium scan, which may reveal the presence of infections, tumors, or other causes of inflammation. Positron emission tomography (PET) scans are now becoming more readily available and are very effective in finding areas of increased cell turnover that could be tumors or infections. Tests such as MRI or ultrasound may be helpful in further evaluation of an area that has been identified as abnormal, but the bone scan and gallium scan have the advantage of evaluating the entire body in order to determine where more precise evaluation may be helpful (see Chapter 25). Urine testing for glycosaminoglycans is a useful screen for mild variants of mucopolysaccharidosis. Blood tests are available for Fabry disease. If you are considering a storage disease, have your ophthalmologist look for corneal clouding and check carefully for an enlarged liver or spleen.

WHEN NOTHING IS FOUND

Families and physicians become frustrated when, despite an entirely normal diagnostic evaluation, a child continues to complain of feeling unwell and is unable to continue his or her normal daily activities. Often the physician-family relationship becomes adversarial. The family *knows* that there is something wrong with the child, but the physician *knows* that he or she cannot find anything wrong. **It is vital for everyone involved to recognize that they are on the same side.** Often in this situation you want to recommend a psychological evaluation. Parents often interpret this as a suggestion that they or their child are crazy or that the child "must be faking it." You should emphasize to the family that you are doing everything possible to get at the root of the problem and restore the child to good health. It is important that they realize that psychological referral does not mean the end of medical evaluation.

To get the best possible outcome, it is important to explain to the family that, while psychological illness may cause chronic complaints of pain, chronic pain may also cause psychological illness. Both issues need to be addressed. The child who is unable to attend school needs psychological support, whether or not the cause is physical. At the same time, referral of the child to a psychologist should not stop the ongoing medical evaluation of the child. **I often explain to families that in medicine we have the luxury of being able to go in two directions at once.** It is easy to ask for a psychological evaluation and an MRI on the same day. Sometimes parents ask me how I can justify doing both. The answer is that it is always justified to do everything possible to find the cause of a child's complaints. Following only one direction at a time may not be in the child's best interest.

If a child is able to attend school and carry out essential activities, it may be necessary to continue to monitor and to repeat the diagnostic evaluation periodically while awaiting the outcome of the psychological intervention. For some families, this situation becomes unbearable. **The family must have complete confidence in the physician. If for any reason the family does not, they should be encouraged to seek a second opinion. We all have the child's best interest at heart. If another physician has a useful suggestion, everyone benefits. If your relationship with the family has foundered and the family can establish a better relationship with a new physician, again, everyone is better off.**

On occasion, I walk into the exam room to meet a new patient and see obvious problems even before I seat the child on the examination table. When the mother says that she took the child X years ago to a doctor who said that nothing was wrong, I wonder how the doctor could have missed the diagnosis.

However, with experience, I know that the initial complaints may have been minor. If every child with minor complaints was labeled with a serious diagnosis, most often the diagnosis would be wrong and the parents would have been made to worry unnecessarily. However, there will be the occasional child who is beginning to develop a serious disease. **The correct answer is to keep an open mind and periodically reevaluate the child rather than either dismissing the complaints as "nothing" or giving a worrisome "possible" diagnosis.**

I often evaluate children who have seen many physicians. Sometimes these children have significant problems that have been overlooked or misinterpreted by other physicians. As a specialist, I am able to diagnose and treat a number of unusual conditions that other physicians might not recognize. Sometimes children have a slowly evolving disease that was not evident initially but becomes more obvious over time. However, some of the families I evaluate are simply looking for the answer they want to hear. **Unfortunately, there are no adequate guidelines that can be listed in a book that will distinguish the child with normal laboratory test results who has an unrecognized illness from the child with a disturbed psychosocial situation. Nor are the two situations mutually exclusive.** Pediatricians must rely on their own experience and judgment in deciding when to go further and when to stop. If the family seems determined to believe that something is wrong, referral to a specialist may provide the needed reassurance for both you and the family.

5

Sports Injuries

I often evaluate children who have significant athletic ability and chronic pain. One of these was a young girl who was training for the Olympics. Tania had grown up in Eastern Europe, and because of her talent she had been selected to come to the United States to work with a famous coach in preparation for the next Olympics. Her family stopped to see me in New York on their way to the training program because she had "minor knee pain." When I took the history, I found that Tania's knee pain had begun over a year ago. At first it occurred only when she worked out, but with time it became more persistent. Her family was very proud, saying, "She works out six days a week, many hours each day despite the pain." Unfortunately, careful evaluation revealed that Tania had permanently damaged the bone in her leg (proximal tibia). Her dedication in continuing to practice despite the pain did not lead to the Olympics; it led to surgery and the end of her career. Had Tania stopped and been evaluated sooner, the diagnosis of benign hypermobile joint syndrome could have been made, the permanent injury could have been prevented, and her athletic career might have been saved.

Sports injuries are the most common causes of muscle, bone, and joint pains in childhood. Most are minor injuries related to trauma, easily recognized because the pain started right after falling, running into another child on the field, twisting an ankle, and so on. Often these are minor muscle and tendon injuries (bangs, scrapes, and sprains) that resolve over a few hours or days at most. Pain that is severe or persists requires medical attention.

Acute sports injuries are not the focus of this book. However, the child who is repeatedly injured or in pain every time he or she participates needs to be carefully evaluated to find out why. Children with chronic or recurrent "sports injuries" are often ignored because they seem to get better with rest. This is a mistake. Children with chronic and recurrent injuries may be suffering from overuse syndromes, unrecognized arthritis, or a variety of other medical conditions. Many children with spondyloarthropathies have been misdiagnosed as having chronic sports injuries by pediatricians and orthopedists unfamiliar with childhood arthritis (see Chapter 9).

The common athletic statement "No pain, no gain" is incorrect. While it is true that muscle pain with activity may be associated with building stronger muscles, **bone and joint pain is never associated with gain.** Continued activity using bones or joints that hurt is causing injury and may be causing permanent damage. Parents and teenagers must remember that athletic coaches and trainers are not physicians. Their primary goal is athletic achievement. Many of the conditions described below are the result of overuse of the bones and joints or imbalance between rapidly increasing muscle strength and more slowly strengthening bones. Some trainers, sports physicians, and orthopedists feel that these conditions should be treated with icing and taping. They commonly recommend that sports be continued unless "the athlete is unwilling or unable to tolerate the symptoms." This is a shortsighted approach. Many adults in their thirties and forties complain of chronic joint pains that they ascribe to high school and college athletics. Are this season's sports worth a lifetime of pain that could have been avoided by simply resting and letting the bones mature?

Just as pediatricians have become concerned about girls who are anorexic in their efforts to become as skinny and beautiful as the models in magazines, we need to be concerned about the girls and boys like Tania who are causing permanent damage to their bones and joints in an effort to excel. High-impact activities and sports associated with repeated trauma to any part of the body are not in the child's best interest, no matter how good the accomplishment makes them feel. There is increasing recognition of the chronic brain damage suffered by professional boxers, football players, and hockey players—their orthopedic problems are well known. But children are also at risk of chronic injuries, which will persist throughout life. Parents, coaches, and children need to recognize that while athletic activity is clearly beneficial, overemphasis on achievement is not.

Many children with enthesitis-associated arthritis are misdiagnosed as having chronic sports injuries by physicians who are unfamiliar with childhood arthritis (see Chapter 9). If you examine a child with left ankle pain but fail to ask questions or examine the rest of the body, you will probably not recognize that there are problems in other joints as well. But it is easy to make the correct diagnosis if you take a complete history and examine the entire child. I often see children with arthritis in multiple joints who come in complaining only about their knees or ankles. Neither they, nor their families, nor their physicians had recognized that they were suffering from arthritis rather than multiple independent injuries. When questioned, however, most gave a history of morning stiffness and other signs of arthritis. With proper diagnosis and treatment, we can often make many problems disappear and allow the resumption of full activity.

SPECIFIC INJURIES

The emphasis in this book is on children with chronic or recurring problems, and the proper evaluation and differential diagnosis of these conditions are discussed in the following sections. This book does not deal with specific fractures or acute injuries, but it is important to realize that some problems that seem to begin as acute injuries are in fact chronic conditions. For example, a child with Lyme disease may notice a swollen knee and pain after a soccer game. The parents and the family physician may assume that the child's knee had been twisted, failing to consider a chronic condition. It is important that medical as well as orthopedic conditions be considered when, after an "injury," a child's pain does not resolve as expected.

Stress Fractures

Overview

Stress fractures are one of the most common chronic injuries associated with sports activities in children and adolescents, occurring because of overuse and abuse of the bones. Typically, these fractures are caused by repeated impact. Stress fractures of the metatarsals are a common injury in runners, tennis players, and other athletes. However, stress fractures may occur in many different locations. Most often they occur in the legs, but tennis players and baseball players may experience stress fractures in the arms and shoulders as well. Most stress fractures usually occur early in the athletic season because the child tries to do too much too soon. But older children who are participating in team sports may overuse their bones with continued efforts and develop more severe stress fractures later in the season.

Diagnosis

Stress fractures usually first become evident when a child reports pain in a specific location following activity. If ignored, the pain will gradually become more severe and begin to occur earlier in the course of activity. Children with severe stress fractures of the metatarsals may have pain while walking. Because the pain of a stress fracture is right at the location of the fracture, it is often easy to diagnose on physical examination. However, other conditions can cause the gradual onset of worsening bone pain at a specific site, and proper radiographic evaluation is important. Most stress fractures occur in the shaft of the bone, not near the ends, but in growing children there can be stress fractures at the growth plate. These can be diagnosed by characteristic changes on the X-rays. Immediately after the injury the X-rays may be negative, but in any child with chronic pain they should be diagnostic. Magnetic resonance imaging studies are more sensitive and will help to exclude other possible causes of pain. Although much less common than stress fractures, both infections of the bone and bone tumors may begin with similar symptoms. Some children with arthritis are also initially misdiagnosed as having stress fractures that "did not show up on the X-ray." If the child has complained of pain for more than two weeks and the X-ray does not show a fracture, it is very unlikely that there is one.

Treatment

Children with stress fractures who are diagnosed quickly often will recover with ten to fourteen days of rest. However, it is recommended that children not begin to resume activities until they have had no symptoms for three weeks or more. Full activity should be avoided for several months. Continued participation despite pain may result in permanent disability. In more severe cases, casting is necessary. If rest and casting do not provide relief, surgery may be required. Any child with a presumed stress fracture who does not begin to recover as expected should undergo a thorough evaluation to exclude other causes of bone pain.

Tendonitis and Sprains

Overview

Tendonitis is usually the result of overuse of the muscles or an imbalance between the strength of the muscles and the bones. Bones and the attachments of tendons to bones strengthen slowly with growth and activity. Muscles strengthen much faster. As a result, children who begin vigorous activity at an early age strengthen their muscles and put excessive force on the bones and tendons before these structures are able to adapt. This often results in inflammation

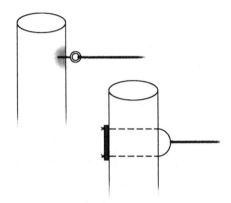

Figure 5-1 *On a working farm or ranch, you will never find a rope attached to a post by a single screw. Because the rope is often yanked on, it has to be carefully secured. Most often there is a U-shaped attachment through the post with solid supports on the other side. A rope attached to a fence post by a simple eyelet screw will rapidly be pulled out. By analogy, as children grow, it takes time for the tendons to become firmly anchored to the bones. If they are repeatedly jerked with physical activity such as jumping or kicking a ball, the insertion becomes irritated and may never develop normally.*

at the tendon insertion (see Fig. 5-1). This should be treated with rest and, if necessary, NSAIDs. Continued activity may result in long-term injury.

Diagnosis

Most commonly, tendonitis occurs in the shoulders and elbows of children who are participating in throwing sports (e.g., baseball, basketball, football) or around the ankles of children who are participating in activities that involve a lot of running. Tendonitis around the knee is relatively rare, with the exception of Osgood-Schlatter disease (see Chapter 3). Since tendonitis is most often associated with overuse, its occurrence should be regarded as a warning to decrease the intensity of training until the child's body is able to mature further. In older children who are skeletally mature, it is a clear indication of overuse.

Treatment

The key to resolving this situation is to enforce rest so that the inflamed tendon and bone can heal Although the inflammation can be reduced by local injections of corticosteroids, this does not correct the fundamental problem. Reduction of the activity causing the inflammation is the wiser approach.

Children with enthesitis-associated arthritis (spondyloarthropathy; see Chapter 9) have excessive tendonitis as part of their disease. Any child with multiple episodes of tendonitis or tendonitis in multiple joints should be carefully evaluated to exclude these conditions.

BACK PAIN

Back pain is not a common complaint in childhood. Children with back pain should be carefully evaluated, and chronic back pain should never be dismissed as growing pains (see Chapter 3). The most common cause of chronic back pain related to sports in adolescents is **spondylolysis**. This is a stress fracture of the pars interarticularis (see Fig. 5-2). It is often the result of excessive stress on the low back with dancing, running, weight lifting, or other activities. Female gymnasts are prone to this injury. As with stress fractures in other locations, the pain is usually exacerbated by activity and relieved by rest. X-rays may reveal the fracture, but in some cases an MRI or bone scan may be required. Children with this type of pain should be carefully questioned about pain in other joints or morning stiffness. Children with involvement of multiple joints or morning stiffness may have arthritis.

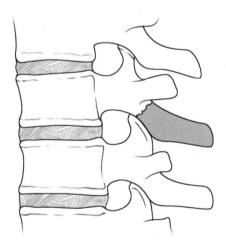

Figure 5-2 *Stress fracture of the pars interarticularis (darkened segment) causing back pain.*

Other causes of back pain that may become evident in association with physical activity are **disc herniation** and **spondylolisthesis.** Significant disc herniation is readily apparent on proper physical examination. Any child with pain when the straight leg is raised while lying flat on the back requires a thorough evaluation (see Fig. 5-3).

Spondylolisthesis is a progression of spondylolysis to the point where the vertebral body slides forward. This causes chronic back pain and is readily evident on radiographs. Many other chronic back conditions are not the result of sports injuries but may become more obvious when they limit a child's ability to participate. These conditions are discussed in the section on back pain in Chapter 3.

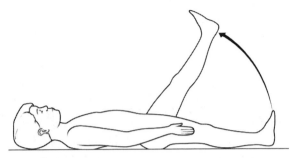

Figure 5-3 *Any child with pain when the straight leg is raised while lying flat on the back requires prompt medical evaluation.*

ELBOW PAIN

Chronic elbow pain often results from overuse. Younger children are very vulnerable to damage to the ligaments and growth plate of the elbow. Excessive pitching or throwing exercises and climbing on overhead bars (such as monkey bars) are common causes of elbow pain in children. Even if a child is well within the recommended level of activity for his or her age (e.g., 200 pitches per week for Little League), pain is an indication of ongoing injury. The child should stop and rest the joint. If the pain recurs after a period of rest, further medical evaluation is indicated and the activity must stop until it is completed. Other causes of elbow pain are discussed in Chapter 3.

Direct trauma to or overuse of the elbow can lead to **osteochondritis dissicans,** a dense area of damaged bone along the edge of the joint line. Osteochondritis dissicans is a common injury in children who have, despite pain, continued their throwing activities. It may respond to extended rest and immobilization of the limb, but in some cases the fragment of damaged bone will cause mechanical blockage. If this happens, the elbow may lock and surgery may be required to remove the fragment.

SHOULDER PAIN

Overuse is again the most common cause of pain in the shoulders. The shoulder is a relatively unstable joint that has a large range of motion. There is relatively little bony reinforcement. Without bony reinforcement, significant additional stress is put on the muscles and tendons of the shoulder. **Little Leaguer's shoulder** is the result of repeated stress to the humerus. Chronic pain and weakness in the shoulder are accompanied by widening of the growth plate at the proximal humerus. Rest, enforced by immobilization in a sling or cast in more severe cases, will usually result in full recovery if the activity is stopped.

Excessive stress to the shoulder can lead to **rotator cuff inflammation** and **impingement syndromes.** Acute tears are typically sudden in onset and easily recognized, but chronic inflammation evolves more slowly. Over time children complain of increasing pain with activity, especially with overhead throwing or swimming. These overuse syndromes are best treated with rest and modification of activity; NSAIDs may be helpful. Every child with chronic pain of this type should be carefully evaluated for symptoms in other joints. Children with spondyloarthropathies may first come to medical attention because of chronic shoulder pain, and only when specifically questioned will they admit to having pain in other joints. Even then, they often attempt to "explain away" these pains.

WRIST AND HAND PAIN

Wrist and finger injuries are common in sports activities. Fractures are usually immediately apparent. However, fractures of the scaphoid bone may not be immediately recognized. Scaphoid fractures usually occur after a fall on the outstretched hand. Following the fall, there is continued pain in the wrist but no pain at the ends of the long bones in the forearm (radius and ulna). If there is a fracture of the scaphoid, pressure on the anatomic snuff box (see Fig. 3-10) produces a dramatic increase in pain.

Another fracture that may not be immediately recognized is the **boxer's fracture** at the end of the fifth metacarpal. This fracture frequently occurs when adolescents strike something hard, often a wall or a locker. There is marked pain over the distal metacarpal. Failure to correct the injury may result in deformity.

Swollen and "jammed" fingers should be regarded with suspicion. A diffusely swollen finger is often thought to be due to an injury. However, dactylitis is a common finding in children with psoriatic arthritis and other spondyloarthropathies. A swollen finger that does not improve within ten to fourteen days should be thoroughly evaluated from both medical and orthopedic viewpoints. I have seen many children treated for months or years for chronic finger tendon injuries who were found to have obvious arthritis when other joints were examined as well.

HIP PAIN

Acute fractures and dislocations of the hip are immediately evident. Avulsion fractures are usually associated with the sensation of a snap or pop and immediate pain. X-rays typically confirm the diagnosis. Stress fractures in the femur or pelvis may develop more slowly, with children complaining of progressively increasing groin pain with activities. Although stress fractures in the femur are not always evident on X-rays, they are usually obvious on bone scan or MRIs.

Stress fractures of the pelvis are seen in adolescent runners. This is an uncommon injury that causes steadily increasing pain in the lower groin with activity that is relieved by rest. Like stress fractures elsewhere, they may be diagnosed by bone scan before they become evident on X-rays. The treatment is rest.

A number of chronic conditions in the hip may initially become evident during physical activity. These are described in detail in the section on hip pain in Chapter 3. Hip pain is a common complaint of children with spondyloarthropathies. Any child with chronic or recurrent hip pain that does not resolve with a period of reduced activity should be carefully evaluated. Continued activity in a child complaining of hip pain may result in permanent disability.

KNEE PAIN

The most common cause of knee pain in athletic children is **Osgood-Schlatter disease**. A disease similar in cause is **Sinding-Larsen-Johansson disease.** The condition is common among teenagers who do a lot of jumping in sports such as basketball and volleyball. Jumping increases stress on the knee with sudden pulling on the patellar tendon where it arises on the inferior pole of the patella. These children complain of knee pain whenever they jump, and examination reveals pain at the inferior pole of the patella (see Fig. 5-4). Treatment consists of resting the knee and avoiding jumping activities. **Jumper's knee** is a more severe injury occurring in older children. The mechanism of the injury is the same; excessive jumping repeatedly jerks the tendon where it inserts on the inferior pole of the patella. In jumper's knee there is a deep tear of the tendon itself that may ultimately require surgery to relieve the pain.

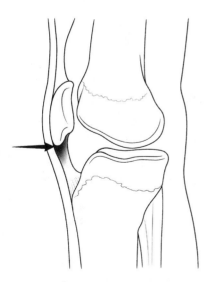

Figure 5-4 *Irritation where the tendon attaches to the bottom of the knee cap (patella) causes pain with jumping, which can be reproduced by pressing on the bottom of the patella in teenagers with Sinding-Larsen-Johansson disease.*

Knee pain with sports may also be the result of osteochondritis dissicans. This is a common injury in children who have continued running and jumping activities despite pain. It may respond to extended immobilization, but in some cases surgery may be required to remove the fragment.

Another common condition is **chondromalacia patella** or **patellofemoral dysfunction**. Knee pain that worsens when going downhill or downstairs is a very frequent problem with this condition. Despite the large number of children and young adults who suffer from this condition, it is poorly understood. No one has been able to demonstrate its cause convincingly. It typically responds to physical therapy and strengthening of the quadriceps musculature. Children incorrectly diagnosed with chondromalacia patella or patellofemoral dysfunction may have easily treated enthesitis. Although there are many proposed treatments for patellofemoral dysfunction, only two are generally agreed upon. The first is to avoid the activities that aggravate the condition. The second is a program of straight-leg raising exercises, which increase the strength of the quadriceps muscles. Several weeks of such exercises, if properly done, often restore the ability to resume normal activities without pain.

The iliotibial band is a band of tissue that runs along the lateral edge of the leg and anchors to the knee. If the band becomes tight, it will produce pain along the outside edge of the knee and in the outer aspect of the thigh. Although this condition occurs most commonly in joggers, iliotibial bands may also tighten in children who are active in other sports. The typical finding is chronic pain along the thigh and the outer edge of the knee. The pain comes on with running, but only after an extended period. It is often aggravated by going upstairs, in contrast to chondromalacia patella, which is worsened by going downstairs. A program of proper stretching and leg-strengthening exercises is often sufficient to correct this problem.

Plicae are folds of synovial tissue that may be seen in the knee on MRI. They are a normal finding and not usually a cause of pain. If a child has vague unexplained knee pains and a plica is noted on MRI, orthopedists may suggest arthroscopic surgery. However, there is a good chance that the plica is not the cause of the pain. Proper diagnosis of children with plicae centers on excluding other causes of the pain. Once that has been done, most children are advised to avoid the activities causing pain. If the pain persists despite these measures or the activity cannot be reasonably avoided, consider surgery. However, early arthritis is accompanied by thickening of the synovium, and it is not rare for a child with arthritis to be misdiagnosed as having plicae.

Meniscal tears are typically acute injuries that occur when the foot is fixed in position and the leg twists excessively, compressing the meniscus. Meniscal injuries during sports activity often are associated with damage to the cruciate ligaments and dramatic pain and swelling. Chronic knee pain due to meniscal injury usually is the result of a fall or a twisted knee that initially responded to rest. These are less severe injuries that may not come to immediate medical attention. Children with these injuries often report a grinding sensation or a sudden catching feeling deep in the knee. If the cruciate ligaments have been injured, there will also be instability. Instability of the knee often results in complaints of the knee suddenly giving out or locking. These symptoms always necessitate orthopedic evaluation and may require arthroscopy or an MRI.

True meniscal tears and cruciate ligament tears often require surgical intervention. Partial tears may be treated conservatively or operatively. When MRI testing first became routinely available, some children were found to have irregularities in the meniscus that did not extend to the surface. The explanation for these MRI findings remains controversial, but most authorities agree that surgery is not indicated.

LOWER LEG PAIN

There are relatively few conditions that cause pain in the tibia or fibula. Overuse may result in stress fractures. These present as chronic pain that recurs whenever the child attempts to resume physical activity. Infections and tumors are less frequent. These conditions often are easily detected if routine X-rays are obtained when a child has persistent complaints.

Shin splints are a common complaint of children who do a lot of running. They typically occur in children who are trying to do too much too fast. Often the problem disappears with additional conditioning. Children with continuing pain should be evaluated radiographically to be sure that there is not a more serious problem (stress fractures, infections, etc.). Arch supports and orthotics may be helpful in chronic cases.

Chronic compartment syndrome may be a cause of pain in the calf that recurs whenever the child is very active in sports. These children often feel well but complain of pain in the calf region after playing on the field for a significant period. The pain disappears with rest but recurs with activity. Often these children complain of tenderness when the calf is squeezed; typically, the problem is one-sided and occurs in the dominant leg. The pain results from enlargement of the muscles with exercise to the point that they are constricted by the surrounding tissues. If the problem does not resolve with a period of rest, surgery may be required.

Blount's disease is a condition in which the growth plate of the tibia becomes damaged along its inner aspect, resulting in unbalanced growth. The outside edge grows more than the inside edge, resulting in genu varum. This condition seems to occur more often in children who are obese and may be related to the stress that the excess weight places on the growing bone. The diagnosis can usually be made on a routine X-ray. Surgery may be necessary to correct the condition. (See the section on knee pain in Chapter 3.

ANKLE PAIN

The ankle is particularly vulnerable in growing children. Missteps and falls that place excessive force on the ankle joint are common injuries, but most ankle sprains are easily recognized and treated. More severe injuries should be evaluated to exclude the possibility of a fracture; this is especially important if there is evidence of bruising. Chronic or recurrent ankle injuries require careful evaluation. Some of these are due to partial tears of the ligaments that support the ankle. Others may be caused by damage to the growth plates of the bones.

A child with recurrent ankle pain without obvious injury should be investigated fully. Some children with recurrent ankle sprains in fact have inflamed tendons from arthritis. Children with enthesitis-associated arthritis may have marked tendon swelling and tenderness, especially around the ankle. On careful examination, many of these children are found to have tendon inflammation around multiple joints. With appropriate diagnosis and treatment, they are often able to resume full activity.

FOOT PAIN

There are many bones and joints in the foot, and all are subjected to substantial stress with normal walking and running that is greatly increased by competitive athletic activities. Because the foot is heavily reinforced mechanically and typically protected by shoes, acute injuries are relatively uncommon. When they do occur, they usually are the result of obvious direct trauma. Chronic foot pain may result from a variety of conditions.

The most common serious cause of chronic foot pain in athletes is a **stress fracture of the metatarsals**. These are overuse injuries found in many different sports, ranging from football and soccer to dance and gymnastics. These cause severe local pain, often over the lateral aspect of the foot. They are typically treated with casting and rest. Although the initial X-ray may not show the fracture, follow-up X-rays should demonstrate callus formation to confirm the diagnosis.

Mild **mechanical foot pain** is quite common. Often children with mechanical foot pain are found to have flat feet, and their pain is attributed to this finding. However, "flexible" flat feet are a common normal variation and are not thought to be a cause of significant foot pain. An orthopedist should evaluate all children with chronic foot pain. Some children obtain relief from the use of pads and other shoe inserts. Although relatively uncommon, there are more serious causes of flat feet that do require surgical correction. (See Chapter 3.)

Tarsal coalition may cause frequent foot pain, ankle sprains, and other foot discomfort. Although the condition begins early in life, many children become symptomatic only in the teenage years. This is also a time when the symptoms of enthesitis-associated arthritis may develop (see Chapter 9 for a full discussion). Children with chronic foot or ankle pains should be carefully evaluated. Tarsal coalition should be easily recognized on a CAT scan.

Heel pain is another symptom that can have multiple causes. Children with enthesitis-associated arthritis often have heel pain that has been unsuccessfully treated as a sports injury. A proper history and careful physical examination of the entire child are the keys to making the proper diagnosis. Many children with heel pain are given the diagnosis of **Sever's disease**. Sever's disease may be clinically diagnosed in children with pain at the sides of the heel but not at the base of the heel. X-ray diagnosis of Sever's disease on the basis of darkening of the growth plate at the back of the foot (calcaneal apophysis) is unreliable; many children without heel pain have identical findings (see Chapter 3).

PART II

THE RHEUMATIC DISEASES AND RELATED CONDITIONS

6

Why Do Children Get Rheumatic Disease?

Fill a football stadium with 100,000 random children, and the rheumatic diseases are rare. Fill that same football stadium with 100,000 children who have relatives with rheumatic disease, and children with rheumatic disease will be ten or twenty times as common. Researchers believe there is a genetic contribution here. While most of the rheumatic diseases clearly occur more frequently in relatives of people with rheumatic disease, not all parents with a family history of rheumatic disease need to worry. But these diseases occur in relatives often enough that investigators have to notice.

Since rheumatic disease is not good for your health, **why don't genes that contribute to it disappear over time?** As an explanation, I ask my patients to imagine a bank of ten switches that regulate the power to your town. Each switch provides 10 percent of maximum power. If all the switches are turned off, nothing works. One switch on helps, but two or three switches turned on are better. Everything works very well if five or six switches are turned on. However, maximum power is too much, and things will start to overheat or short out if seven switches are turned on, especially if there is a thunderstorm. Eight switches on causes many more problems if it is too hot or too cold or if there are storms. Things always go wrong if nine or ten switches are on. Now imagine what happens if the number of switches that are turned on for any given town is controlled by rolling dice. Most towns will do fine. Some towns will have problems only in special situations, such as thunderstorms. However, a few towns will have trouble all the time. But since each switch is independently controlled and some of them must be turned on or there is no power, everyone has to take the chance that too many switches might be turned on.

Then I ask my patients to imagine that instead of power switches, we are discussing genes that regulate the ability to fight infection. You are born with them either on or off. If you are born with none turned on, you are very likely to get an infection and die. If too many are turned on, you develop a rheumatic disease if the wrong things happen. Most people end up in the middle and do fine. You can't get rid of the switches because you never know which ones will be turned on in any given child at birth.

> How does the body's ability to fight infection relate to autoimmune disease? Rheumatic diseases appear to be the result of the immune system caus-ing damage to normal tissues as if an infection existed. Does this mean that the immune system is too strong or too weak? Imagine that your work requires you to go into a bar in a tough part of town. You were selected for this job because you are big and strong. If someone starts a fight, you will win, but if the person who attacks you is also big and strong, there may be damage to the bar and some of the innocent patrons may be injured. That happened not because you wanted to hurt them. The damage to the other patrons is *bystander damage*—an inadvertent side effect of what you had to do to protect yourself. So, a strong immune system can cause unintended damage.
>
> If a weak person has to go into a tough bar, he is in big trouble. Either he will be quickly done away with or he will carry a shotgun for backup. If someone picks on him and he starts firing the shotgun, a lot of people will get hurt and a lot of furniture will be damaged—again, a great deal of bystander damage. People with weak immune systems who survive do so because the immune system overreacts to any threat.

There is scientific evidence that this crude bar story is actually a good framework for understanding how autoimmune diseases come about. From the immune system's point of view, there are all sorts of bad guys out there. We need a strong immune system, but not one that is too strong. That's why the drugs we use for serious cases of rheumatic disease are immunosuppressive drugs. Survival depends on maintaining the delicate balance between overreacting to an infectious agent and not reacting adequately to protect yourself from the infection.

One of the key elements in pediatric practice is to get a good family history from the parents of newborns and other children. It takes a few extra minutes, but it can be very helpful in knowing what to look for if problems occur later. Many physicians rely on simple questionnaires to be filled out in the waiting room, but a quick verbal listing of diseases often causes parents to remember things they overlooked when filling out the form. Psoriasis, diabetes, thyroid disease, and inflammatory bowel disease all may be indications of an increased familial predisposition to autoimmune disease. More information on genetic factors can be found in Chapter 22.

7

Juvenile Arthritis

Juvenile Rheumatoid Arthritis, Juvenile Chronic Arthritis, Juvenile Idiopathic Arthritis

Whenever the diagnosis of juvenile arthritis is considered, two important points must be remembered. First, fever and rash should not be present in children with juvenile arthritis except in those with systemic-onset arthritis. If a child with arthritis has fever or a rash, a strong effort must be made to exclude infectious causes. Fever, rash, and arthritis may be present in Lyme disease, reactive arthritis, and a variety of other diseases that are not juvenile arthritis, including sarcoid, lupus, and IBD.

Second, it is important to differentiate between arthritis with painful, swollen joints and bone pain. Children are sometimes thought to have arthritis because they hurt all over. As a general observation, children with arthritis do not cry in pain when they are not touched or have an inflamed joint. Children who cry in pain when not being touched are obviously in distress, and this usually indicates a fracture, an infection, or a malignancy such as leukemia, lymphoma, or neuroblastoma.

NOMENCLATURE

Names may not seem very important, and indeed, in many ways they are not. It does not matter what you call a disease—it's still the same disease. However, nomenclature is very important when you are trying to learn more about a disease or discuss the care and treatment of a child. While most orthopedic conditions are well defined and only occasionally have more than one name for the same condition, the nomenclature of the rheumatic diseases of childhood is less clear.

According to the criteria of the American College of Rheumatology, juvenile rheumatoid arthritis (JRA) is the proper diagnosis for any child with the onset of arthritis before sixteen years of age, if the arthritis lasts for at least six weeks in more than one joint or three months in a single joint, without any other explanation. Thus, every child with chronic arthritis has JRA. However, it is very clear that not every child with arthritis has the same condition. If you told a rheumatologist specializing in adult arthritis that every adult with arthritis lasting for at least six weeks in more than one joint or more than three months in a single joint had rheumatoid arthritis, you would be told that you were poorly informed. There are more than fifty causes of chronic arthritis in adults, only one of which is rheumatoid arthritis. Nothing magic happens on the child's sixteenth birthday. There are probably just as many (if not more) causes of arthritis in childhood. But everyone assumes that all children with arthritis have JRA. This has resulted in a lot of confusion and misinformation.

Children with JRA are traditionally divided into three major groups: those with **pauciarticular onset** (fewer than five joints involved during the first six months), **polyarticular onset** (five or more joints involved during the first six months), and **systemic onset** (daily spiking fevers and rash; the number of joints does not matter). This system of nomenclature is unsatisfactory because a little girl with a swollen knee and inflamed eyes does not have the same disease as a teenage boy with a swollen knee and ankle pain, even though both would qualify for pauciarticular onset. It is important to recognize that they do not have the same disease because they have a different prognosis, different responses **to medications**—the best medicine for the little girl is unlikely to be the best medicine for the boy, and vice versa—and **most likely a different cause**. If both children are grouped together in a drug study as cases of pauciarticular JRA, the study may conclude that the drug does not work. However, if the study is done only with little girls or only with teenage boys, the doctors may find that the drug works very well. Even the most clearly written criteria are subject to confusion when applied in new situations.

CLASSIFICATION

I would like to describe a common fruit. It begins green, and while some remain so, many varieties turn red or yellow in color as they ripen. It has a prominent stem, is somewhat juicy, and has an obvious core with seeds that people normally discard. Some eat this fruit with the skin on, while others prefer to peel and section it before eating it.

This sounds like a clear description of an apple, and we are all familiar with apples. However, it would also describe a pear. To those of us who are familiar with these fruits, the distinction is obvious when we have one in our hand. However, for someone unfamiliar with them, this description could easily lead to misidentification of a pear as an apple or vice versa. Imagine attempting to follow an apple pie recipe using pears or a constantly varying mixture of apples and pears. Not only would you never get the expected results, but if you had a constantly varying mixture, you would never get the same results twice.

Arthritis is defined as pain, swelling, or limitation of motion in a joint. The official definition of JRA is any arthritis starting before sixteen years of age that persists as above without any other explanation. (The persistence is important because many viral and bacterial illnesses can cause arthritis that lasts for only a few weeks; see the section on reactive arthritis.) The arthritis may not necessarily have been noticed by a doctor for the previous six weeks or three months; there simply must be convincing evidence that it has been present for at least that long.

Most children with arthritis do not have a disease that is in any way related to the rheumatoid arthritis seen in adults. To reflect this difference, it has been proposed that the terms *juvenile chronic arthritis* (*JCA*) or *juvenile idiopathic arthritis* (*JIA*) replace *juvenile rheumatoid arthritis*. However, children suffer from many different forms of arthritis with many different causes and courses. It must be clearly recognized that these names refer not to a single disease but to a variety of diseases that share arthritis as a prominent symptom. To minimize confusion, I use the following nomenclature in this text: **Juvenile arthritis** (**JA**) will refer to *idiopathic* inflammation of the joints in a child. I use this term as *juvenile rheumatoid arthritis* was originally used, that is, to refer to all children with unexplained arthritis beginning before the age of sixteen, with the requirement that the arthritis is present for an extended period, as described above. Juvenile arthritis does not refer to a single disease with a single cause. It is not a disease at all; it is a group of signs and symptoms with many different causes and outcomes. Thus, to say that a child has JA is no more meaningful than to say that a child has a broken bone. Much depends on which bone is involved and how badly it is broken.

A number of subgroups of JA have been proposed. None of these is truly definitive, and there may well be several distinct diseases within each subgroup. Three important points must be remembered: First, unless we attempt to identify and investigate subgroups, we will never advance our current knowledge. In the end, some of the subgroups may need to be divided further, while others may be incorporated into the larger group. Second, if we insist on lumping groups together until someone has proven that they are different, we risk attempting to make apple pie with varying combinations of apples and pears and wondering why our results are inconsistent. Virtually every published article on the treatment of JRA suffers from this fault. Third, while it may be possible to memorize the entire American Kennel Club classification of breeds of dogs, there will always be mixed breeds that do not fit any classification. We are dealing with biologic phenomena occurring in nature, not a predetermined system. Diseases do not read or write textbooks and are not bound by what is written in them.

PAUCIARTICULAR-ONSET JUVENILE ARTHRITIS

Diagnosis

The first key distinction is between children with arthritis in a few joints (pauci- or oligoarticular-onset JA) and children with arthritis in many joints (polyarticular-onset JA). As originally defined, this categorization refers to the number of joints involved during the first six months of illness. Thus, a child who originally has only one joint involved but develops arthritis in four more joints during the next three months has polyarticular-onset disease. But a child who originally has only one joint involved and develops more joint involvement, but does not have a total of five joints involved until eight months later, still has pauciarticular-onset disease.

The distinction between pauciarticular-onset and polyarticular-onset JA is based only on the number of joints involved during the first six months after onset. This is both confusing and of limited utility. After all, who knows exactly when the arthritis started and can accurately date the six months? However, the classification persists because it is generally useful, and these flaws are easily dealt with by recognizing that children with involvement of the small joints of the hands and feet, with or without involvement of the large joints, have a different prognosis (and probably a different disease) than children with only large joint involvement. Since there aren't that many large joints (JA tends to spare the hips at the beginning), children with only large joint involvement typically have pauciarticular-onset JA. In contrast, involvement of the fingers or toes rapidly becomes polyarticular. Further, even if children have only one finger involved (two or three small joints), they have an entirely different prognosis (and a different disease) than children with two or three large joints involved. Understanding this flaw in the nomenclature makes it clear why a child who had been diagnosed with pauciarticular-onset JA may have disease that does not behave like the textbook description.. The proper classification should be onset with only large joints involved versus onset with small joints involved, with or without large joints.

Older children with disease only in large joints often have a spondyloarthropathy. This is a completely different group of diseases with different outcomes and different best therapies. Thus, they are discussed separately in Chapter 9. Children with involvement of fingers or toes (*dactylitis*) also must be considered separately, even if fewer than five joints are involved during the first six months of disease.

Pauciarticular-onset arthritis has a variety of forms. This is most often a disease of young girls and some boys that starts between one and seven years of age. In the most typical cases, there is a single swollen knee. Frequently, there is no history of pain and the parents are unaware of the problem until a friend or relative points out the swollen joint. When asked, the parents cannot tell you when the problem began. There may be awareness that the child walks oddly when he or she first gets up, but because the child walks normally after a little while, the parents often think that he or she "just sleeps on it in a funny way." Some physicians have referred to this as "painless JRA" because the child does not complain. However, if you squeeze the joint or attempt to put it through the full range of motion, it is painful. The child does not complain because the child does not recognize that the condition is abnormal.

Children with the acute onset of a painful swollen knee should not be considered as having pauciarticular JA. Among the conditions that may cause the acute onset of this swelling are infections (including Lyme disease), reactive arthritis, foreign body synovitis, and injuries. On rare occasions, a child with a chronically swollen knee (i.e., pauciarticular arthritis) that has gone unnoticed will be brought to the doctor complaining of acute pain in conjunction with an infection. The chronically swollen knee was noticed only with the increased problems brought on by the infection. This can be determined by a careful history and physical examination. Frequently, bony overgrowth is present and there is atrophy of the surrounding musculature. These are clear indications that the disease has existed for a prolonged period, since bony overgrowth and muscle atrophy take months to develop.

Children who begin with pain in the hip also should not be considered as having pauciarticular JA. Although polyarticular arthritis and systemic-onset arthritis may ultimately involve the hip, this is never the first joint involved and it is never involved in pauciarticular arthritis. I have seen cases of toxic synovitis, Lyme disease, osteoid osteoma, occult fractures, and tumors misdiagnosed as JA starting in the hip. Spondyloarthropathies may start in the hip, but these occur most often in children over the age of ten years. Any young child with hip pain must be thoroughly investigated, and an explanation other than pauciarticular-onset arthritis should be found. (There are exceptions to every rule, but never accept the idea that your case is the exception without very careful evaluation.)

Monitoring

Laboratory findings in children with pauciarticular-onset disease are usually entirely normal. They should have a normal complete blood count (CBC), normal metabolic panel, and normal erythrocyte sedimentation rate (ESR). Rheumatoid factor (RF) should be negative, but antinuclear antibody (ANA) may be present (see Chapter 25 for a full discussion of these tests). Mild abnormalities of the CBC and ESR are common, but children with significant laboratory abnormalities during the first six months of treatment should be regarded with suspicion.

During the first six months of disease, children with true pauciarticular disease should not have a hemoglobin level below 11 gm/dl without an explanation or an ESR greater than 40 mm/hr. Those who do are more likely to have further arthritis in the future. Other findings that increase the risk of continuing or recurrent arthritis are IgA deficiency or the genetic marker HLA B27. A family history of psoriasis or IBD also increases the risk of further arthritis. It is most likely that children with these findings do not have the same disease as those with true pauciarticular-onset JA. The prognosis for children with well-defined pauciarticular-onset disease is good. This is the form of JA responsible for the myth that "most children grow out of it." Children with pauciarticular-onset disease who do not do well are often distinguished by the exclusions indicated above.

Complications

There are two typical complications of pauciarticular-onset disease. These are limb length discrepancy and uveitis.

Limb Length Discrepancy

Limb length discrepancy is the result of persistent inflammation in one knee. The inflamed knee develops an increased blood flow as a result of mediators produced by the inflamed synovium, bringing more nutrients to the bones around the knee. With additional nutrients the bones will grow more rapidly, causing increased growth on that side. Yes, the arthritic leg will actually grow longer. This is not always easy to see, but it is easy to detect by properly measuring the leg. This is best accomplished by doing a CAT scan and using the computer to measure the exact length of each bone in the leg. In the past, it was done with a special radiograph called a *scanogram*, an X-ray including a visible ruler so that the bones can be directly measured. Either technique can be used, but the CAT scan is faster and more accurate.

One may not be aware of a difference in leg length just by watching a child walk. This is because children with arthritis in the knee often develop a flexion contracture that makes the leg appear shorter. Bending the knee decreases the pressure in the inflamed joint, and it hurts less. Unfortunately, at the same time, the pain causes the muscles around the knee to spasm. With prolonged muscle spasm, a flexion contracture develops, and it becomes impossible to completely straighten the leg.

As the inflammation improves with treatment, the flexion contracture may not resolve as expected. Children with a leg length discrepancy often continue to hold the longer leg bent in order to keep both legs functionally the same length when walking. This can be corrected by putting a lift in the shoe on the shorter side. Many parents don't like to put lifts in their children's shoes, but failure to correct the situation makes it difficult to correct the flexion contracture and may lead to hip damage in later life. Occasionally, children with involvement of the elbow may develop a discrepancy in the length of the arms or a flexion contracture at the elbow. In these children, the condition is noticed when they cannot fully extend the elbow.

Box 7-1   Testing for a knee flexion contracture

If you as a parent are concerned that your child may have a knee flexion contracture, you can easily evaluate this by having the child sit on the floor. A normal child can put the knee flat on the floor so that you cannot even slip a piece of paper underneath it. If you can see a space under the knee or slip your fingers under it, a flexion contracture exists (see Fig. 7-1).

When evaluating a child with pauciarticular-onset disease for joint swelling or a limb length discrepancy, you may be misled by the fact that in addition to the leg growing longer, the distal femur and proximal tibia are growing larger. When the arthritic leg is compared with the normal one, muscle atrophy will make the situation look even worse. You need to examine the knee carefully to differentiate between bony overgrowth and continued swelling. Bony overgrowth makes the knee look bigger, but excessive joint fluid is not present. This does not require a change in medication. If the knee is swollen because of extra joint fluid, then it does need to be treated. Sometimes a knee with bony overgrowth becomes inflamed and there is extra joint fluid as well.

The key to preventing muscle atrophy, limb length discrepancies, and flexion contractures is to bring the inflammation under control quickly. Once these problems have developed, the child should be given extensive physical therapy to correct the weakness and contracture as quickly as possible. Leg length

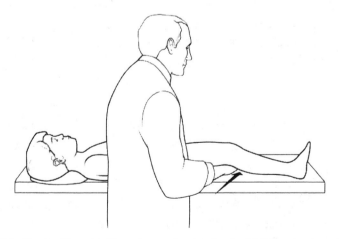

Figure 7-1 *You should **not** be able to slip your hand under the child's leg when he or she is sitting on the floor with the knee flat.*

discrepancy may not persist if the inflammation is brought under rapid control. If it does persist, it should be corrected as the child nears adult height.

Uveitis

Uveitis is the other significant complication of pauciarticular JA. Although the reason for its occurrence has not yet been fully determined, the presence of a positive ANA is strongly correlated with the risk of eye disease. Children with pauciarticular-onset disease who are ANA-positive are much more likely to have eye disease than those who are ANA-negative. The eye disease takes the form of inflammatory cells

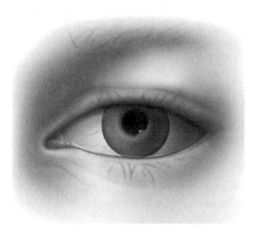

Figure 7-2 *Synechiae in the eye of a child with uveitis.*

in the anterior chamber of the eye called *uveitis* or *iridocyclitis*. The inflammation can lead to damage to the iris with scarring and irregularity of the pupil. These scars are called *synechiae* (see Fig. 7-2). Because the eye disease is usually painless and may go unnoticed for a long period, it is recommended that an ophthalmologist screen such children every three months. ANA-negative children should be screened every six months. Although the risk of eye involvement is lower in ANA-negative children and in children with polyarticular-onset disease, it may still occur. For more information, see Chapter 8.

Stiff Neck

On occasion, I see children who were diagnosed with pauciarticular-onset disease many years earlier and who now have stiff necks. It is well recognized that children with polyarticular-onset disease may develop cervical fusion over time that causes a stiff neck. Often there is no complaint from the child, and the finding is noted only on X-rays. Usually, at the time I see these children, it is because they have developed more arthritis. It is unclear whether cervical fusion is a complication of true pauciarticular-onset arthritis or whether these children should have been characterized as polyarticular initially.

Jaw Pain

Temporomandibular joint pain (jaw pain) and a decreased ability to open the mouth wide also occur years later in some children with pauciarticular-onset arthritis. It can present as difficulty opening the mouth wide, difficulty chewing, or chronic headaches on one side of the head. Often this occurs in the same children who have neck pain. How these two findings are interrelated, and how they are related to true pauciarticular-onset arthritis, is unclear. Temporomandibular joint involvement also occurs in some children with spondyloarthropathies.

Medical Treatment

Treatment for pauciarticular-onset arthritis usually consists of NSAIDs. These drugs are discussed in detail in Chapter 23. Since this is primarily a disease of young children, medications in liquid form are preferred. Ibuprofen and naproxen preparations are widely available as liquids. Indomethacin is also available in liquid form but has more frequent side effects and should be reserved for difficult cases. Celecoxib is another NSAID that has been approved for use in children and comes in liquid form. Nabumetone is available only in pill form but dissolves easily in warm water and can be drunk by children who do not know how to swallow pills.

I often use diclofenac for children with pauciarticular-onset disease who do not respond adequately to the readily available liquid medications. Although it is not stocked in liquid form, a compounding pharmacist can easily provide liquid diclofenac. Naproxen, celecoxib, nabumetone, and diclofenac have the advantage of being required less frequently than ibuprofen.

For children who meet my definition of true pauciarticular arthritis, additional medications will rarely be necessary. Corticosteroids (prednisone), methotrexate, cyclosporine, and other immunosuppressive drugs should not be needed (remember, there are exceptions to virtually every rule, but they are rare). Occasionally, there are children who have persistent swelling of one or two joints despite an adequate trial of NSAIDs. For these children, it is reasonable to consider intra-articular injection of corticosteroids.

Intra-articular corticosteroids rarely have side effects and often provide rapid and dramatic relief (see Chapter 23). Unfortunately, it is impossible to predict who will respond and for how long. The majority of children get a good response for months, if not longer. Some physicians will inject multiple inflamed joints in an effort to avoid increasing the medications. I will consider injecting two joints, but if more than two joints are persistently inflamed, I prefer to alter the medication rather than subject the child to multiple injections. Multiple inflamed joints suggest that this is polyarticular disease, not pauciarticular JA (even if only four joints are involved), and systemic medication is more likely than multiple intra-articular injections to give the desired long-term response (note: because some steroids leak out of the joint following injection, a brief dramatic improvement following multiple joint injections is common, but this is a short-lived effect).

If only one joint is to be injected, the majority of children can be easily talked through the procedure without requiring anesthesia and without undue distress. If multiple joints are to be injected, anesthesia may be necessary. Most pediatric rheumatologists believe that appropriate use of intra-articular corticosteroids will decrease the frequency of leg length discrepancy by bringing the inflammation under control more rapidly. Intra-articular corticosteroids in conjunction with **night splints** or **serial casting** and physical therapy often make it easier to correct flexion contractures. Physical therapy is a valuable adjunct for children with arthritis. In children with pauciarticular-onset disease, physical therapy can help to restore lost strength and to correct or prevent flexion contractures. In many cases, children with flexion contractures will benefit from night-resting splints or serial casting without intra-articular injections.

Surgery

Surgical therapy for true pauciarticular-onset arthritis is rarely necessary, but if it is, surgery to correct leg length discrepancy is a minor procedure. Most small children who develop leg length discrepancies as a result of pauciarticular-onset arthritis will self-correct with growth and remodeling over time. However, the arthritis must be under good control for this to happen.

In children who reach the age of ten with a significant persisting leg length discrepancy, an orthopedic appointment should be scheduled. With CAT scans or scanograms for leg length measurement and an X-ray called a *wrist for bone age*, the orthopedist can predict the amount of future bone growth using standard tables. In general, orthopedists will not intervene unless they expect a leg length difference of greater than one inch. If it is likely that there will be a significant difference, the orthopedist will monitor the child to determine how long it will take the short leg to catch up to the long one. When appropriate, a staple is placed in the distal epiphysis of the longer leg. This signals the bone to stop growing. Now that the excessively long bone has stopped growing, the shorter one keeps growing: If the child fulfills the predictions in the table, there will be little or no difference in the length of the legs once full size is attained.

There are two other situations in which surgery is considered for children with pauciarticular-onset arthritis. If a very severe flexion contracture has developed and it cannot be corrected with physical therapy and intra-articular corticosteroids, the orthopedist may consider doing tendon releases. In addition, there are exceptional cases of children with chronic active synovitis unresponsive to multiple medications or intra-articular corticosteroids. These children probably do not have true pauciarticular-onset arthritis. It may be necessary for the surgeon to explore the joint and do a synovectomy and/or a biopsy to exclude other diseases, such as plant thorn synovitis (see Chapter 3).

Prognosis

The prognosis for true pauciarticular arthritis is very good. Most children become well within a few months. My normal standard is to treat a child until there is no evidence of active disease for six months. This often means nine months to a year of treatment. At that point, I will discontinue the NSAIDs and watch carefully. Most children (about 80 percent) will remain well without medication. In a few children the disease will flare up shortly after medication is stopped, and a few more children will develop new episodes of arthritis over the next few years. The explanation for this is unclear.

When pauciarticular-onset arthritis flares up, the child should be carefully reinvestigated to exclude other problems. Children with a well-documented history of JA may develop Lyme disease, bone infections, or other problems that at first look like a recurrence of JA.

There is no reason to expect that children with true pauciarticular-onset disease will be unable to lead fully functional lives. There is nothing about pauciarticular-onset disease that should limit the ability to play sports, have families, or participate in all other normal activities. The prognosis for children with significant eye disease will depend on their ultimate visual status; this is best discussed with the treating ophthalmologist (see Chapter 8). It should be noted that it is rare for children with pauciarticular arthritis to develop new eye disease after ten years of age.

Children who do not have true pauciarticular arthritis may ultimately be recognized as having several different diseases. As previously indicated, any child with a hemoglobin level below 11.0 gm/dl, an ESR greater than 40 mm/hr, IgA deficiency, HLA B27, a family history of psoriasis, or a family history of IBD should not be considered as having pauciarticular arthritis. Many of these children will develop arthritis in additional joints before six months and fulfill criteria for polyarticular-onset disease.

I commonly see children for a second opinion because the parents were told that the child had pauciarticular-onset disease and would grow out of it. A few months later, the disease is spreading and their physician is recommending aggressive therapy. The parents consider the possible side effects and ask, "Why should we take these risks if our child is going to grow out of this?" If the physician had recognized that the child was at increased risk, this situation could have been avoided. Not all children who fulfill the criteria for increased risk do poorly. However, the percentage of children who have continuing problems is higher. If the parents and physicians are aware of the increased risk, they will not be lulled by false expectations. These children should be treated like children with polyarticular-onset disease, a condition discussed in the next section.

POLYARTICULAR-ONSET JUVENILE ARTHRITIS

Overview and Diagnosis

Polyarticular-onset disease is defined as arthritis involving more than four joints during the first six months of disease. In my opinion, any involvement of small joints indicates polyarticular-type disease, even if initially fewer than five joints are involved. Polyarticular-onset disease may occur in any age group but is found more often in girls than in boys. This is a very heterogeneous group of diseases. There are two major peaks in the age at onset of disease; in young children between eighteen months and eight years of age and in teenagers after eleven years of age. Some children start with only one or two arthritic joints, the arthritis slowly spreading to other joints, while other children rapidly develop arthritis of multiple joints.

Most pediatric rheumatologists make distinctions based on the presence or absence of RF—it is normally absent. They may also subcategorize according to whether the disease is symmetric or asymmetric. Children with tendon insertion inflammation (enthesitis), a family history of psoriasis, a family history of IBD, or the presence of HLA B27 are included in this group by some physicians but excluded by others. I exclude children with these findings because I believe most of them have spondyloarthropathies that behave differently (see Chapter 9). Even when all the children with these findings are excluded, the remaining children are a diverse group and most likely have several different diseases.

Laboratory findings in children with polyarticular-onset arthritis are highly variable. Some have entirely normal laboratory test results, while others have elevated ESR and low hemoglobin. A small percentage of children with polyarticular-onset disease are RF-positive and should be considered as having early-onset adult-type rheumatoid arthritis. However, RF may be found in a number of other conditions (see Chapter 25) and should not be relied on to establish this diagnosis. A positive test for RF in a child less than ten years of age is far more likely to be a false-positive result or an indication of another illness than a sign of early-onset RF-positive polyarticular arthritis. The test for ANA may also be positive in children with polyarticular-onset disease. Although their risk of eye disease is lower than that of ANA-positive children with pauciarticular-onset disease, ANA-positive children with polyarticular disease also have an increased risk of uveitis and should be sent to the ophthalmologist for a screening examination every three months.

Several diseases need to be distinguished from polyarticular-onset arthritis. Children with rheumatic diseases such as systemic lupus erythematosus, dermatomyositis, polyarteritis nodosa, sarcoidosis, and mixed connective tissue disease often have polyarticular arthritis in addition to their other conditions. A variety of less frequent diseases also may begin with polyarticular arthritis. These diseases should be excluded by an appropriate history, physical examination, and laboratory evaluation. Children with chronic pains in their hands or feet without obvious synovitis should be evaluated for the possibility of conditions such as Fabry disease or mucopolysaccharidosis.

The disease most often confused with polyarticular-onset JA is **reactive arthritis** (also called **infection-associated arthritis**). Reactive arthritis often begins with the rapid onset of disease involving the large and small joints (see Chapter 9). The key to suspecting this diagnosis is a history of an infection usually ten to fourteen days before the onset of arthritis. Children who rapidly develop polyarthritis should be evaluated carefully for evidence of either a recent infection or an infection that is still present and may need to be treated. Parvovirus B19 infection and Lyme disease are just two examples of many infections that cause an acute reactive arthritis with an elevated ESR and an ill-appearing child. Reactive arthritis can often be differentiated by the history or the laboratory findings. This is important because reactive arthritis typically resolves over a period of a few weeks to several months. In some cases, it appears that an infection that is known to cause reactive arthritis initiates chronic polyarticular arthritis in a susceptible individual (this arthritis is discussed in detail in Chapter 9).

Children with early-onset polyarticular disease often seem to improve, then worsen repeatedly over a period of years. As a result of repeated episodes, they develop progressively more joint involvement and are a difficult group to bring under continued control. It is usually possible to bring their arthritis under reasonable control with medications, but it is unlikely that their arthritis will ever completely disappear, never to return.

Treatment

Children who have continuing smoldering disease activity should be treated relatively aggressively. Often the parents and children become tired of all the medicines and doctors' appointments. However, the outcome is generally much better for children who are consistently treated than for those who take medication only when they are uncomfortable (see Chapter 27). With the availability of medications such as etanercept and adalimumab, we can provide sustained relief of symptoms and slow or prevent joint damage.

Children with later onset of polyarticular disease have highly varied outcomes. Some have arthritis that seems to resolves without explanation, while others develop progressively severe joint involvement. Therapy with methotrexate, etanercept, or adalimumab should be considered for any child who is not obtaining nearly complete symptomatic relief from NSAIDs. And any child with evidence of erosions or other indications of long-term joint damage should be given methotrexate, etanercept, or adalimumab.

Complications

The complications of polyarticular-onset arthritis are primarily those of the arthritis itself. Pain, swelling, and limitation of motion may result in weakness, bone loss (osteoporosis), and difficulty in performing activities of daily living. This type of arthritis may spread to involve the hip, and hip replacement surgery is sometimes necessary. Involvement of the wrists and fingers may also limit function. Cervical spine fusion and foot deformities are additional complications seen in some children with chronic active disease. Fortunately, the majority of children experience substantial relief when treated aggressively. Usually, the need for joint replacement surgery diminishes substantially with the increased utilization of etanercept and adalimumab.

The key to minimizing complications in children with polyarticular disease is early and aggressive medical intervention. Once it is recognized that a child has progressive polyarticular disease, every effort must be made to suppress the inflammation. With the availability of agents such as etanercept and adalimumab, pediatric rheumatologists are able to keep polyarticular arthritis under nearly complete control in a large majority of children.

Medical Treatment

A few children with mild polyarticular-onset arthritis will respond well to NSAIDs. Most need the more effective NSAIDs (diclofenac is usually my first choice), but some find nabumetone, naproxen, or ibuprofen adequate. For children with persistent or more severe disease, sulfasalazine is often an effective second-line agent. If further medication is necessary, the standard answer has been methotrexate, but the tumor necrosis factor (TNF) inhibitors etanercept and adalimumab are more efficacious, with a faster response and fewer potential side effects. Tumor necrosis factor inhibitors are given by injection, which makes some parents uncomfortable, but they often produce dramatic, rapid, and sustained improvement (see Chapter 23). For children who do not respond to TNF inhibitors, additional agents that block T-cell signaling (abatacept) or interleukin-1 (IL-1) (anakinra and others) or IL-6 (tocilizumab and others) have become available. There is extensive experience with the long-term safety and efficacy of TNF inhibitors (etanercept, adalimumab, infliximab) and anakinra. Other agents are still undergoing evaluation. Fortunately, few children fail to respond to TNF inhibitors.

Rituximab is a monoclonal antibody to CD20, which is a marker on the surface of B cells. Adults with rheumatoid arthritis have shown dramatic benefit with rituximab. This drug has also been beneficial for children with polyarticular arthritis who have not responded to other medications. A second and new agent is abatacept. This agent blocks T-cell signaling, which is important in driving the immune response. It too has proven effective in adults with rheumatoid arthritis and in children with polyarticular disease. A large number of additional agents are in the late stages of clinical evaluation and may become available before the next edition of this book is published.

Aggressive Medical Treatment

I am often confronted by parents who are concerned that their child is taking too much medicine. "Why can't we just wait and see what happens?" they ask. If the disease is mild and the child appears to be doing well, this is a perfectly sensible question. However, the reason for being a specialist in a field of medicine is to gain greater experience in that area and then bring that experience to bear on the problem. As a practicing pediatric rheumatologist, I pay a lot of attention to my sense of whether or not things are going well. If they are not, I will strongly encourage families to move forward before the damage becomes obvious. Here's one way to explain to a parent why aggressive therapy might be necessary:

> Imagine that you are having a party and a guest reports that he smells smoke. No one will be too concerned if no one else smells smoke, but you'd better investigate, just in case. At the first indication that there really is smoke, you want to call the fire department. Imagine explaining to the firemen that you did not call sooner because you did not want to upset everyone or disrupt your party. They will then tell you that they can put out fires, but once the fire has gotten out of control, they cannot repair what has already been damaged. Anti-inflammatory drugs work the same way. They can suppress inflammation to prevent joint damage, but they cannot repair joint damage once it has occurred. Don't let your child develop permanent damage before deciding to accept more aggressive therapy. The whole point of aggressive therapy is to prevent the damage.

Steroids will make a child with arthritis feel better rapidly, but if they are used for a prolonged period, they are frequently associated with major side effects. For children with polyarticular-onset arthritis, steroids should be viewed like a fire extinguisher next to the stove. They may be very useful if things suddenly flare out of control, but they certainly are not intended for repeated or continuing use. This doesn't mean that we never use them—only that we try to minimize their use.

I reserve steroid-containing drugs primarily for children with severe disease impairing their daily activities. I will nearly always begin a second-line agent shortly after I begin the corticosteroids with the intent that the second-line agent will help me stop the steroids as quickly as possible. With the ready availability of newer biologic agents such as etanercept and adalimumab that block TNF-α activity, the use of steroids is rarely necessary.

Treating Pain

I occasionally see children with arthritis who are taking pain killers. Excessive use of codeine and its derivatives or similar drugs is often associated with abnormal behavior and in some cases can lead to addiction. Some physicians feel that judicious use is warranted. Unfortunately, everyone's definition of judicious is different. For most children with arthritis, acetaminophen is an appropriate and adequate addition to help control pain. There are children who require tramadol or propoxyphene on occasion.

Surgery

Surgical therapy for children with polyarticular-onset arthritis is primarily limited to joint replacement surgery. Specific examples include the following:

- Children with severe involvement of the shoulder may benefit from replacement of the glenoid. Upper extremity joint replacement below the shoulder is generally unsatisfactory.
- Children with fused elbows may benefit from elbow replacement.
- Children with severe involvement of the wrist or fingers may benefit from fusion of troublesome joints. Replacement of finger joints is not generally helpful. When there is significant wrist subluxation, surgery to fuse the wrist in a functional position is often helpful. In addition, it is sometimes necessary to remove the distal ulna to prevent damage to the extensor tendons.

Lower extremity joint replacement surgery is much more effective. If a child is losing the ability to walk because of hip pain, it is important to replace the hip. Twenty-five years ago, children with severe hip pain were given a wheelchair, and most are still using them. Now we replace the hip joint, and arthritic children in wheelchairs are no longer frequently seen in major treatment centers.

As soon as the hip begins to prevent the child from walking outside the house, it is time to replace the hip joint.Many parents are worried and want to wait. This does not make sense. As soon as the child's walking becomes limited, strength and range of motion are lost. This makes recovery after surgery much more difficult and complete functional recovery much less likely. Many children who have had total hip or total knee replacement could walk right by, and you would never notice (see Chapter 26). Fortunately, appropriate use of TNF inhibitors has made childhood joint replacement surgery infrequent.

Physical and Occupational Therapy

Physical and occupational therapy play an important role in children with polyarticular-onset disease, even though parents may complain that their children do all sorts of physical and occupational (not to mention medical) therapy and never seem to get better. Exercises and stretching play an important role in maintaining strength, endurance, and range of motion in children. It is important to realize that children with arthritis who are left untreated steadily get worse. Sometimes in the face of very active disease, successful therapy slows down the problem until new medications take effect or the disease itself slows down. These children are much better off because of their therapy, even though they may have gotten worse while being treated.

Splinting is an important part of physical and occupational therapy. Children with pain often hold their joints in the position of maximum comfort. This is not the position of maximum function. Over time, the tendons contract and the child progressively loses range of motion and function. Knee flexion contractures can be sharply reduced or prevented by the appropriate use of night-resting splints. Children do not like them because they cannot walk with the splint on and it is uncomfortable to sleep with the leg held straight all night. But splints are also important to prevent flexion contractures and subluxation at the wrist. They substantially improve the long-term outcome.

Prognosis

The long-term prognosis for children with polyarticular-onset disease is highly variable. Most long-term complications can be prevented by early use of TNF inhibitors and additional agents if necessary. If significant joint damage has occurred prior to or despite proper therapy, surgical intervention may be helpful. Tumor necrosis factor inhibitors are very effective in preventing disability and joint destruction, but for most children the drugs cannot be withdrawn. These drugs suppress the disease, not cure it.

SYSTEMIC-ONSET JUVENILE ARTHRITIS

Diagnosis

> **Quick Summary**
>
> - The fever must disappear at least once each day. If it does not, the diagnosis is probably wrong.
> - The rash should have the characteristic salmon pink appearance. It is never ecchymotic or purpuric.
> - Positive ANA and uveitis are rare in systemic-onset JA.
> - Rheumatoid factor should not be present.

Systemic-onset JA refers to the onset of arthritis with fever and a characteristic rash. Systemic-onset JA has no relationship to adult-onset rheumatoid arthritis or the other forms of JA. It is an entirely separate disease.

Although all children with systemic-onset arthritis share key characteristics, the outcome of this disease is varied. There are several key points to remember when making the diagnosis of systemic-onset arthritis. First, the fever must disappear at least once each day. Second, the rash should have the characteristic salmon pink appearance. The rash is never ecchymotic or purpuric, but it is occasionally pruritic. Some children have onset of fever and rash before the arthritis becomes evident. These children should always be followed carefully for the possibility of another diagnosis, especially an infection.

Pauciarticular and polyarticular arthritis affect girls more frequently than boys, but in systemic arthritis the sex ratio is equal. In pauciarticular and polyarticular disease, ANA is commonly present and eye disease is frequent. Eye disease and ANA are both rare in systemic-onset JA. Rheumatoid factor should not be present in children with systemic-onset arthritis.

The typical presentation of systemic-onset arthritis is a child who has recurring fevers and rising ESR, WBC, and platelet counts but falling hemoglobin. The child frequently looks extremely ill. Most often the child is thought to have an infection, and the possibility of systemic-onset arthritis is considered only when there has been no response to antibiotics.

The first real indication that the diagnosis is systemic-onset arthritis may be the appearance of the characteristic rash. If the rash is not obvious, look for it in the axillae and around the waist. The rash is often visible only when the child is hot (e.g., after a bath or after playing sports). If the child is left with the shirt off, the rash may disappear before you can show it to someone else. It is often possible to make the rash more evident with a warm bath. Textbooks describe the Koebner phenomenon, in which a line made by pressure on the skin will spread beyond the area that was initially touched. In clinical practice, this test is rarely positive. Arthritis may be present even at the earliest stages of the disease. Often it is present but has been overlooked.

A helpful finding in establishing the diagnosis of systemic-onset arthritis is dramatic improvement during the period when the fever disappears each day. Often I will be called in the afternoon to see a child who looks very ill and might have systemic-onset arthritis. The child has been in another hospital and was not getting better. After transfer to my hospital, pediatric rheumatologists have been called in as part of the evaluation. Typically, after evaluating the child carefully for other explanations, we discuss the possibility of systemic-onset arthritis and wait for new test results. While waiting for these results, it is common for the physicians on the ward to change to new antibiotics.

The next morning, the ward physicians are happy to announce that the fever is gone, the child looks much better, and by changing the antibiotics they are curing the infection; pediatric rheumatology isn't needed. In the late afternoon I get a phone call saying, "Please come back right away." The fever has returned and the child looks sick again. This is a typical case of systemic-onset arthritis. Children with reactive arthritis, infections, or leukemia may be misdiagnosed as having systemic-onset disease. However, these diseases rarely have periods without fever during which the child looks nearly normal.

In children with reactive arthritis, the fever usually does not disappear every day. Children with infections also tend not to have a normal temperature every day. These children may have a rash, but not the classic salmon pink rash of systemic-onset disease. Children with leukemia also may appear very ill and in pain, with an elevated ESR suggesting the possibility of systemic-onset JA. These diseases can often be differentiated by their laboratory findings, in addition to the child's failure to look better at any point during the day. A significant elevation of the platelet count is characteristically associated with systemic-onset arthritis, while a decreased platelet count is more likely seen in children with reactive arthritis, leukemia, and infections . If a child is thought to have severe systemic-onset arthritis, a low or even low-normal platelet count should be considered suspicious.

Until the diagnosis of systemic-onset arthritis is clear, it is far better to continue to look for infections and treat with antibiotics if necessary. It is also far better to do a bone marrow aspiration to exclude the possibility of leukemia than to delay that diagnosis, thinking that the child has systemic-onset arthritis. Children sent to me for possible systemic-onset arthritis have been found to have cancers, infections, polyarteritis nodosa, Kawasaki disease, IBD, and many other illnesses.

In addition to the high WBC count, high platelet count, high ESR, and low hemoglobin, laboratory evaluation of the child with systemic-onset arthritis may show mild elevation of the liver enzymes (AST/ALT; see Chapter 25). Significant elevation of these test findings in a child with systemic-onset arthritis is a cause for concern. It may signal that (*1*) the diagnosis of systemic-onset arthritis is incorrect, (*2*) there has been drug toxicity, or (*3*) a severe complication called *macrophage activation syndrome* (*MAS*) has begun to develop.

Complications

The complications of systemic-onset arthritis take many forms. In addition to fever, rash, and arthritis, many children will have a small **pericardial effusion** on an echocardiogram. These effusions are often insignificant, but if they become large, they may cause difficulty. Hepatomegaly or splenomegaly may be significant. **Proteinuria** may herald the onset of **amyloidosis**, but this is almost never seen in North America and it is rare in other populations.

There are reports describing damage to the heart or heart valves, lung involvement including pleural effusions, central nervous system problems such as seizures, and a number of vasculitic complications. Whether these are true complications of systemic-onset arthritis is uncertain, because many times what is reported as an "atypical complication" of systemic-onset arthritis is really a typical complication of systemic vasculitis with arthritis or another disease in a child mistakenly thought to have systemic-onset arthritis.

Macrophage activation syndrome (**MAS**) is the most worrisome acute complication of systemic-onset arthritis. If a child with typical systemic-onset arthritis seems to be responding to therapy but the ESR, platelet count, and WBC count begin to fall rapidly while the liver enzymes are increasing, this should spark great concern. When they see the ESR come down and the WBC count and platelet count decrease, many physicians assume that the patient is getting better. The physician may suspect that the elevated liver enzyme levels are an indication of mild liver irritation caused by the medicine. However, this may instead be the beginning of MAS. This is especially true if the child appears ill.

Most often MAS begins early in the course of systemic-onset arthritis, but it may occur at any time. The typical presentation is in a child with systemic onset arthritis who rapidly appears ill with fever, abnormal liver enzyme levels, and liver enlargement. The condition frequently occurs shortly after a change in medication or in conjunction with a viral illness. However, the cause is not always evident. In the early stages of MAS, the fibrin degradation products (FDP) test or fibrin split products (FSP) test may become abnormal—some laboratories now use D-dimers to test for early stages of MAS—and the prothrombin time (PT) may be prolonged (see Chapter 25 for an extended discussion). This will not be the case if the child's systemic-onset arthritis is improving.

A definite diagnosis of MAS is made by demonstrating the presence of macrophages that are destroying erythrocytes in the bone marrow (the macrophages are eating red blood cells and their precursors). This requires a bone marrow aspiration. However, it is rarely necessary to perform this test, as the clinical picture is quite striking. This can be a severe and life-threatening problem because of the clotting abnormalities and liver damage that occur. It is treated with high doses of intravenous corticosteroids and fresh frozen plasma. Some children with MAS have improved with cyclosporine therapy. Macrophage activation syndrome has been reported infrequently in children with other types of arthritis. New research suggests that there may be predisposing genetic factors. Under the right circumstances, MAS may occur in any child with the genetic predisposition, even if he or she doesn't have systemic-onset arthritis.

Severe arthritis and the complications of chronic corticosteroid therapy are major long-term problems for children with systemic-onset arthritis. While some children have little or no residual arthritis, as noted above, those who progress to chronic destructive disease may have severe damage to both large and small joints. Hips and knees are frequently affected and may require replacement. The cervical spine is another frequently affected area, and fusion of the vertebrae in the neck may occur. In some children the wrists are also significantly involved.

As in treating children with polyarticular-onset disease, the physician's first goal must be to prevent joint destruction. When this cannot be accomplished, total joint replacement and reconstructive surgery for systemic-onset arthritis are similar to reconstructive surgery for children with polyarticular-onset arthritis (see Chapter 26). Many children with systemic-onset arthritis receive corticosteroids to control the fever and rash. As a result, osteoporosis is a common complication and avascular necrosis of the hips may also occur. This can be corrected by total hip replacement. Short stature is another common complication of prolonged use of corticosteroids. This cannot be corrected by surgery and may lead to a lifetime of social difficulty. However, short stature has also been reported in children with severe systemic-onset disease who never received corticosteroids.

Medical Treatment

The medications used in the treatment of systemic-onset arthritis are essentially the same as those used to treat polyarticular-onset disease. However, there are a number of key differences. It is important to remember that virtually all of the medicines used to treat JA may irritate the liver. In children with systemic-onset arthritis, the disease itself often causes irritation of the liver as well. But it is difficult to avoid these medications, as corticosteroids are the only readily available alternative. As a result, children with systemic-onset arthritis must be monitored carefully for signs of liver irritation, especially after any change in medication (see Chapter 23 for recommendations regarding monitoring).

Indomethacin is uniquely effective in treating the fever of systemic-onset arthritis and may be effective when other NSAIDs have failed. However, indomethacin is associated with irritation of the stomach, the kidneys, and the liver more often than the other NSAIDs. It also may cause headaches and depression. In young children, indomethacin is associated with an increased incidence of inexplicable temper tantrums. Experienced physicians frequently use indomethacin in children with severe systemic-onset JA when none of the other NSAIDs has been adequate. If a child is very ill, it may be necessary to use corticosteroids to provide immediate relief, but they are not desirable long-term treatment.

For children who fail to respond adequately to NSAIDs, methotrexate is the traditional next choice. However, recent studies have demonstrated that IL-1 and IL-6 play a major role in the manifestations of systemic-onset arthritis. Anakinra is dramatically effective in some children but fails to provide relief for others. Children with continuing active disease, despite taking these medications, are difficult to treat. Tocilizumab, a monoclonal antibody that blocks the IL-6 receptor, is in clinical trials and has been very effective for children with systemic-onset disease. It does have worrisome side effects and as of this writing is not yet licensed in the United States. Thalidomide may dramatically improve the symptoms of children with systemic-onset arthritis, but it should only be prescribed by experienced physicians. Additionally, cyclosporine, adalimumab, etanercept, and infliximab have all been used with success in some children.

A few children with severe systemic-onset arthritis can be controlled only with long-term use of corticosteroids, but every alternative should be considered. None of the remaining medications is consistently effective, but there are several, and it is rare for a child not to respond to any of them. None of these agents work for every child. Additional agents utilized in the care of polyarticular-onset disease, such as abatacept and rituximab, have not yet been tested in systemic-onset arthritis.

I have cared for children who failed to improve with every medication I tried until I added thalidomide. The fever and rash subsided, and the child was "perfect" in ten days. However, the next child who seemed to have the identical condition did not respond to thalidomide at all. It is clear that there is no single uniformly effective drug for children with systemic-onset arthritis except corticosteroids. Leflunomide, azathioprine, mycophenolate mofetil, and cyclophosphamide have all been used with limited success. All have significant potential risks (see Chapter 23).

As with medical treatment for all forms of arthritis, the key to caring for the child with systemic-onset arthritis is to eliminate the symptoms and relieve the inflammation associated with the disease with the least possible toxicity. Many parents are disturbed by the possible side effects of immunosuppressive medications recommended for the treatment of systemic-onset arthritis, but it is important to remember that significant side effects of these medications are rare. In contrast, every child experiences side effects from corticosteroids, which may have severe emotional and physical consequences (see Chapter 27).

Bone Marrow Transplantation and Other New "Cures"

Bone marrow transplantation and other dramatic therapies have been proposed for children with the most severe disease. When parents hear that children with severe disease have been "cured" by these treatments, they get very excited. There are a number of interesting experimental therapies for children who have failed to respond to all other alternatives.

We could eliminate systemic-onset arthritis if we eliminate the immune system. But of course, the immune system is how we fight infection. Elimination of the immune system for even a short period (as is done in bone marrow transplantation) carries a high risk. Nearly 20 percent of the children who undergo bone marrow transplantation for systemic-onset arthritis die. It is true that some transplant patients remain well without taking medication, but others relapse. So, this is not a miracle cure. It is an experimental procedure that should be reserved for the very worst cases. This doesn't mean that bone marrow transplantation is wrong. I have suggested it for some of my most severe cases. The best way to perform bone marrow transplantation in children with severe arthritis continues to be investigated.

Good results have been reported for small numbers of patients with a variety of very potent medications. Again, unless you are treating one of the worst cases, you should not take the risk until these new medications have been proven safe and effective. We will have better therapy for children with arthritis in the future—some of the new treatments you hear about will turn out to be major advances. But others will be failures, and the children will not benefit. Until we know more about these new therapies, they should be reserved for the most severe cases, and these children should receive their care at the most advanced centers.

Physical Therapy and Surgical Treatment

Physical and occupational therapy are very important in maintaining strength and range of motion in children with systemic-onset arthritis, just as they are in each of the other subtypes of JA. Without proper therapy, these children may develop widespread weakness, muscle atrophy, and flexion contractures.

Surgery has little direct role in the treatment of children with systemic-onset arthritis. But once the systemic manifestations have come under control, these children may be left with significant polyarthritis. Reconstructive surgery, as discussed for children with polyarticular-onset arthritis, is appropriate for children with systemic-onset arthritis. Because many of these children have required extended periods of therapy with corticosteroids, they often have avascular necrosis of bone and require joint replacement surgery (see Chapter 26).

Prognosis

The normal course of systemic-onset arthritis is highly varied. Some children make a complete recovery in a short period of time and never have further problems. Other children have chronic debilitating disease that leaves them with permanent limitations. There are three key groups of children with systemic-onset arthritis, but not all children fit one of these descriptions.

- The first group consists of children who have an acute onset of fever, rash, and arthritis that responds quickly to treatment with NSAIDs. Because these children have a fever that disappears every day and the characteristic rash, they are classified as having systemic-onset arthritis. However, in many cases, the duration of disease is less than three months. Some have argued that these are unusual viral infections mimicking systemic-onset arthritis. An outbreak of what was initially thought to be an epidemic of systemic-onset arthritis in a boarding school was found to be due to parvovirus infection when it was carefully investigated. All of these children recovered. Perhaps all of the children who rapidly recover never really had systemic-onset arthritis. We don't know.

- The second group of patients with systemic-onset arthritis consists primarily of teenage boys. Although their disease may be significant initially, it most often comes under control with NSAIDs. A few require the addition of a second-line agent, but their primary problems are fever and rash with relatively little arthritis. Many of these teenagers do well except for the recurrence of rash whenever they become very hot in physical education class or during other activities. Some have mild persisting arthritis or limitation in their wrists, but they do not have major arthritic problems.

- The third group is a much more problematic group of children who begin with systemic-onset disease early in life. In many of these children the disease comes under control with multiple medications, but some require continuing treatment for years. Most of these children are brought under good control long before there is significant damage to the bones and joints, but a few suffer from chronic destructive arthritis. Others are ultimately limited by the side effects of the chronic corticosteroid therapy used to control their fever and arthritis. The key to an improved prognosis for this group is early recognition and aggressive intervention while avoiding chronic high-dose corticosteroid therapy whenever possible.

The long-term prognosis for most children with systemic-onset disease is very good. The systemic symptoms usually disappear over time, and the remaining problems are those of polyarthritis. Only a small percentage of children develop prolonged, unresponsive arthritis or life-threatening complications of the disease itself. With the advent of newer therapies and increasing recognition of the importance of intervening early to minimize the use of corticosteroids, the long-term complications of corticosteroid usage are becoming less frequent. Most children with systemic-onset arthritis will be able to live full, productive lives. To achieve the best possible outcome, the small group of children with severe resistant disease should be cared for by very experienced specialists as soon as their disease is recognized.

STATE-OF-THE-ART CARE FOR CHILDREN WITH JUVENILE ARTHRITIS

State-of-the-art care for children with pauciarticular-onset, polyarticular-onset, and systemic-onset JA requires that physicians and families make sure that the inflammation is promptly brought under control and not allowed to cause continuing joint damage. In the past, physicians believed that children who had evidence of low-grade active disease but were "doing well" should not be treated aggressively. We now know that this is wrong. Smoldering disease means continuing bone and joint damage and a continuing risk of further disease flares.

Children whose disease comes under good control within six months of starting therapy will generally do well. Children with any type of JA whose disease is not under good control within six months of starting **appropriate** therapy are at increased risk of a poor outcome. While this may seem obvious, it is a very reliable guideline. Appropriate therapy is difficult to define. To me it means the right NSAID in the right dosage. It also means monitoring carefully and changing the NSAID if it does not appear to be having the desired effect.

Because there are studies that indicate that NSAIDs may not be fully effective until they have been taken consistently for three months, some physicians will not consider changing therapy until three months after the first dose. Indeed, some physicians will prescribe an NSAID and then not see the child for several months. We must not allow growing children to have continuing joint damage for any longer than is absolutely necessary. **If a child is not beginning to improve within three or four weeks of starting an NSAID, another should be tried.**

Any child who is not clearly improving after six months of therapy may need to be on a second-line agent, but before I conclude that a child needs a second-line agent, I want to try two or three first-line agents (see Chapter 23). Different children have different responses to these medications. For this reason, I want to see the child at least monthly at the beginning and more frequently if he or she is not making good progress. You should not change NSAIDs at every visit. If the child is clearly improving, you should continue to use the medication. But if the child has obviously stopped improving or is getting worse, appropriate changes should be made. The best possible care requires careful monitoring by both the parents and the physician so that any problems are promptly dealt with and appropriate adjustments are made as needed.

In addition to getting routine checkups, every child should be carefully reevaluated six months after starting therapy. Is the disease under good control? Are the remaining problems simply weakness, contractures, or bony overgrowth? These require physical therapy and time, not more medicine. However, if there is evidence of active disease with an elevated ESR, unexplained anemia, morning stiffness, joint swelling, or pain, more aggressive therapy with a second-line agent should be considered. For children with pauciarticular-onset arthritis, this might be the time to consider an intra-articular corticosteroid injection.

For children with continuing active polyarticular- or systemic-onset JA six months after diagnosis, a second-line agent should be added if one has not been added already. Sometimes I'll wait a little longer if the child still seems to be almost completely well. These are not absolute rules—there aren't any. But if the fire is not clearly out, there is ongoing bone and joint damage. This should not be tolerated for an extended period. You cannot rely on X-rays to detect joint damage early in the disease in childhood, since the earliest damage is to the rapidly growing cartilage, which does not show up on X-rays. These changes may not show up as bone damage on X-rays until years later.

The second-line agents most commonly used for resistant JA are methotrexate, sulfasalazine, etanercept, adalimumab, and infliximab. Cysclosporine, leflunomide, and azathioprine are less commonly used. Thalidomide and anakinra are used primarily in children with systemic-onset arthritis. Some children improve dramatically with one of these agents, while others don't respond. Studies are underway to help determine who will or won't respond. Rituximab and abatacept are becoming the agents of choice for children with polyarticular disease who don't respond to the conventional second-line agents. Both have shown promising results and are likely to see increasing use as our experience accumulates. Tocilizumab remains under active investigation and may be licensed for children with severe systemic-onset disease by the time you read this book. Oral corticosteroids should be avoided except for children who are having serious problems and cannot function without them. With appropriate use of second-line agents, the need for corticosteroids is becoming rare, except in children with systemic-onset disease. All of these medications are discussed in detail in Chapter 23.Few children fail to respond adequately to some combination of these agents. Those who do should be under the care of experienced pediatric rheumatologists in major centers, where they have access to ongoing investigation of the newest therapies.

MEDICATIONS NO LONGER ROUTINELY USED FOR JUVENILE ARTHRITIS

The medications used in the treatment of children with arthritis have changed dramatically in the past thirty years. Three medications that were commonly used in the past are no longer routinely used by pediatric rheumatologists in the United States. When I began my career, aspirin and "gold shots" were the mainstays of therapy. In the intervening years, other medications have replaced them. Aspirin remains a useful medication for children with arthritis, and it is very inexpensive. However, it needs to be given three or four times a day and has frequent side effects. Aspirin remains a mainstay of therapy when the expense of other medications is a major barrier to care (mostly in third world countries).

Gold shots are injections of gold-containing compounds given initially once each week. They are extremely effective for some children but are given much less often now because of their inconvenience and side effects (see Chapter 23). Many other medicines are as effective as gold shots and are available in more convenient form.

D-Penicillamine is another medicine that is now rarely used. Although this medication was beneficial for some children, it has been replaced by other medications that have a more rapid onset of action with a lower incidence of side effects.

8

Uveitis

Eye Complications of Juvenile Arthritis and Related Conditions

Virginia was a nine-year-old girl who had pauciarticular-onset JA. Her arthritis began when she was two years old but was well controlled with medication. She had a flare-up of arthritis in her knee at six that was easily controlled. Because she was ANA-positive, her eyes were checked every three months, as recommended. There were never any eye problems. Shortly after her seventh birthday, her parents separated and Virginia moved out of state with her mother. Her father brought her in for a routine checkup of her arthritis when she returned to visit him two years later. Virginia said she was doing fine and had had no problems with her arthritis. However, when I examined her, I could not see into her right eye. It was quickly apparent that she could not see out of that eye. When asked, she admitted that she had noted slowly decreasing vision in the right eye, but she had not said anything because she did not want to upset her mother. Her mother had had many other things on her mind after the divorce and had not arranged for a new ophthalmologist to monitor Virginia. By the time I discovered the problem, the vision in her right eye could not be saved.

It is important that the parents of children with JA and related conditions understand that the eyes may be involved even when there is no evidence of active joint disease. Ocular complications may take several forms. Children with pauciarticular-onset, polyarticular-onset, and psoriatic JA are all at risk of developing chronic anterior uveitis (silent, painless eye inflammation). In this condition, inflammatory cells accumulate in the eye, and the resultant irritation may cause damage to the iris, the lens, and other structures (see Fig. 7-2). The most worrisome aspect of this inflammation is that it does not produce pain or redness. As a result of its gradual, painless progression, the inflammation may cause serious eye damage without being detected. The key to preventing serious eye damage in children with JA is careful screening for the presence of inflammatory cells by an ophthalmologist. A trained ophthalmologist can detect the earliest signs of inflammation with a slip lamp examination and begin treatment.

DIAGNOSIS

Since we cannot rely on children to tell us when there is inflammation, pediatric rheumatologists insist on routine screening as described in Box 8-1. An additional quick and easy test recommended by some ophthalmologists is for parents to shine a flashlight in the child's eyes at bedtime one night each week. If you shine a light in a normal child's eye, you will see the pupil shrink dramatically. It should shrink in a perfect circle. If one eye does not shrink or the circle is irregular, this may be evidence of eye involvement. This test may detect the onset of inflammation in the eye occurring between screening tests by the ophthalmologist, but it is not a substitute for the screening tests.

Box 8-1   Frequency of routine screening ophthalmologic examinations for children with juvenile arthritis (pauciarticular-onset and polyarticular-onset disease)*

Disease	Disease duration	Frequency of routine screening
ANA-positive		
Age at onset less than seven years	Less than four years	Every three months
	More than four years	Every six months
	More than seven years	Yearly
Age at onset over seven years	Less than four years	Every six months
	More than four years	Yearly
ANA-negative		
Age at onset less than seven years	Less than four years	Every six months
	More than four years	Yearly
Age at onset over seven years		Yearly
Systemic-onset JRA		Yearly

*These are recommendations for routine screening of children who are not known to have uveitis. If the child has uveitis, the frequency of follow-up should be determined by the ophthalmologist.

We do not yet understand why some children develop eye disease and others do not. There are certain genetic factors that seem to increase the risk. However, many children with these factors do not get eye disease, and some children without these factors do. Attempts to understand why having ANA increases the risk have failed.

If you look carefully at the joint of a child with arthritis, the inflammation is found to be centered in the synovium, the lining tissue that functions to keep the joint clean of debris. Examination of the eyes of children with uveitis has shown that the inflammation is centered in the ciliary body, a tissue that serves to keep the fluid in the eye clean of debris. Since the two tissues serve a similar function, it is easy to understand how the same disease process might involve both of them. But if it were that simple, we would expect all children with arthritis to develop eye involvement. In fact, less than half ever have any evidence of eye inflammation.

TREATMENT AND MONITORING

If uveitis is present, it should be treated aggressively. The normal first-line therapy is steroid eye drops. Often a short course of this treatment is enough to bring the disease under control. Unfortunately, steroid eye drops will damage the eye if used for an extended period. The prolonged use of steroid eye drops is associated with an increased risk of both cataracts and glaucoma. Because of these complications, if it appears that a short course of treatment with steroid eye drops is inadequate, many ophthalmologists will recommend switching children with severe eye disease to immunosuppressive medications taken by mouth. Often methotrexate is the first medication used after corticosteroids have proven inadequate. Adalimumab and infliximab are also used in this situation with good efficacy. I prefer to use adalimumab, which seems to have a faster onset of action and produce a better and more sustained response. Some children respond best to the combination of methotrexate and adalimumab. Since adalimumab works faster, I usually add methotrexate only when it is apparent that adalimumab alone is not enough. Additional agents that have been reported to be effective in some children with eye disease include mycophenolate mofetil, daclizumab, and abatacept.

Many children with JA are found to have mild uveitis, but when treated appropriately, they do very well. However, if the uveitis is very severe, very resistant to therapy, or not found until very late, there is a risk of permanent blindness. Uveitis may occur in only one eye or in both eyes and may appear at a time where there is no evidence of active arthritis. This is why routine monitoring is so important. Routine monitoring will find eye disease that is not suspected to be present, and will allow the ophthalmologist to begin therapy before too much damage accumulates.

EYE COMPLICATIONS OF OTHER RHEUMATIC DISEASES

Eye involvement may also occur in children with spondyloarthropathies. However, these children usually develop acute, painful eye disease (see Chapter 9). Because it is painful, it is usually rapidly detected. Frequent monitoring of children older than ten years of age with spondyloarthropathies who do not have eye symptoms is not required. In contrast, young children with psoriasis-associated arthritis are at high risk of inflammatory eye disease and must be monitored just as if they had typical JA (see Box 8-1).

Eye involvement may also complicate a variety of other rheumatic diseases in childhood, including sarcoidosis, SLE, and Sjögren's syndrome. Children with these conditions should have their eyes checked by an ophthalmologist routinely. In some cases, they will have symptoms of eye disease; in other cases, the eye disease may occur without the parents or child being aware of it. This is why routine checkups by the ophthalmologist are so important.

UVEITIS WITHOUT PREVIOUS EVIDENCE OF RHEUMATIC DISEASE

Some children develop uveitis without evidence of a rheumatic disease. Since this eye disease looks the same as the eye disease in children with JA, it is treated the same way. However, the first step in evaluating a child with uveitis is a careful evaluation to make sure that he or she does not have a rheumatic disease. Sometimes I find children who cannot bend one knee all the way or who have one leg longer than the other. Although there are other possible explanations, these findings suggest that the child may have had arthritis that was never noticed. However, the list of diseases that may cause uveitis in childhood is quite long and contains many diseases unrelated to rheumatology that must also be considered.

9

Spondyloarthropathies

Enthesitis-associated Arthritis

Fifteen-year-old Samantha began to complain of hip pain after a skiing accident. When repeated evaluations of her injury were negative, she was told
that the hip was "bruised." Although she improved with physical therapy, her
parents became concerned when she awoke a few months later with pain in
the opposite hip. A family friend told them that the pain was a symptom of
Lyme disease. However, visits to several doctors confirmed that all of the tests
for Lyme disease were negative. Samantha began experiencing intermittent
pain in both hips and occasional knee pain. When she went for long car rides,
she could barely get out of the car. When she did, she walked like "a little
old lady" for ten to fifteen minutes until she loosened up. She was diagnosed
with fibromyalgia by an adult rheumatologist. On physical examination, she
was found to be tender in several fingers. She nearly jumped off the table
when I percussed her sacroiliac joints. She had pain in the tendon insertions
around her knees and her ankles.

Spondyloarthropathy is not a specific disease. Instead, it is a pattern of arthritis
or inflammation that may occur in adults or children with a variety of underlying conditions. Conditions that are associated with this pattern of arthritis in
childhood include enthesitis-associated arthritis, ankylosing spondylitis, juvenile
ankylosing spondylitis, seronegative enthesitis-arthritis (SEA) syndrome, reactive arthritis, infection-associated arthritis, Reiter's syndrome, psoriatic arthritis,
arthritis associated with gastrointestinal diseases (including IBD and celiac disease), and a variety of miscellaneous conditions (e.g., recurrent "toxic synovitis,"
hypogammaglobulinemia-associated problems, or IgA deficiency).

Spondyloarthropathy means "arthritis involving the back." Adult rheumatologists first used this term when they began to recognize different forms of
arthritis in adults. In adults, rheumatoid arthritis rarely involves the back, while

spondyloarthropathies often involve the back and sacroiliac joints. Recognition that these were different conditions was an important step in increasing our understanding of the different diseases causing arthritis.

Children with spondyloarthropathies confuse some physicians and parents because damage to the back and sacroiliac joints often does not become obvious on X-rays until the children reach adulthood; sacroiliac joint involvement may be evident on MRI years before it can be detected on routine radiographs. For many years, children with spondyloarthropathies were included in JRA. Currently, the official term for this group is **enthesitis-associated arthritis**. (Although enthesitis-associated arthritis is a subtype of JA or JIA in the newest nomenclature, it is important to recognize that this is a very different disease from typical JRA. Remember, *juvenile arthritis* and *juvenile idiopathic arthritis* are being used as umbrella terms encompassing a large number of different conditions.) In contrast to typical JRA, the spondyloarthropathies have a different pattern of joint involvement, a different prognosis, different recommended medications, and a different underlying cause. Nonetheless, an awareness of these integral differences is a new development in our understanding of the spondyloarthropathies.

The first widely recognized group of children with spondyloarthropathies were teenage boys with swollen knees and low back pain. They stood out because under the old nomenclature they were classified as having pauciarticular-onset arthritis. However, typical pauciarticular-onset arthritis occurs in young girls. Teenage boys with swollen knees have spondyloarthropathies, and their disease differs in many ways. Unlike young girls, who usually get better, the boys often have persistent chronic arthritis. The boys are rarely ANA-positive, and if they develop eye disease, it is acute and painful, not the silent eye disease seen in younger children. In addition, their disease may start in the hip and is often associated with back pain.

When rheumatologists began to look more carefully at this group of teenage boys, they discovered that they often had inflammation in the tendons around the joint (enthesitis) as well as in the joint. Recognition that these boys were different was hastened by the discovery of HLA B27. This is a genetic marker that is found in about half of this group (discussed later in this chapter) but only infrequently in young girls with arthritis. Spondyloarthropathies are common in childhood, but often go undiagnosed or are misdiagnosed as frequent sprains or "growth plate fractures" that don't show up on X-rays because there often is no associated joint swelling.

DIAGNOSIS

Spondyloarthropathies do occur in girls, but rarely in severe form. They typically begin in the early teenage years and are often mistaken for recurrent athletic injuries. Many of the children who come to me have been treated extensively for repeated ankle or knee sprains with exercise, casting, and, in some cases, even surgery. Other children with spondyloarthropathies who have a lot of tendon pain but no swollen joints or abnormal laboratory test results have come to me after having been labeled "complainers." Unlike typical pauciarticular arthritis, in which another affected family member is uncommon, family members of children with spondyloarthropathies are frequently found to be symptomatic. However, the affected relatives often do not know that they have this problem. The chronic back or knee problems they have had since they were teenagers are attributed to injuries or other vague causes.

The key findings in children with spondyloarthropathies often relate to tendon inflammation rather than arthritis. Enthesitis often causes pain around the wrists, knees, ankles, or heels. Frequently, physicians are confused because the child complains of a lot of pain, but nothing is broken and the joint is not swollen. Careful palpation around the joint will often reveal the painful tendonitis. Sometimes the tendons are very swollen and easily noticed on examination. In other cases, the tendonitis is obvious only because the child complains of pain when the tendons are compressed. It is very important that pediatricians recognize that chronic or recurrent pain around joints is not always an injury, nor are these children just complainers or children with fibromyalgia. Enthesitis as part of a spondyloarthropathy is a very real condition that can be easily treated.

Periarticular pain (pain around the joint), is the hallmark of spondyloarthropathies. The key to recognizing that the child is not suffering from recurrent athletic injuries lies in a careful examination that often reveals the presence of multiple tender joints (i.e., it's not just the left ankle that hurts; the right ankle, the heel, the low back, and the wrist may also be tender when examined). Discovering that there are similarly affected family members when taking the family history also may speed recognition of a spondyloarthropathy.

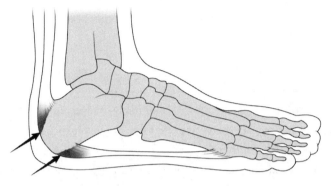

Figure 9-1 *Pain in enthesitis-associated arthritis commonly occurs at the back of the heel (Achilles tendon insertion) or the bottom of the heel (plantar fascia insertion).*

If questioned carefully, most of these children report pain and inflammation in at least two locations. It is common for them to have low back pain or stiffness. Surprisingly, asking about this often produces resistance: "Why are you asking about my back? It's my knee that hurts!" or "Of course, my back is stiff for ten to fifteen minutes every morning. Isn't everyone's?" Another common finding is pain at the Achilles tendon insertion on the back of the heel or at the insertion of the plantar fascia on the bottom of the foot (see Fig. 9-1). This can be detected by percussion or deep palpation at either point.

Dactylitis (sausage digit) may be the first manifestation of a spondyloarthropathy in both young children and teenagers. Instead of swelling being limited to the joints, the entire finger or toe appears swollen, like a sausage. This is because of swelling around the inflamed tendons as well as the joint. At first, the child complains of only a single affected finger or toe and is commonly thought to have injured it. However, on careful examination, you may find evidence of pain and tenderness around multiple joints. Often there is unrecognized inflammation in toes on the same side as the finger (or in fingers on the same side as the toe that was noticed) that can be found by careful examination. It is also common to find unsuspected wrist involvement on the affected side. These children do very well when properly treated for arthritis, but I have seen a number who have undergone unnecessary surgery for suspected tumors or torn tendons, among other things. These children may be ANA-positive and may have unsuspected uveitis. It is important that they be properly screened for eye disease (see Chapter 8).

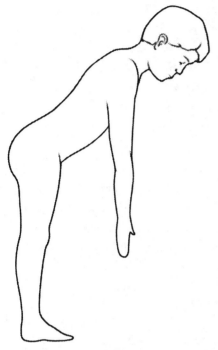

Figure 9-2 *Flattening of the back with limited anterior forward flexion in a child with enthesitis-associated arthritis.*

In teenagers, **limited anterior forward flexion** is an additional finding that assists in making this diagnosis. Typically, these children are unable to touch their toes (see Fig. 9-2), and frequently, their parents and physical education instructors have noted that they are not flexible. Sacroiliac joint tenderness on percussion is another common finding. Laboratory test findings may not be helpful: Although in severe cases there may be an elevated ESR, all test results are often normal in children with mild spondyloarthropathies. HLA B27 is present in only about one-half of these patients. Rheumatoid factor should never be present. Antinuclear antibody is present in some cases (see Chapter 25). The key to making this diagnosis is recognition of the recurrent pain and stiffness associated with decreased range of motion in the back and the pain on compression of tendon insertions (most often the Achilles tendon insertion).

ASSOCIATED CONDITIONS

Once a child is diagnosed with a spondyloarthropathy, it is important to recognize that this pattern of joint involvement may be associated with a variety of other diseases. Ankylosing spondylitis, reactive arthritis, Reiter's syndrome, psoriatic arthritis, infection-associated arthritis (including Lyme disease), and the arthritis associated with gastrointestinal diseases (including IBD and celiac disease) all are associated with a spondyloarthropathy. Many children have a nonspecific spondyloarthropathy, meaning that there is no associated condition. However, the associated condition may not become evident until years after the arthritis begins. This pattern is particularly striking in the case of IBD. Any child with a spondyloarthropathy and recurrent gastrointestinal complaints should be evaluated by a gastroenterologist. I have found that four or more years elapsed between the diagnosis of a spondyloarthropathy and the recognition of IBD even in children I had previously sent to a gastroenterologist for evaluation. In children with a family history of psoriasis, there may also be a delay of several years between the onset of arthritis and the clinical recognition of psoriasis.

Parents of a child with spondyloarthropathies should not be excessively concerned that the child will have other problems; most do not. But if new problems occur, everyone should be aware of the conditions associated with spondyloarthropathies so that the child can be evaluated appropriately. The associated findings and long-term prognosis for each of these conditions are different, so each is discussed separately below.

FORMS OF SPONDYLOARTHROPATHIES

Nonspecific spondyloarthropathy, enthesitis-associated arthritis, SEA syndrome, ankylosing spondylitis, and juvenile ankylosing spondylitis are discussed together because it is rarely possible to separate them reliably in childhood. Most children have a nonspecific spondyloarthropathy. *Seronegative enthesitis-arthritis syndrome* and *enthesitis-associated arthritis* are just different names for the same condition. About half of the children with spondyloarthropathies are HLA B27-positive, as noted above. Often HLA B27-positive boys are labeled as having juvenile ankylosing spondylitis. However, many— probably most—of these children will **not** develop ankylosing spondylitis and should **not** be labeled as having this condition. This is discussed in detail in the section on prognosis below.

Nonspecific spondyloarthropathies are very common. These children have the typical findings of a spondyloarthropathy without a recognized associated condition. The majority of these children, who have enthesitis but little if any joint swelling, rarely develop significant problems. Primary complications are related to the arthritis, if present. But the discomfort and stiffness associated with the enthesitis may result in poor sleep patterns and fatigue. It is not uncommon for these children to be mislabeled as having fibromyalgia. It is important to avoid this misdiagnosis, as the proper medications for fibromyalgia are different, as is the prognosis. For children with abnormal laboratory findings or persistent pain and joint swelling, long-term joint damage is a significant concern. Most often the damage can be minimized by appropriate medical treatment, including second-line drugs. The biologics that block TNF have been shown to be very effective for children with more severe forms of spondyloarthropathy.

Complications

Complications that do not involve the joints (extra-articular complications) are most common in children who have the associated conditions discussed later in this chapter. However, a few specific complications are well recognized to occur in children with nonspecific spondyloarthropathies. **Acute anterior uveitis** is the most common complication. This is a painful disease involving the front of the eye. Often the eye appears very red, and the vision may be affected. This is very different from the silent eye disease of children with pauciarticular-onset arthritis. Although it may be mistaken for conjunctivitis, it will not respond to antibiotic drops and requires care by an ophthalmologist. Acute anterior uveitis may occur in both HLA B27-positive and B27-negative individuals, but it is more common in HLA B27-positive patients.

Cardiac involvement in adults with spondyloarthropathies is well recognized. Fortunately, it occurs in only a small number of children. The most common form of cardiac involvement is inflammation of the root of the aorta, which is called **aortitis**. This inflammation can result in damage to the heart valves and a condition known as **aortic insufficiency**. Children with aortic insufficiency complain of loss of energy and increasing shortness of breath with activity. The condition is easily detected by echocardiography. This complication has been described in teenagers but is rare. Unusual pulmonary or renal findings have been reported in rare cases but may represent the coincidental occurrence of independent conditions.

Medical Treatment

Treatment for children with spondyloarthropathies must be appropriate to their level of discomfort and their risk of developing severe disease. Girls who are at low risk of significant long-term complications infrequently require second-line agents (with the exception of sulfasalazine) unless they have obviously swollen joints or an elevated ESR. Within the family of NSAIDs, it is important to remember that diclofenac, nabumetone, piroxicam, etodolac, oxazepram, and indomethacin are generally more effective for enthesitis than ibuprofen or naproxen. (Sulfasalazine is often remarkably effective for children with spondyloarthropathies, but it contains sulfur and is associated with an increased frequency of allergic reactions.) The majority of children can be treated successfully with these NSAIDs. For children with more severe disease, methotrexate, etanercept, adalimumab, infliximab, and leflunomide all have been used with varying success (see Chapter 23). Because they have a dramatically more rapid onset of action and fewer evident side effects, I prefer the TNF inhibitors (etanercept and adalimumab) in my practice. Skittishness about the need for injections frequently prevents the use of these agents for children whose complaints outweigh their disease involvement, while those with significant disease involvement often report prompt symptomatic relief.

Boys who are HLA B27-positive, with a family history of ankylosing spondylitis and/or MRI- documented sacroiliac joint inflammation, are at risk of progression to true ankylosing spondylitis as adults (discussing what to call them before they satisfy the official criteria is just semantics). These children should be aggressively treated as soon as their condition is recognized. Early addition of TNF inhibitors and methotrexate is the course most likely to alter their long-term prognosis. In adults with ankylosing spondylitis this therapy has been shown to retard bone damage and improve function, and there is no reason to assume that the same is not true for adolescents. It is easier to prevent damage than to repair it.

Other Therapies

Physical therapy is important in caring for children who do not fully respond to NSAIDs. The major concern is their progressive loss of flexibility over time. This loss of flexibility can be slowed, if not completely prevented, by a program of appropriate anti-inflammatory medications, exercises, and strengthening with attention to good posture (see Fig. 9-3). Local inflammatory changes in the wrist may be helped by the use of wrist splints to protect against subluxation and to reduce discomfort. For children with plantar fascia insertion pain or heel spurs, gel-filled heel cups placed inside the shoe may provide substantial relief. Those with more diffuse foot pain may benefit from appropriate referral and the use of prescribed orthotics.

Surgery is rarely necessary for children with spondyloarthropathy. In the small subgroup of children with severe disease, it may become necessary to replace a damaged hip. Occasionally, children develop severe wrist arthritis and may require surgical fusion. Chronic active arthritis may require a synovectomy. With proper physical therapy, it is uncommon for children to need tendon releases. All of these modalities are rarely necessary if children have received appropriate medical therapy.

Long-term Prognosis

The majority of children with spondyloarthropathies do well. When considering the prognosis, it is important to consider boys separately from girls, the HLA B27-positive children separately from those who are HLA B27-negative, and those with an elevated ESR separately from the others. Girls who are HLA B27-negative with a normal ESR do well in the long run but may have recurrent complaints. Many require NSAIDs on a consistent basis, especially in the winter months, but it is rare for this illness to have a major negative impact on their lives. Most of these children have recurrent enthesitis, but

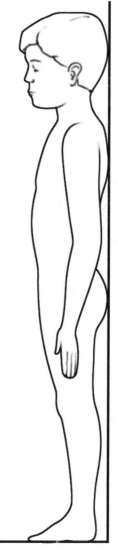

Figure 9-3 *Children should practice standing with their heels, buttocks, shoulders, and head flat against the wall.*

swollen joints are rare. HLA B27-positive girls with a normal ESR tend to have more frequent complaints and more frequently recurring disease than girls who are HLA B27-negative, but they too have a good long-term prognosis.

Girls who have an elevated ESR or recurrent joint swelling are more worrisome. Some of these girls have significant arthritis that will require continuing care and may necessitate the use of sulfasalazine, TNF inhibitors, or other second-line drugs. Nonetheless, I expect these girls to grow up to have jobs and families of their own. The prognosis is a little more guarded for the girls who have an elevated ESR and swollen joints and are HLA B27-positive; this group is more likely to require TNF inhibitors and to have problems that persist into adulthood. However, with proper care, they should have a very acceptable outcome and enjoy a full life.

Most HLA B27-negative boys with a nonspecific spondyloarthropathy also do well. However, their complaints tend to be more frequent and more severe than those of HLA B27-negative girls. They also tend to have more persistent problems with heel pain and back pain. This group may require chronic medication, often TNF inhibitors. These patients generally function well as adults but are typically excluded from the armed forces and emergency services by their lack of flexibility.

Boys with an elevated ESR and swollen joints are at greater risk of an unsatisfactory outcome. They may have more difficulty over the long term and often require TNF inhibitors. Although their outcome is usually quite acceptable, there are HLA B27-negative boys with chronic and persistent arthritis lasting into adulthood. Nonetheless, most have jobs and families and are not limited by their arthritis, with the exception of athletic activities and occupational limitations as noted above.

There are two distinct groups of HLA B27-positive boys. Some have a normal ESR, no swollen joints, and only mild complaints. It appears that they have only a minimal genetic predisposition to arthritis (see Chapter 25). These children do well. Boys who are HLA B27-positive and have swollen joints with an elevated ESR are at greater risk. Some will go on to develop definite ankylosing spondylitis or other associated conditions, which are discussed in the next section.

JUVENILE ANKYLOSING SPONDYLITIS AND ANKYLOSING SPONDYLITIS

In the 1970s, the genetic marker HLA B27 was a new discovery. Since virtually all adult men with ankylosing spondylitis (AS) were HLA B27-positive, there was great concern that all of the HLA B27-positive boys who came to the attention of rheumatologists would ultimately develop AS. However, since most individuals with AS do not fulfill the criteria for the diagnosis until after thirty years of age, at least fifteen years of follow-up are needed to know which teenage boys ultimately develop AS. Keeping track of teenagers is, of course, very difficult, but those who have trouble are more likely to keep in touch with their doctors than those who do not.

No one is sure how great the risk of developing AS is for HLA B27-positive teenage boys with mild or moderate complaints. Diagnosing all HLA B27-positive boys with a spondyloarthropathy as having juvenile ankylosing spondylitis (JAS) is predicting the future without the benefit of a crystal ball. Not only does it cause undue worry for many parents, but it also makes life and health insurance difficult to obtain. Although some will develop AS, labeling all of these children with JAS is unnecessary.

I recommend that the term *juvenile ankylosing spondylitis* be avoided unless there are definite findings of sacroiliac joint involvement on radiographs or MRI scans. Certainly, an HLA B27-positive boy who has swollen joints and an elevated ESR is at risk of progressing to definite AS and should be treated aggressively, but there is no accurate information about how likely he is to develop definite AS. To be diagnosed with definite AS, a child must fulfill a set of criteria that were developed for adults. The specific degree of radiographic evidence of sacroiliitis required by these criteria is rarely present in childhood. Magnetic resonance imaging–documented sacroiliac joint inflammation is worrisome and prompts me to be more aggressive, but we aren't sure that all of these children will progress to AS as adults. Careful studies of adults who were ultimately diagnosed with AS have determined that they often did not fulfill the required radiographic criteria until they reached their thirties. This does not mean that these men did not have arthritic complaints earlier in life. However, they were not diagnosed with definite AS because many individuals with arthritic complaints do not develop full-blown disease. The same is true of children.

Occasionally, I see HLA B27-positive teenage boys who have obvious sacroiliac joint involvement on their X-rays and can be labeled definitively as having AS. However, this is uncommon. More common are teenage boys with HLA B27 and MRI-documented sacroiliitis. At present, I am recommending that they be placed on TNF inhibitors and methotrexate added if they develop changes that are visible on X-rays. I don't label them as having AS because they don't fulfill the official criteria and the label will interfere with obtaining insurance, getting a job, and other aspects of daily life. Hopefully, this situation will ultimately be clarified. When speaking to the parents of a child who is HLA B27-positive, physicians must remember that the child inherited the gene from his or her parents. If neither parent developed AS, why should you assume that the child will? Further, even if one parent has AS, we know that the penetrance of the disease is highly variable. All children who have joint complaints and are HLA B27-positive should be under the care of an experienced rheumatologist who appropriately treats whatever problems develop. This will assure them the best possible outcome, whatever the ultimate diagnosis. Prematurely labeling children with a diagnosis of JAS does not benefit anyone.

REACTIVE ARTHRITIS: INFECTION-ASSOCIATED ARTHRITIS AND REITER'S SYNDROME

Bruce was a sixteen-year-old passenger on a large cruise ship. Due to circumstances beyond his control, one of the dishes served on the ship was contaminated by a bacterium that causes gastroenteritis (vomiting or diarrhea). Some 500 passengers who ate the contaminated food became ill. Most recovered completely within a few days, but fifty of them developed aches and pains in their joints one to two weeks later. Only five of the ill passengers developed persistent arthritis that required treatment. Bruce was one of them. Fortunately, he recovered over a six-month period. However, two other passengers never fully recovered. Although only forty of the passengers who became ill were HLA B27-positive, four of the five who required treatment for their arthritis were HLA B27-positive.

Reactive or **infection-associated arthritis** and **Reiter's syndrome** are important special cases of spondyloarthropathy. Affected children are often very ill, with fever, rash, elevated ESR, and widespread arthritis. Sometimes the arthritis is in only one large joint, but at other times it may be widespread, affecting both large and small joints. It was originally termed **reactive arthritis** because the arthritis frequently begins shortly after a significant viral or bacterial infection. The name was changed to **infection-associated arthritis** to remind physicians that in some cases the infection is still present and may require treatment. Meningococcemia- and gonorrhea-associated arthritis are the two most worrisome infections requiring treatment that are associated with this presentation.

The most common infectious agents that cause these forms of arthritis are bacteria—shigella, salmonella, neisseria, and chlamydia—and viruses, especially parvovirus B19. The arthritis associated with Lyme disease is also a form of infection-associated arthritis. Mild and brief arthritis following a variety of infections is very common. Once the episode has passed, most children recover completely. A typical episode of infection-associated arthritis resolves in three to six weeks. However, some children develop arthritis that lasts for a longer period, as exemplified by the case history above. Occasionally, children have lingering disease that may persist for many months. If the arthritis persists for a year or more, then it is considered arthritis that was initiated by an infection, but it is no longer labeled reactive or infection-associated arthritis.

Although many children with infection-associated arthritis look very ill at the beginning, the majority of them recover completely. Some are initially misdiagnosed as having systemic-onset arthritis, but the fever pattern and rash of reactive arthritis and systemic-onset arthritis are different. The rash with infection-associated arthritis is not the typical fleeting salmon-colored rash of systemic-onset arthritis, and the fever pattern lacks the characteristic return to normal every day that is seen in systemic-onset arthritis. Recurrences of reactive arthritis are rare (if the underlying infection has resolved), but there are children with a strong

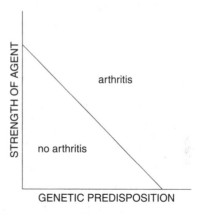

Figure 9-4 *A child with a weak genetic predisposition but affected by a strong environmental agent is much less likely to ever have arthritis again than a child with a strong genetic predisposition. The latter may develop arthritis following infection with a variety of weaker agents.*

genetic predisposition to arthritis who develop repeated episodes of arthritis following exposure to different infectious agents. Some of these children ultimately develop chronic disease. HLA B27 is just one example of a genetic predisposition to arthritis. There are many people with other genetic predispositions to arthritis who are not HLA B27-positive (see Fig. 9-4).

Complications

Since, by definition, infection-associated arthritis resolves within a year of onset, long-term complications are infrequent. There may be complications related to the initial infection, but most children recover fully and do well.

Reiter's Syndrome

Reiter's syndrome is a special case of reactive arthritis. It is distinguished from other cases of reactive arthritis by the occurrence of arthritis, urethritis, and conjunctivitis. Children with Reiter's syndrome sometimes have rashes, particularly on their hands and feet. They may also have severe, painful, acute anterior uveitis. When evaluating a child for the diagnosis of Reiter's syndrome, it is important to remember that the arthritis, urethritis, and conjunctivitis do not all have to be present on the same day. They may occur one after the other without ever overlapping in time. When you are evaluating a child with joint pains, remember to ask if there have been any other problems recently. *Incomplete Reiter's syndrome* is just another term for reactive arthritis. Although Reiter's syndrome with all of the findings is common in adults, it is rare in children.

Treatment

The most important step in treating children with infection-associated arthritis, including Lyme disease and Reiter's syndrome, is to make sure that the infection is properly treated. Once it is clear that the infection associated with the arthritis is no longer active, these children should be treated just like other children with spondyloarthropathies. Most respond well to easily tolerated NSAIDs. In most cases, the arthritis resolves completely over a period of a few months. Tumor necrosis factor inhibitors (etanercept or adalimumab) are sometimes required, while other children benefit from the addition of sulfasalazine. Intra-articular injection of corticosteroids may be useful if only one joint remains troublesome after the infection has been fully treated, but oral corticosteroids are rarely necessary.

Physical Therapy and Surgery

Physical therapy to maintain strength and range of motion is often necessary during the acute phase of the disease. Surgery should not be necessary for a child with infection-associated arthritis unless it is necessary to treat the infection.

Prognosis

Once the infection is properly treated and has resolved, the long-term prognosis for children with infection-associated arthritis is very good. Occasionally, children have recurrent episodes of arthritis with subsequent infections. Rarely, children may have an episode of infection-associated arthritis, recover, and then develop persistent spondyloarthropathy years later.

PSORIATIC ARTHRITIS

Susan is a delightful girl who initially was seen by her pediatrician at the age of two for a stubbed toe that did not heal. There was no obvious explanation for the diffusely swollen toe, and it finally became normal over a four-month period. Susan then did well until she was six years old. At that time, she had a swollen knee and was noted to be ANA-positive. She was diagnosed with pauciarticular JA. Her ESR was elevated to 50 but returned to normal after several months of treatment. Her knee slowly improved, and by age eight she was off all medications. She became my patient at age twelve, when she presented with pain and swelling in both knees and the right wrist. Over the ensuing years she has had continuing polyarthritis controlled by sulfasalazine, methotrexate, and TNF inhibitors. Despite aggressive treatment, she has lost some range of motion in her wrists. Nonetheless, she is currently a successful college graduate in her mid-twenties working for a prestigious firm on Wall Street. Only a careful physician would recognize that she continues to have limitations due to her arthritis. She remains on medication.

Psoriatic arthritis is another spondyloarthropathy that requires special attention. Pediatric rheumatologists continue to debate exactly who belongs in this group, since one does not have to have psoriasis to have psoriatic arthritis and one might have another form of arthritis and coincidentally have psoriasis. It often appears that someone has gone out of his way to make the nomenclature confusing. The situation is further complicated by recognition of two distinct subsets of patients. One group is made up of young children, mostly girls, who are often ANA-positive and may have pauciarticular-onset arthritis. However, these are often the children who have an elevated ESR or low hemoglobin values. Many of them start with a swollen finger or toe (dactylitis). The second group is made up of older children who may start with dactylitis but more often present with polyarticular disease.

The confusing nomenclature results from a lack of long-term follow-up of many children. This is a disease that evolves over several years, just as Susan's did. Most of the children in this group do not have psoriasis when the diagnosis is made. So, why is it called *psoriatic arthritis*? I often think it would be easier to simply call it *Joe's disease*. However, if you follow children who have this type of arthritis for a long period, ultimately (maybe ten or fifteen years later) many of them will develop psoriasis. More importantly, the arthritis behaves like the arthritis associated with psoriasis and responds to the same medications.

There are varied criteria for the diagnosis of psoriatic arthritis. The child is required to have arthritis plus dactylitis or changes in the fingernails of a type often seen in children with psoriasis (onycholysis), as well as a close relative with psoriasis. Some physicians argue over how close the relative must be and how sure the physician is that the relative has psoriasis. These arguments fail to recognize that this arthritis has a characteristic appearance and behavior.

If a child presents with dactylitis or obviously swollen tendons, the condition is most likely psoriatic arthritis. It does not matter whether a relative has psoriasis or whether the child ultimately develops psoriasis. What matters is that the physician recognizes that children with this pattern of arthritis require more aggressive treatment. The same is true for young girls with only a single swollen joint if they have an elevated ESR or low hemoglobin, as noted in the discussion of pauciarticular JA.

It is important for pediatricians to recognize that young children with this form of arthritis need to be treated more aggressively than children with typical pauciarticular arthritis. Most often they are girls, but there are some boys in this group. Except for the laboratory criteria discussed above, they may resemble other children with pauciarticular-onset arthritis. However, their disease is often more difficult to bring under control with NSAIDs, and it recurs much more frequently. Interestingly, they are often ANA-positive and are as much at risk of eye disease as the children with true pauciarticular-onset disease. Some have a family history of psoriasis, and others have a swollen, tender finger or toe that might not have been noticed. In some cases, the swollen toe may have been noticed several months before the knee became swollen and then cleared up. The TNF inhibitors are very effective in treating this group and should be considered early in the therapy of children who are not responding adequately to NSAIDs.

Despite the fact that only a few joints are affected at the beginning, over time these children often develop polyarticular disease. A typical child might have had a swollen toe that rapidly improved at eighteen months of age, then a swollen knee at thirty-six months of age that improved over six months, and then swollen wrists at six years of age that are still causing trouble at age twelve. The key to obtaining a good outcome for these children is aggressive therapy to bring the disease under control. This often requires entanercept or adalimumab. Once the disease is under control, the children typically need prolonged suppressive therapy with a medication such as sulfasalazine. I have cared for children who had no evidence of arthritis while being maintained on sulfasalazine for several years whose disease flared within a few months when the sulfasalazine was discontinued.

The second group with psoriatic arthritis is made up of children who often first see a rheumatologist between twelve and sixteen years of age. Again, girls are more common than boys in this group. Often they give no history of earlier problems. Their problems may begin with a swollen finger or toe, and they are invariably thought to have suffered recurrent athletic injuries. Some present with a swollen wrist without evidence of any other joint involvement. They often have an elevated ESR, and about half of them have a family history of psoriasis. Sometimes the arthritis is difficult to control. In other children it seems to come under control easily, but it keeps coming back. It is unlikely that this form of arthritis ever truly disappears. A significant number of these children develop widespread arthritis over time. However, most respond well to aggressive therapy. As with all forms of arthritis in childhood, early intervention is essential to prevent the accumulation of significant long-term joint damage. Since this arthritis frequently recurs, continued follow-up even when the child seems well is also important. I frequently have parents return after having skipped appointments for a year or two because the child recently has begun to complain of pain. Careful examination often reveals long-term changes that take months to appear. If the family had kept the scheduled follow-up appointments when the child was not complaining, the problem could have been detected sooner and much of the damage prevented.

Because of its destructive potential, it is important that this form of arthritis be recognized promptly. This is the most likely diagnosis for any child presenting with dactylitis or predominantly upper extremity involvement (i.e., elbows, wrists, and shoulders). Although the neck is rarely the first joint involved, it frequently becomes affected over time. Involvement of the jaw is also more frequent in these children than in children with other forms of spondyloarthropathy. Unfortunately, lower extremity involvement is not uncommon. Early and aggressive therapy is the key to a good outcome.

Complications

The primary complications of psoriatic arthritis are related to recurrent arthritis in both the upper and lower extremities. Some children develop significant joint damage over the course of their disease, and every effort should be made to prevent this. Serious eye involvement can occur in young children, and children with ANA-positive psoriatic arthritis must be monitored just as carefully as those with ANA-positive pauciarticular-onset JA. Fortunately, eye involvement is less common in teenagers, but it is still possible. Persistent wrist and finger involvement is often prominent. In some children, this seems to be the only evidence of disease. However, children may begin with only wrist involvement but years later develop problems in other joints. Elbow, neck, and jaw involvement is more common in children with this form of arthritis and must be looked for. Hips, knees, ankles, and toes may also be involved. Because the arthritis can become widespread, it is important to do everything possible to bring it under control quickly and, if possible, to prevent it from returning.

Medical Treatment

Initial treatment for this group is the same as the treatment for other children with spondyloarthropathies. Again, it is important to remember that diclofenac, nabumetone, piroxicam, etodolac, oxazepram, and indomethacin are generally more effective for enthesitis than ibuprofen or naproxen. I am much quicker to use sulfasalazine and/or TNF inhibitors such as etanercept and adalimumab for children in this group. They are often remarkably effective. I favor the TNF inhibitors because they act faster and provide superior relief. However, studies have suggested that children who take sulfasalazine as well are likely to have a better long-term outcome than those taking TNF inhibitors alone. I have cared for a number of children who did very well for several years on sulfasalazine but then had recurrent disease within a few months of stopping the drug. As a result, in the absence of side effects, I continue to use sulfasalazine as long as possible. As with all medications, children on long-term therapy with sulfasalazine or TNF inhibitors require routine monitoring of their laboratory tests (see Chapter 23). Most often, problems with sulfasalazine occur at the beginning of treatment.

Methotrexate is often used in the treatment of children with psoriatic arthritis. It is effective, both alone and in combination with TNF inhibitors. However, its onset of action is slower than that of the TNF inhibitors, and it has additional side effects. I tend to reserve methotrexate for children with severe disease who are not responding adequately to TNF inhibitors alone. Thalidomide has been effective in children who have failed all other therapies, but it must be used only by physicians with extensive experience with this medication (see Chapter 22 for more details). Except for occasional intra-articular injections, corticosteroids are rarely necessary and should be avoided if possible.

Physical Therapy

Physical therapy plays an important role in maintaining strength and range of motion for these children. Since this form of arthritis has a propensity to involve the wrists and fingers, occupational therapy is often an important part of their care as well.

Surgery

Surgery is rarely necessary for children with psoriatic arthritis. For children with severe disease, it may be necessary to replace a damaged hip. Occasionally, children develop severe, painful wrist arthritis that may require surgical fusion. With proper physical therapy, it is uncommon for children to need tendon releases or any other surgical procedures.

Prognosis

The long-term prognosis for children with psoriatic arthritis is more guarded than that for children with a nonspecific spondyloarthropathy or typical pauciarticular-onset JA. Young children who have only dactylitis that resolves quickly may nonetheless, years later, develop arthritis in other joints. With aggressive therapy and careful monitoring, most children with psoriatic arthritis will have a very acceptable, if not perfect, outcome. Over a period of years, some children with this arthritis develop progressive changes in their fingers and wrists despite aggressive therapy. Fortunately, the routine use of TNF inhibitors has reduced the frequency of these complications.

Children with psoriatic arthritis and a significantly elevated ESR should be treated aggressively even if it appears that only a single joint is involved. It is common to see a teenager who initially complained of only a single swollen finger or tender wrist with an elevated ESR ultimately develop widespread polyarthritis. These children frequently require NSAIDs, sulfasalazine, methotrexate, etanercept, adalimumab, or infliximab. With aggressive therapy, the majority of them are able to function normally as adults.

ARTHRITIS ASSOCIATED WITH BOWEL DISEASE

Ulcerative colitis and **regional enteritis** (Crohn's disease) are collectively referred to as **inflammatory bowel disease (IBD)**. It is well known that some children with these diseases have arthritis. This arthritis typically takes the form of a spondyloarthropathy and may become evident before IBD develops. The complete explanation for this association is lacking. Careful studies have demonstrated that many individuals with spondyloarthropathy have a gastrointestinal mucosa with an unusual appearance. But exactly how this relates to developing arthritis is uncertain. Children with IBD are often on strong immunosuppressive medications for the IBD. They also may be receiving corticosteroids. In most cases, the therapy for their IBD is sufficient to control their arthritis. However, occasionally, children require NSAIDs in addition to the therapy for their IBD. Infliximab and adalimumab are beneficial for children who don't respond to NSAIDs.

In evaluating a child with a spondyloarthropathy who has gastrointestinal complaints, testing for the antibody pANCA may speed recognition of the child with IBD. Two skin findings, erythema nodosum (large, tender, painful, red or purplish bumps over the shins) and pyoderma gangrenosum (large areas of skin breakdown with weeping sores), in a child with a spondyloarthropathy should spark careful consideration of possible IBD. Many children with arthritis and IBD are HLA B27-positive. Children with IBD who are HLA B27-positive are more likely to have significant and persistent arthritis than those who are HLA B27-negative.

Medical therapy

Adalimumab has recently been approved as therapy for IBD. This agent is extremely effective for the arthritis of IBD as well as for the disease itself. Use of adalimumab is increasing, as there is increasing hesitation on the part of gastroenterologists to use NSAIDs in children with IBD.

Complications

The long-term complications of children with IBD are primarily related to their gastrointestinal disease and its treatment and are not discussed here. Complications of the arthritis of IBD are similar to those of children with spondyloarthropathy. With the exception of hip and sacroiliac joint involvement, the arthritis rarely is of long-term significance.

Physical Therapy

Physical and occupational therapy for these children is the same as for children with other spondyloarthropathies.

In addition to IBD, children who have abdominal pain, rash, and arthritis may have **reactive arthritis, Henoch-Schönlein purpura, Kawasaki disease, polyarteritis nodosa, dermatomyositis, SLE, or other vasculitic diseases,** as well as many other conditions (discussed in other chapters). Most often the correct diagnosis is evident, but I have seen children with IBD initially misdiagnosed with these illnesses, and vice versa.

One special situation that deserves attention is that of the child with a complaint of severe abdominal pain, fever, arthritis, and a limp. If a child has been ill with severe abdominal pain and developed a limp on the right side, the physician should consider the possibility of undiagnosed **appendicitis**. Most children with appendicitis develop fever and severe abdominal pain and are promptly diagnosed. However, over the years, I have seen several children with a limp referred for evaluation. On careful examination, these children were found to have right lower abdominal pain on deep palpation. The limp and the findings "in the right hip" were the result of abdominal pain because there was an abscess around a ruptured appendix that was not diagnosed at the time it occurred. This situation can often be suspected from a careful history and physical examination. It can be confirmed by a CAT scan of the abdomen or perhaps abdominal ultrasound.

Celiac disease (gluten-sensitive enteropathy) is another gastrointestinal disease associated with arthritic complaints that typically takes the form of a spondyloarthropathy. Celiac disease most often begins with poor growth during the first years of life. However, it is being increasingly recognized in teenagers with nonspecific joint complaints or spondyloarthropathies and chronic upset stomachs. When questioned, many of these children complain of disliking pasta, pizza, and other high-gluten foods. A definite diagnosis of celiac disease requires the characteristic findings on small intestinal biopsy, but the diagnosis is strongly suggested by the presence of anti-endomyseal antibodies (IgA anti-tissue transglutaminase) in the blood. The treatment for celiac disease is a gluten-free diet. With this diet, the arthritic complaints will normally subside. Untreated celiac disease is associated with a number of autoimmune conditions, including thyroiditis, and may be associated with a positive ANA.

Nonspecific arthritic complaints may also be seen in children who have recovered from a severe insult to the gastrointestinal tract. The most common examples are children who suffered **necrotizing enterocolitis** during the neonatal period. *Bypass arthropathy*, in which individuals with surgically induced short-bowel syndromes developed arthritis, was well recognized when this surgery was briefly popular for the treatment of morbid obesity. Because of the very high rate of complications associated with this procedure, it is now rarely done.

Since there are a variety of conditions that affect the gastrointestinal tract and cause arthritis, it is natural to wonder how the two problems are associated. There are no studies that answer this question to everyone's satisfaction. It appears that a damaged or atypical intestinal tract will allow elements of the diet to enter the bloodstream. In some people (perhaps because of a genetic predisposition), these elements may reach the joints and initiate arthritis. If the damage to the intestinal tract can be corrected, the arthritis may disappear. This association has led to the hope that dietary changes may relieve the arthritis. This is true for children with celiac disease, who improve if they avoid foods containing gluten. However, it does not appear to be true for other conditions (see Chapter 24).

MISCELLANEOUS CONDITIONS RELATED TO SPONDYLOARTHROPATHIES

Hypogammaglobulinemia-associated Problems

IgA Deficiency

Immunoglobulin A deficiency is a low level of immunoglobulin A (see Chapter 25 for a full discussion of immunoglobulins). Children with IgA deficiency develop rheumatic diseases much more frequently than the normal population. While this often takes the form of a spondyloarthropathy, studies have shown an increased frequency of IgA deficiency in virtually every child with rheumatic disease. There are two important issues to be aware of regarding a child who is found to have IgA deficiency. The first is that this is a permanent condition that makes recurrent arthritis more likely, even in a child who otherwise appears to have pauciarticular-onset disease.

The second problem is that individuals who are IgA-deficient are vulnerable to *transfusion reactions*. These are not due to incompatibility with the transfused red blood cells, but rather are the result of a reaction to the IgA in the serum transfused with the red blood cells. Routine laboratory cross-typing will not detect this problem. Parents of children who are IgA-deficient must inform any treating physician of this condition. A clue to the presence of IgA deficiency is a strong history of recurrent ear infections or similar problems. However, many children who have had many ear infections have no identified abnormality.

Common Variable Hypogammaglobulinemia

This is a condition in which children with immature immune systems do not have completely normal levels of immunoglobulin. As the immune system matures, the problem frequently disappears. Children in the three- to seven-year-old age group who limp whenever they have a viral infection often have low immunoglobulin levels. This group is not well described in the literature. On evaluation, they often have very mild periarticular pain and no other obvious findings. The complaints typically disappear in a day or a few days, when the infection has resolved. However, the limp or other joint pains may recur with subsequent infections. I have seen a number of children with six, seven, or even eight such episodes.

Routine laboratory evaluation of these children is usually completely normal. When serum immunoglobulin levels are measured, they are found to be clearly abnormal for an adult but are considered at the low end of normal for the children's age. I have cared for several dozen of these children over the past twenty years. As their immune system matures, the immunoglobulin levels rise and the problem ceases. No detailed reports of the long-term outcome of these children are available. No child that I have cared for has developed significant rheumatic disease. Since the immunoglobulin levels in these children are at the low end of normal for their age, they are not officially immunodeficient. Many have been misdiagnosed as having JRA.

Children with definite common variable hypogammaglobulinemia and IgG subclass deficiencies may also have an increased incidence of arthritis. These are children with low immunoglobulin levels of varying specific types. The arthritis these children develop also generally follows the pattern of a spondyloarthropathy. Many investigators feel that this situation is similar to that of children with abnormal gastrointestinal tracts. In children with mild immune deficiencies, proteins or other molecules that are normally kept out of the body by the immune system are able to enter and cause mild arthritis. In most children these episodes are short-lived and without serious complications, but there are exceptions. In addition, it is important to recognize that the defect in their immune systems leaves them vulnerable to bone or joint infections that require treatment with antibiotics.

Children with more severe forms of immunodeficiency are occasionally found to have arthritis. In this group, the immunodeficiency and the resulting infections are usually more significant problems than the arthritis. However, these children may benefit from treatment with NSAIDs. Often the underlying immunodeficiency is treated with intravenous immunoglobulin (IVIgG), and this leads to resolution of the arthritis as well.

"Recurrent" Toxic Synovitis

Toxic synovitis is a transient inflammation of the hip that most often occurs in young children (see Chapter 3). I occasionally see children diagnosed with "recurrent" toxic synovitis. This diagnosis should be regarded with suspicion. Some of these children have Legg-Calve-Perthes disease that has not been recognized. In others, recurrent episodes of synovitis in the hip may be the first manifestation of what ultimately becomes an obvious spondyloarthropathy. Toxic synovitis should never be diagnosed in a child over nine years of age. Isolated synovitis of the hip in children over this age is usually the initial manifestation of a spondyloarthropathy. However, other causes of hip inflammation must be excluded.

Poststreptococcal Reactive Arthritis and Rheumatic Fever

Poststreptococcal reactive arthritis is another form of infection-associated arthritis. It differs in that this form of infection-associated arthritis is initiated by a group A streptococcal infection. Poststreptococcal reactive arthritis behaves just like the other forms of infection-associated arthritis. Sometimes the arthritis is located in a single large joint such as the hip; at other times, it can affect multiple joints.

Box 9-1   Jones criteria for the diagnosis of acute rheumatic fever

Major criteria

- Carditis (inflammation of the heart valves or muscle)
- Migratory polyarthritis (swollen, tender joints with involvement shifting from one joint to another)
- Sydenham's chorea (a condition consisting of uncontrollable movements)
- Subcutaneous nodules (bumps under the skin)
- Erythema marginatum (a red rash with dramatic red outlines)

Minor criteria

- Elevated C-reactive protein (CRP), ESR, or leukocyte levels (laboratory results)
- Arthralgia (joint pain without swelling or limitation of motion)
- Fever

The diagnosis of acute rheumatic fever requires two major criteria, or one major and two minor criteria, and evidence of a recent streptococcal infection.

There is a lot of confusion regarding the relationship of poststreptococcal reactive arthritis to acute rheumatic fever. Since acute rheumatic fever is associated with possible damage to the heart and requires penicillin prophylaxis, this is an area of great concern. **Acute rheumatic fever** is defined according to the Jones criteria (see Box 9-1). Children who develop a nonmigratory (not moving from joint to joint) arthritis after a streptococcal infection do not fulfill these criteria. As a result, many physicians do not treat these children with penicillin prophylaxis. However, some of these children go on to develop heart damage due to rheumatic fever following a later streptococcal infection.

Medical therapy

Since no large-scale studies have been carried out to determine how much risk there is for children with poststreptococcal reactive arthritis who do not fulfill the Jones criteria, there is no definite answer regarding penicillin prophylaxis for these children. In families with a history of acute rheumatic fever or in children in whom the arthritis associated with the streptococcal infection was severe, I prefer to use penicillin prophylaxis to prevent recurrences and reduce the risk of future rheumatic fever–related heart damage. Some physicians insist that this should not be done unless the child fulfills the Jones criteria. I would point out two facts to these physicians. First, the Jones criteria are guidelines, not laws; they were drawn up by a committee. Second, several physicians who were practicing medicine when rheumatic fever was common treated many children who did not fulfill the Jones criteria. **Our concern should be to prevent children from developing heart disease, not slavishly applying written guidelines.** However, this must be balanced against the risks of penicillin allergy and the appearance of bacteria that are resistant to penicillin.

The arthritis in children with poststreptococcal reactive arthritis is treated with NSAIDs, as in other forms of spondyloarthropathy. Although aspirin was the traditional therapy for acute rheumatic fever, the other NSAIDs are safer, more convenient, and equally effective.

Prognosis

The prognosis for children with poststreptococcal reactive arthritis and for children with acute rheumatic fever is primarily related to heart involvement. By definition, children with poststreptococcal reactive arthritis do not have heart involvement. If they have heart involvement, they fulfill criteria for rheumatic fever. (Our concern is that they will develop heart involvement with a future streptococcal infection.) For children with acute rheumatic fever, severe inflammation of the heart can lead to permanent heart damage or even death. However, the arthritis is short-lived and rarely of long-term significance. Any child with heart damage secondary to acute rheumatic fever should be under the care of a cardiologist.

10

Lyme Disease

Frankie was a delightful twelve-year-old who loved to play sports. Halfway through football season, he began to complain of knee pains. When his symptoms didn't improve, he was taken to his pediatrician. At first, the pediatrician thought that Frankie had simply twisted the knee. When Frankie was unable to continue football because the knee was swollen and painful, he was referred to an orthopedist. Three months later, Frankie continued to have pain in the knee that prevented him from playing. With activity the knee often became swollen but then improved over a week to ten days. He was sent to me to treat his "JRA." The father was sure that he had been tested for Lyme disease, but careful review of the records revealed that the test had never been done. The orthopedist was sure that the pediatrician had checked, and the pediatrician was sure that the orthopedist had done so. When I did the Lyme test it was strongly positive, and Frankie improved dramatically when we treated him with antibiotics.

Sam was a five-year-old from an area where Lyme disease was quite common. Although he had played happily outdoors all summer, he seemed to be dragging in the fall. When he began to complain of pain, his mother took him to the pediatrician. The blood tests were negative for Lyme disease, but the ESR was moderately elevated. Since Lyme disease was common in the area where Sam lived, the pediatrician treated him for that disease despite the negative test. When the prescribed oral antibiotics did not work, Sam was given intravenous antibiotics for two more months. He still didn't improve. Finally, Sam was sent to me for treatment of his difficult Lyme disease. X-rays revealed that Sam had a large tumor in his pelvis, necessitating surgery, radiation therapy, and extensive chemotherapy. Sam was left with permanent damage after the surgery. He had never had Lyme disease. Had the tumor been found sooner, the outcome might have been better.

Lyme disease is a chronic infection caused by *Borrelia burgdorferi*. This is a spirochetal organism that is carried by mammals such as deer and deer mice and spread by very small deer ticks (*Ixodes scapularis*). The ticks bite an infected animal and pick up the spirochete with their blood meal. They then transfer the spirochete to people or animals they feed on, infecting them with Lyme disease.

Lyme disease in humans is often only an acute flu-like illness. However, some adults and children develop rash and arthritis. The key to understanding Lyme arthritis in children is to recognize that it is in many ways a typical infection-associated arthritis; the major difference is that Lyme disease follows a much more protracted course. Typical infection-associated arthritis develops within a few weeks of the original illness, and the fever and rash (erythema migrans, or EM) of Lyme disease also occur early. However, the arthritis of Lyme disease usually does not appear until two to four or more months after the initial infection.

Ticks found in the spring and early summer are young ticks (nymphs) that are not as likely to carry Lyme disease. But as they feed repeatedly on different animals, the likelihood of their being infected dramatically increases. Many of the children I see in my office are infected during late August or early September, developing arthritis in November, December, or January, when parents and physicians aren't thinking about Lyme disease. Children who present with arthritis in the early summer often have been infected the previous fall. (It is rarely possible to prove exactly when a child was infected. The Western blot test detects a specific number of bands, which gradually increases over time as the infected individual mounts an immune response to the spirochete. A child diagnosed with Lyme disease in the early summer who has more than ten positive bands on the Western blot test was most likely infected the previous year.)

Some parents understand that their children are at risk because they live in areas where deer are common. Other families have visited such areas but the parents have never found a tick on their children. It is important to realize that the deer tick that carries Lyme disease is extremely small—no larger than the head of a typical pin. Ticks are often recognized only after the area surrounding the bite becomes red and irritated or when a parent notices a "moving freckle." While it is a disadvantage that these ticks are so small, parents who find a larger dog tick on their child (about the size of lentil) can be confident that this tick does not carry Lyme disease. Even people who live in areas where Lyme disease is common are often surprised to learn that arthritis that appeared in January is the result of a tick bite the previous summer.

In children, the flu-like symptoms of early Lyme disease are often dismissed as a virus. The child may develop the characteristic rash of EM a few weeks after the original illness. This is most often a series of large circles the size of a quarter or even much bigger. The outer edge of the circle is red and inflamed, while the center is usually pale. Anyone with the characteristic rash should be tested for Lyme disease and treated if positive. (There are other illnesses that may produce a rash with central clearing. If the Lyme disease test is negative, make sure that other possible explanations are carefully considered.) Children do not usually have arthritis when the rash first appears. However, the rash can recur later in the illness at a time when the child does have arthritis. This rash does not come and go rapidly, like the rash associated with systemic-onset arthritis. In addition, in children with Lyme disease, the individual lesions are typically far fewer but much larger.

A number of nonspecific symptoms, such as headaches, are often seen at the beginning of Lyme disease. Their significance is uncertain. It is clear that Lyme disease does involve the nervous system in some children, although most children with headaches do not have central nervous system Lyme disease. Bell's palsy is often a symptom of Lyme disease in endemic areas. If the facial nerve is not functioning properly, the child may have difficulty or be unable to open the mouth, to smile, or to close the eye tightly on the involved side. While there are many possible causes of Bell's palsy, it is well recognized that Lyme disease is a common cause in Lyme-endemic areas.

Lyme arthritis usually begins dramatically. It can affect any large or small joint and often suddenly affects many joints. Children with Lyme disease are often in significant pain. This is very different from the pain of typical childhood arthritis, which comes on gradually. Although EM is a typical manifestation of early Lyme disease, it is rarely present when the arthritis develops.

Since the arthritic symptoms develop months after the initial tick bite, children with Lyme disease are easily diagnosed only if the physician remembers to check a Lyme titer. However, it is important to remember that children with other serious illnesses may also have been exposed to Lyme disease in the past and have a positive titer that is not the explanation for their symptoms. Some children with Lyme disease present with only a single swollen joint. These children differ from children with typical JA in that the arthritis often comes on rapidly. In addition, like other forms of infection-associated arthritis, Lyme arthritis can begin in the hip. (However, I have never seen dactylitis due to Lyme disease.)

Children with Lyme disease who have gone untreated for a long period of time may have recurrent episodes of joint swelling. This most often takes the form of recurrent knee swelling, which may have been dismissed as an athletic injury or sprain. It is important that any child with swollen joints who lives in or has visited an area where Lyme disease occurs be appropriately tested. This is particularly important for children who may be known to have JA. I have cared for several children with JA whose symptoms unexpectedly worsened dramatically. When tested, they were found to have become Lyme-positive even though, when I began treating them several years previously, they had been Lyme-negative. These were not children with JA due to Lyme disease. They were children with JA who, because they lived in an endemic area, also developed Lyme disease. Most children who develop Lyme disease are detected because of the new onset of symptoms. Because the children I follow have chronic arthritis, I systematically check their Lyme titers in the fall each year.

DIFFERENTIAL DIAGNOSIS

Lyme disease is a typical infection-associated or reactive arthritis. As a result, it may be confused with any other infection-associated arthritis. The key differences in children with arthritis due to Lyme disease are the absence of a recent infection (most children develop infection-associated arthritis two to three weeks following a recognized illness) and the presence of a positive Lyme titer. In any child being evaluated for Lyme arthritis, it is important to consider the other causes of infection-associated arthritis, including streptococcal and other bacterial infections and parvovirus and other viral infections.

Systemic lupus erythematosus and other forms of collagen vascular disease may also begin with the rapid onset of arthritis involving the large and small joints. The key to distinguishing these diseases is their different clinical appearance and the use of appropriate laboratory tests. I have seen many children with these illnesses misdiagnosed as having "seronegative" Lyme disease. In areas where there is a high frequency of exposure to Lyme disease, the situation may be complicated by a positive Lyme test in a child who is suffering from another illness. **All children with positive Lyme tests should be treated for Lyme disease, but if there is no quick and dramatic response, physicians should investigate carefully other possible causes of the child's symptoms.**

There is much debate about the occurrence of Lyme disease in children who do not have positive titers (see Chapter 25). Most of this debate stems from the period when Lyme testing was not well standardized. At present, it is extremely unlikely that a child with a negative Lyme titer has the disease. While it is always possible for the laboratory to make a mistake in reporting a result, this problem can be easily resolved in a suspicious situation by simply repeating the test, perhaps using a different laboratory. I have seen many children treated extensively for Lyme-negative Lyme disease. More unfortunate than the fact that they were treated with unnecessary antibiotics is that they were not properly treated for their real disease. In children with bone or joint pains due to infections, JA, or cancer, this mistake can have tragic consequences.

LABORATORY FINDINGS

Children with Lyme disease almost invariably have a positive Lyme titer and a positive Western blot test result (see Chapter 25 for a discussion of these two tests). In addition, they have elevated ESRs and WBC counts. While the elevated WBC count and ESR are commonly present in children with polyarticular-onset arthritis, they are infrequent in children with pauciarticular-onset disease. Some children with Lyme disease have positive tests for ANA. They should not have RF, antibodies to double-stranded DNA (dsDNA), or complement abnormalities.

Some physicians and laboratories have developed specialized tests for the detection of Lyme disease. If these tests had stood up to careful evaluation, we would all be using them. However, strategies such as giving a child antibiotics and then collecting the urine to look for evidence of spirochete antigens are unlikely to detect subtle Lyme disease that did not show up on regular testing. These tests and polymerase chain reaction (PCR) tests are not considered reliable by the Centers for Disease Control (CDC). It is important to understand that all humans have normal spirochetes in their mouths. That is why the Western blot test was developed. Screening tests for spirochete antigens do not distinguish between the response to the spirochetes that are normally present in the body and the Lyme spirochete—only the Western blot test does this. While it may be recommended that a child in whom there is a strong suspicion of Lyme disease and a positive enzyme-linked immunosorbent assay (ELISA) but a negative Western blot test result take antibiotics for two weeks, continued treatment in the face of continued symptoms is unwise. Such children need a complete and thorough evaluation for other possible causes of the symptoms.

COMPLICATIONS

Fortunately, serious complications of Lyme disease are rare. The vast majority of children with Lyme disease–related arthritis recover promptly (within a few weeks) and, with treatment, completely. In children with Lyme disease who have a large number of bands on their Western blot (e.g., nine or more), it is likely that the infection has been present for a prolonged period. Some of these children will have continuing arthritis after the first thirty days of antibiotic treatment. It is important to recognize that, like other causes of infection-associated arthritis, Lyme disease tends to provoke arthritis in those who have an underlying "arthritic predisposition." If the arthritis persists after appropriate treatment for Lyme disease, the emphasis must be on treatment of the arthritis, not continued antibiotics. As is typical of infection-associated arthritis, the majority of these children become well within a year of diagnosis. Any child with arthritis persisting after a year must be treated with the assumption that Lyme disease provoked an underlying arthritic disease. There is no evidence that further antibiotics are beneficial.

Bell's palsy and other neurologic symptoms of Lyme disease typically respond well to antibiotics. There are some who argue that Lyme disease has many chronic symptoms in childhood, including attention deficit disorder and other unexplained conditions. It is important to recognize that Lyme disease is common, and therefore it will be found in a significant number of children with a wide variety of coincidental problems unrelated to it. The issue seems clear-cut if the child's problems resolve with medical treatment. However, if the problems are not related to Lyme disease, months or even years of antibiotic treatment are unlikely to provide real relief. There are many children with these complaints who live in areas where Lyme disease never occurs. Beware of colleagues who think that these problems are always due to Lyme disease. **While every child with a positive test for Lyme disease should be given appropriate treatment, this disease should not eliminate the need for attention to other potential causes of the child's complaints.**

Another possible complication of Lyme disease is the **Jarisch-Herxheimer reaction**. This was initially described in the treatment of syphilis (another spirochete infection) when penicillin first became available. When the first dose of penicillin was given to a patient who was heavily infected, a very large number of spirochetes would die and release their contents into the blood. This would produce an acute toxic reaction with fever, rash, and severe malaise. Although it could occur in someone with a large number of Lyme spirochetes as well, I have never seen this reaction in a child under my care.

MEDICAL TREATMENT

Optimal treatment for Lyme disease is dependent on the age of the child, the manifestations of the disease, and whether the child has any allergies to drugs. Young children are typically treated with amoxicillin, while children over the age of ten are typically treated with doxycycline. Doxycycline is not used in younger children because it will become incorporated in the enamel of developing teeth and may cause a permanent grayish stain. Some physicians feel that it is acceptable to use doxycycline in children as young as eight years of age if the adult teeth appear to be fully formed in the gums. In children who are allergic to amoxicillin and doxycycline, cephalosporins or erythromycin derivatives may be considered.

The duration of therapy for Lyme disease also depends on the manifestations of the disease. The majority of the medical community agrees with the recommendations shown in Box 10-1.

Box 10-1   Duration of antibiotic therapy for the manifestations of Lyme disease

- Children with a positive test for Lyme disease in the absence of arthritis or neurologic symptoms should be treated with **twenty-one days** of an appropriate antibiotic. The vast majority will respond well to oral antibiotics.
- If a child has arthritis, **thirty days** of antibiotic therapy are recommended. Again, this may be done orally. However, therapy is often begun intravenously for a possible bacterial infection of the joint and oral therapy used only after bacterial infection has been excluded. This decision will depend on the clinical situation and how strongly the physicians suspect that a bacterial infection might be present. The child should also be treated with NSAIDs for as long as the arthritis continues. This will control the inflammatory response in the joint, minimizing the damage from inflammatory enzymes and providing significant pain relief.
- Children with **neurologic manifestations** of Lyme disease also require **thirty days** of antibiotic therapy. However, in this situation, many physicians prefer to begin with intravenous therapy, since this provides better assurance of a

---

Box 10-1   (Continued)

---

high level of drug reaching the central nervous system. In the majority of children who do not have a long-standing infection (as evidenced by the number of bands on the Western blot), the neurologic manifestations resolve completely within thirty days. Further treatment of children with neurologic manifestations that have not completely resolved after thirty days of intra- venous therapy will depend on the nature of the manifestations and the degree of improvement that has occurred.

- Children who have arthritis that has not fully resolved with thirty days of oral therapy represent a challenge. Since this is infection-associated arthritis, it is well recognized that the arthritis may persist long after the infection is gone; thus, further antibiotics may not be necessary. For children who have only a moderate number of bands on the Western blot, I recommend a month of continued NSAID therapy. Almost all children are well at the end of this additional month.

- Children with a large number of bands on the Western blot may be difficult to bring under complete control. Most often these are children who have had arthritic symptoms for months before being diagnosed with Lyme dis- ease and did not receive appropriate treatment. Since the arthritis frequently lingers in this group, I recommend an additional thirty days of intravenous therapy so that both the parents and I can be sure that the Lyme disease has been adequately treated. Some of these children will continue to have active arthritis after the additional thirty days of antibiotic therapy. I do not treat these children with further antibiotics. Over time they will respond to NSAIDs.

Many disagree over the best first response to a child found with an embedded deer tick. In my experience, a Lyme titer should be obtained immediately. It will not reflect infection from the tick just found, but it may indicate that there is a preexisting infection that requires treatment. If this titer is negative, it needs to be repeated in six weeks to determine whether it has turned positive. If it has, the child should be treated appropriately.

Some experts recommend an alternative approach. If a child is found with an embedded tick, a Lyme titer is performed and two weeks of oral antibiotic ther- apy are begun immediately. If the titer is negative, treatment is stopped at two weeks. If the titer is positive, treatment is continued for an additional week. It has been shown that this may prevent Lyme infections and is more cost effective than repeated testing. One new study suggests that one day of treatment may work as well as two weeks. However, if a child lives in an area where Lyme dis- ease is common, how often should he or she be treated? There is no unanimous answer to this question. Often parents will bring a tick to the physician to be tested for Lyme disease. This is useless because of the small size of the deer tick. If the child had one tick that the parents found, there is a significant risk that the child had other ticks that the parents didn't find. The child—not the tick—must be tested, and the child will need repeat testing in six weeks.

Many family physicians ask how they will know if a child they care for gets a second Lyme infection and needs an additional round of treatment. This is another question for which there is no satisfactory answer. In most infections, the assumption is that either the bacterium can be cultured if it is present or, in the case of viruses, a single infection provides immunity that prevents further infection. In the case of Lyme disease, it is virtually impossible to culture the spirochete from tissues to prove that an infection is present. At the same time, it appears that a single Lyme infection does not provide lifelong protection. The Lyme vaccine was withdrawn from the market because it had side effects and did not guarantee protection from future infection.

In my patients, I periodically monitor the Lyme titer and Western blot. During the first few months after diagnosis and treatment, both the Lyme titer and the number of Western blot–positive bands may increase. This represents *immunologic recruitment* (the immune response is gathering strength over time), not continued infection. After six or more months, the Lyme titer should begin to decrease. The number of positive bands on the Western blot may not. If a child develops signs of possible repeat infection a year or more after initial treatment, I will compare the results with those found six months after the initial treatment (to account for the immunologic recruitment). If the response is stronger, I will retreat with oral antibiotics. There is no proof, and there are no controlled studies to guide us. Each physician must recommend what he or she thinks is most logical in this situation.

There are some physicians who firmly believe that Lyme is a more chronic infection and may require years of therapy. There is no convincing evidence that they are correct, and prolonged antibiotic therapy has been associated with serious side effects. Many children come to me after long periods of antibiotic therapy without sustained improvement. Often it is because Lyme disease is not the cause of their complaints. Once a proper diagnosis is made and they are begun on appropriate therapy, they often promptly improve. I have seen children who came to me after many months of antibiotics for "Lyme disease" who turned out to have tumors, infections, arthritis, or regional pain syndromes.

11

Systemic Lupus Erythematosus

Margaret was fourteen years old when I met her. She did well in junior high school but seemed lazy over the summer before starting high school. When high school began, she did not seem to be making new friends and complained of being tired. School was hard. Her family just assumed that she needed to get used to high school. As the semester progressed, she seemed to be spending more time in her room. Her parents got phone calls reporting that she was not performing well in school, and her grades were poor. She was losing weight, irritable, and disinterested. By December there were questions about drug use, difficulty adjusting to the new school, and so on.

In January the school requested a psychiatric evaluation. The psychiatrist asked for a pediatric evaluation. Fortunately, the pediatrician ran a full set of blood tests and found that Margaret was anemic, with an elevated ESR and a positive ANA test. She was referred to my office. When I walked into the room and shook her hand, she cried because her hands hurt when I squeezed. She had not realized that she had arthritis. She had no rash, but her blood and urine tests confirmed the presence of systemic lupus erythematosus. As I write this, I saw Margaret yesterday. It's eight years later, and she is finishing college and doing very well. She wants to teach English.

WHAT IS SYSTEMIC LUPUS ERYTHEMATOSUS?

In textbooks, systemic lupus erythematosus (SLE) is defined as a complex autoimmune disease with protean manifestations. In plain English, the key to understanding SLE is to recognize that the disease begins with a breakdown in the regulation of the immune system. In a normal immune response, the immune system identifies an invader and mounts a response against it. To protect itself, the body uses every possible type of immunity (e.g., antibodies, complement, innate and cell-mediated immunity). Once the invader has been controlled, the system turns off and everything goes back to normal. In children with SLE, the immune system is constantly responding to an invader. No one has found an indication of what the invader is. Because decades of research have failed to find an invader (despite many false leads), we now believe that in SLE the regulatory system breaks down and the body is unable to turn off the immune response after the initial attack (by any one of many different invaders) is over.

Investigation of a number of these illnesses suggests that they involve a two-step process. It is now thought that SLE occurs in children and adults who have a genetic abnormality that makes it more likely that their immune system will become deregulated. However, the genetic abnormality is harmless unless a related infection occurs at a vulnerable time. Although various answers have been suggested, it appears that there is no single genetic abnormality, no single related infection, and no single vulnerable time.

Typically, SLE is a disease that affects teenage girls and young adult women. Less frequently, SLE occurs in both older and younger individuals and in boys. It often begins with fevers, rash, joint pains, and fatigue. Although these symptoms are worrisome, it is the ability of SLE to affect many different internal organs that makes this a serious illness. Serious involvement of the pulmonary system, the central nervous system, or the kidneys can lead to permanent disability or even death. It is important that children who have SLE be promptly recognized so that they can be treated and internal organ damage prevented whenever possible. Some children are found to have evidence of internal organ damage with no complaints of obvious symptoms.

Because in children and adults with SLE the body fails to turn the immune response off, patients develop fevers, ache all over, and often have a rash. When these symptoms occur as part of a normal infection, the infecting virus or bacterium does not directly cause the problems. The fever and aches and pains are the result of the body's immune response to the infection. Just as different infections can damage different parts of the body, in children with SLE the uncontrolled immune response can produce many different types of damage. Problems can occur anywhere, including the central nervous system, cardiac system, pulmonary system, muscles, kidneys, skin, joints, liver, or intestine.

Typically, when areas are damaged by SLE, antibodies, complement, and inflammatory cells are present, and the local tissue has been damaged by the resulting inflammation. We are beginning to understand more clearly why the immune system fails to turn off in children with SLE, but we do not understand why certain children develop one set of problems and other children develop completely different problems. In animal models, genetics seems to be an important factor in determining which problems develop.

Sun Exposure and Systemic Lupus Erythematosus

One of the most difficult issues for the families of children with SLE is sun exposure. Everyone wants to play outside, go to the beach, get a tan, and participate in normal outdoor activities. However, it is well documented that ultraviolet light exposure damages cells and causes cell death. "Programmed" cell death is called *apoptosis*. This process allows damaged cells to self-destruct in an orderly fashion and be cleaned up and disposed of by the body with minimal difficulty. In patients with SLE this process is defective, and the damaged cells remain as stimulants to the immune system for a prolonged period. This is thought to promote the formation of not only ANA but also other antibodies directed against important cellular elements that drive SLE as well. As a result, significant sun exposure may lead to a severe flare of the underlying SLE. It is essential that children with SLE wear an appropriate sun block and avoid significant sun exposure. A single trip to the beach (or the tanning salon) can cause life-threatening complications.

DIAGNOSIS: WHEN TO SUSPECT SYSTEMIC LUPUS ERYTHEMATOSUS

Systemic lupus erythematosus most often affects girls in the teenage years, but it may affect both boys and girls at any age. Although the typical butterfly rash on the face is considered a characteristic feature of the disease, it is found in only one-third of children when they first come to the doctor's office. Since many doctors do not think of SLE unless they see the butterfly rash, many children have symptoms of SLE for months before the proper diagnosis is made. The key to a prompt diagnosis of SLE is for primary-care physicians to consider this diagnosis whenever they are evaluating children who appear to be chronically ill or have unexplained damage in organs that are frequently affected by SLE (e.g., the kidneys).

Box 11-1 American College of Rheumatology criteria for a *definite* diagnosis of systemic lupus erythematosus

1. Malar rash: a red rash over the cheeks (often crossing over the nose)
2. Discoid rash: a scaly red rash (uncommon in children)
3. Photosensitivity: easy sunburning, rashes and sensitivity to light
4. Mucosal ulcers: sores in the mouth or nose
5. Serositis: inflammation of the lining of the chest or abdomen producing pain
6. Arthritis: pain, swelling, or limitation of motion of a joint
7. Renal involvement: abnormalities on urine tests or blood tests (see this chapter)
8. Neurologic involvement: seizures or difficulty thinking normally
9. Hematologic involvement: abnormalities of the red cells, white cells, or platelets (see this chapter)
10. Immunologic disorder: abnormal blood tests characteristic of SLE (see this chapter)
11. Antinuclear antibodies

A child is considered to have definite SLE if he or she has any four of the eleven criteria.

Many physicians are confused by the American College of Rheumatology criteria for a definite diagnosis of SLE (see Box 11-1). They often assume that these criteria are the most common symptoms of SLE. This is completely incorrect. The criteria were written not to aid in making the diagnosis, but to help distinguish SLE from other diseases. They are intended to make sure that everyone included in a study of patients with SLE really has SLE. The most common symptom of SLE is fever. The second most common symptom is a chronic complaint of not feeling well (malaise). The third most common symptom is arthritis of the small joints of the hands and feet, often described as "hurting all over."

Prompt diagnosis of SLE in children requires parents and physicians to consider SLE whenever a child is not doing well. For very young children who are failing to thrive, there is a standard evaluation to look for problems such as cystic fibrosis and hypothyroidism. There should also be a standard workup for older children who are failing to thrive (see Chapter 4). Although SLE is only one of many possible causes, it is important to include ANA testing in this evaluation. Many diseases may be associated with a positive ANA test in children and teenagers (see Chapter 25). However, SLE should be carefully excluded when evaluating any child with a positive test. A negative test for ANA makes SLE very unlikely.

Although the onset of SLE typically occurs between the ages of twelve and twenty-five years, I have seen SLE patients as young as three years of age. In a pediatric rheumatology practice, it is not unusual to see SLE starting at the age of eight years. The incidence of SLE varies by sex and race; however, no one has ever sampled a completely homogeneous population to determine the precise number of children with SLE by race. It is estimated that among 100,000 girls of each race between the ages of nine and nineteen years, there are 31 Asians, 20 African Americans, 13 Hispanics, and 4 Caucasians with SLE. There should also be 1 or 2 boys with SLE for every 100,000 male children.

Although chronic failure to thrive is the most common presentation, SLE can also begin in many other ways. Chronic swelling of the hands and feet, easy bruising (with or without thrombocytopenia), joint pains, hematuria or proteinuria, photosensitivity, seizures, altered personality and depression, and poor school performance all may be initial findings in children with SLE. However, it is important to remember that these are nonspecific symptoms that may occur in many different illnesses.

Some children with SLE reach my office after a long history of being evaluated for problems such as anemia, fatigue, fever, and weight loss without explanation. Less often the onset of SLE is sudden and dramatic, with pulmonary hemorrhage, renal compromise, sepsis, or multiple-organ involvement. Again, it is important to remember that SLE is not the only disease that may cause these findings. Even when a positive ANA is present, SLE may not be the correct diagnosis. This is why it is very important that all such children be evaluated by a physician experienced with SLE.

Once the diagnosis of SLE is suspected, proper evaluation begins with testing for ANA. If the ANA test is negative, it is extremely unlikely that the child has SLE. (A variety of other rheumatic diseases may mimic the symptoms of SLE.) If the test for ANA is positive, further evaluation should include complete routine testing, such as a complete blood count (CBC), metabolic profile, clotting studies, urine analysis, and testing for Ro, La, Sm, RNP, and anti-DNA antibodies (see Chapter 25). Complement C3 and C4 should be measured. It is also useful to screen these children for thyroid function abnormalities, antithyroid antibodies, anticardiolipin antibodies, and RF. Sometimes it is clear at the completion of these studies that a child has SLE. In other cases, there are several abnormalities but not enough to make a definite diagnosis of SLE.

One of my patients is a young woman who complained of aches and pains when she was fifteen years old. There were no significant findings on examination, but her pediatrician was quite surprised when she tested positive for ANA. She was referred for evaluation, but her aches and pains had resolved by the time she came for her appointment. Her examination was entirely normal, but on repeat testing she remained ANA-positive and was also positive for Sm antibody. The remaining tests were normal. I did not make a diagnosis of SLE, but I continued to examine and test her periodically. She remained well until four years later, when she called to tell me that she had developed a rash and joint pain. On examination, she was found to have arthritis and a facial rash with an ulcer on the roof of her mouth. Blood tests again revealed a strongly positive ANA and Sm antibodies, but now anti-DNA antibodies and decreased serum complement C3 and C4 levels as well. She had developed definite SLE, but we caught it very early. Today, years later, she is doing fine.

The diagnosis of definite SLE requires that the child fulfill four of the eleven American College of Rheumatology criteria. However, there are many children with SLE who initially fulfill fewer than four criteria. **If several findings suggest SLE but the children do not fulfill four criteria for a definite diagnosis, they should be monitored carefully.** It does not matter whether they are believed to have SLE, possible SLE, or probable SLE. The key to proper care for these children is to treat their problems appropriately. If this is done, it won't matter if the ultimate diagnosis is SLE or another condition—they will have received appropriate care either way. I sometimes see children with only three criteria who have been told that because they do not have definite SLE, they do not need to be treated. This is incorrect.

Children with uncertain symptoms and relatives who have SLE are often of great concern to their families. Up to one-third of the relatives of a patient with SLE will be ANA-positive but have no disease. However, relatives of someone with SLE are at greater risk of developing SLE than members of the normal population. On one occasion, I examined all the relatives of more than ninety children with SLE. When I tested everyone, I found that there were thirty ANA-positive sisters among the relatives. Two had unrecognized SLE and were treated. I personally examined the remaining twenty-eight repeatedly for several years, and no one developed disease during the first few years of follow-up.

However, several developed definite SLE between three and five years after I first evaluated them. This group was clearly at increased risk relative to the normal population, but most of the twenty-eight ANA-positive sisters did not develop SLE.

Children who have nonspecific symptoms and a positive ANA require routine follow-up to look for evidence of disease. Their physicians must remain aware of the possibility of SLE. Simply dismissing these children as not having criteria for definite SLE and never needing to be seen again is incorrect. Some physicians simply instruct the parents to bring the child back if more problems develop. I prefer to be proactive and periodically look for problems. This often allows me to begin therapy before the problems become more serious. It is well known that children with SLE may develop renal disease without initially complaining of pain or discomfort. It is important to detect these problems as early as possible and to minimize the damage to vital organs.

CLINICAL MANIFESTATIONS OF SYSTEMIC LUPUS ERYTHEMATOSUS

The patterns of disease involvement in children with SLE range from fever, rash, aches, and pains but no serious organ damage to a lack of complaints but serious renal or hematologic involvement found on routine screening tests. Serious internal organ involvement most often affects the kidneys, but the central nervous system, cardiac system, pulmonary system, and other internal organs also may be seriously affected.

Many children with SLE have mild disease that is easily treated, but others have serious internal organ involvement. As early as possible, it is important to recognize which children have mild disease and which ones have severe disease. This cannot always be done with absolute certainty. Some children start out with mild disease that worsens. Others start out extremely ill, respond well to therapy, and improve. The challenge for physicians is to find the proper balance between the side effects of medications and the risks of damage from the disease (see the section in this chapter on treatment). When they can be recognized, children with severe disease should be treated aggressively *before* there is a lot of organ damage, not afterward. "Let's wait until we are sure that the house is burning down before we call the fire department" is not a good approach.

Renal Involvement

Recognizing Potential Problems

Renal involvement is one of the most worrisome aspects of SLE. However, there are varying degrees of involvement, from very mild to very severe. Approximately two-thirds of children with SLE will have at least mild renal involvement at the time they are diagnosed. Most but not all children with significant renal involvement have evident abnormalities on a urine analysis when they are first brought to the doctor. In some cases, hematuria or proteinuria is detected on a routine exam and leads to the diagnosis of SLE. Other children are brought to the doctor because of swelling of their feet and are found to have proteinuria. Red blood cells (RBCs) in the urine, WBCs in the urine, urinary casts, and protein in the urine all may be manifestations of SLE (note again that there are many other possible causes of these problems).

Diagnosing And Treating Renal Complications

In a child with obvious SLE, the physician may elect to treat with corticosteroids and do a renal biopsy only if the child does not respond to this treatment. Other physicians will biopsy every child with SLE, and some biopsy every child with SLE who has abnormal urine test results. There is no single correct answer. A World Health Organization (WHO) class I or class II biopsy is not a cause for major concern. A class III, IV, or V biopsy is worrisome. In addition to reporting the WHO classification, the biopsy report should contain immunofluorescence study results.

Box 11-2   World Health Organization classification of renal biopsy pathology in systemic lupus erythematosus.

- Class I: normal kidney
- Class II: mild glomerulitis
- Class III: focal segmental glomerulonephritis
- Class IV: diffuse proliferative glomerulonephritis (DPGN)
- Class V: membranous glomerulonephritis

It is worrisome if the immunofluorescence studies show a lot of immunoglobulin or complement in the glomeruli. This is especially important if the biopsy is reported as WHO class III. Class III is focal segmental glomeru-lonephritis, which means that most of the glomeruli seen under the microscope are normal but some (less than half) show evidence of inflammation. This has long been thought to be a less serious degree of renal involvement that does not require the same aggressive treatment as WHO class IV. However, this assumes that the damage has stopped. All too often, children with a class III initial renal biopsy progress to class IV disease over time. In WHO class IV (DPGN), more than half of the glomeruli are damaged. Everyone agrees that children with class IV disease are at significant risk of serious renal damage and, ultimately, renal failure. As a result, these children must be treated aggressively. Most physicians now look carefully at any biopsy interpreted as class III and treat the child aggressively if the immunofluorescence is strongly positive, since this suggests that the disease is likely to become worse over time.

A child with class IV renal disease needs to be treated aggressively. Some children with class IV disease do well, but others do not. It is important to know the *activity* and *chronicity* scores. Activity is a measure of the amount of cellular inflammation in the kidney. The pathologist looks at the glomeruli and determines how inflamed they are and whether there are large collections of inflammatory cells (these are often referred to as *crescents*). The presence of crescents means that there is very severe, very active inflammation in the kidney. A high **activity index** means that a lot of damage is being done. At the same time, the pathologist will report a chronicity index, another very important number. The **chronicity index** is an estimate of the amount of scarring in the kidney. The greater the percentage of sclerosed glomeruli present in the kidney and the greater the damage to other structures, the higher the chronicity index.

If the chronicity index is very high, it does not make sense to treat the child aggressively. Badly scarred kidneys are not going to recover, no matter how hard you try. These children will ultimately need renal dialysis and renal transplantation. The key to a successful outcome is to catch the involvement early and prevent the chronicity index from rising over time. **Although many different treatments have been recommended for children with lupus renal involvement, only the systematic use of intravenous cyclophosphamide has been shown to prevent a rise in the chronicity index over time.** Thus, it is very important that all children with a worrisome class III biopsy and all children with a class IV biopsy receive appropriate treatment. Some physicians do favor other therapies, but only intravenous cyclophosphamide has been proven to work over the long term in published studies.

World Health Organization class V renal biopsies are a special case. These biopsies show membranous glomerulonephritis, which has a characteristic "wire loop" lesion on the renal biopsy. It is associated with significant proteinuria. If the kidneys are losing too much protein, the body cannot compensate by making more. The level of albumin and the osmotic pressure drop. When that happens, water starts leaking out all over the body. Excessive water accumulates in the feet when the patient is sitting or standing or around the buttocks if he or she is lying down. In an effort to correct the problem, the body starts making more of components that do not leak easily; normally, this takes the form of cholesterol. Children with nephrotic syndrome may have cholesterol levels in the 600 or 700 mg/dl range. This partially helps to solve the problem of water leaking out of the blood vessels, but these very high cholesterol levels often lead to early cardiac disease and need to be treated with statins.

In addition to the problems resulting from edema and high cholesterol levels, the prolonged proteinuria in children with class IV or V disease is damaging to the glomeruli. As a result, if children with proteinuria are not properly treated, the glomeruli will eventually fail. This can be partially prevented by the use of angiotensin-converting enzyme (ACE) inhibitors (a class of drugs used to treat high blood pressure). Many doctors will treat children with class V disease with cyclophosphamide, which works, but not as well as it does for class IV disease. However, we do not have anything that is clearly better. Children with mixed class IV and class V disease should be treated aggressively with intravenous cyclophosphamide. There is also increasing evidence that rituximab is beneficial for these children.

All children with serious renal involvement due to SLE need to be treated aggressively. All too often, I see children who have been followed for "mild" renal involvement for a long period of time. The treating physician did not become concerned until the serum creatinine level began to exceed 2.0 gm/dl. Unfortunately, many of these children are found to have serious damage when a new renal biopsy is done. Things may not have looked bad on the first renal biopsy or maybe the condition was not bad enough initially to do a renal biopsy. The disease was allowed to smolder. The new biopsy shows a lot of scarring and a high chronicity index. It is now too late to do anything to prevent the kidneys from ultimately failing. These children require renal transplants and will be on antirejection medicine for the rest of their lives. Many people tell me that they fear the side effects of intravenous cyclophosphamide. However, the side effects of intravenous cyclophosphamide and rituximab are far less serious than the side effects of chronic renal dialysis or the lifetime of immunosuppression required following renal transplantation.

New drugs and new combinations of drugs are beginning to be used in the treatment of renal involvement. In the section on treatment that follows, there are discussions of rituximab, abatacept, and mycophenolate mofetil. These drugs can be used alone or in varying combinations in addition to or as a replacement for cyclophosphamide. As yet, there is no best answer. In my own experience, the combination of cyclophosphamide and rituximab appears to give superior results and allows a reduction in both the amount of prednisone needed and the number of treatment courses of cyclophosphamide.

Central Nervous System Involvement

Recognizing Potential Problems

Children with SLE may exhibit a wide variety of central nervous system abnormalities. Seizures, strokes, and other serious abnormalities are obvious but relatively infrequent. However, subtle problems due to central nervous system involvement in children with SLE vary from difficulty with fine motor skills and poor penmanship to suddenly worsening grades and severe depression. These problems are common. There are many psychological effects of chronic illness. There are also many psychological effects of having to take a lot of medicine, visit the doctor all the time, and endure frequent blood tests.

I often listen to doctors arguing over whether a child's poor school performance and behavior problems are due to central nervous system involvement, medicines, or the situation. They want to decide that the answer is exclusively one or the other. In real life, this is like arguing about the word *cat*. Is *cat* a small furry animal because of the *c*, the *a*, or the *t*? After all, if I change the *c* to *b*, it's *bat*. But if I change the *t* to *p* it's *cap*, but changing the *a* to *o* makes *cot*. Well, this is ridiculous! All three letters act together in a specific order to make *cat*, and they cannot be separated or assigned individual responsibility. In real life, the disease, the medications, and the situation all act together as well. It is never all one or the other. If a child's behavior is not normal, do not look for a single answer; assume that the disease, the medicines, and the situation all need to be evaluated and corrected as well as possible.

Involvement of the central nervous system in children with SLE has at least three primary forms. Some children have clotting disorders that lead to strokes resulting in central nervous system damage. There is also evidence that the antibodies causing the clotting disorders may directly damage nerve cells in the central nervous system. Other children suffer central nervous system damage because their lupus results in chronic inflammation of the blood vessels in the brain or spinal cord, and the inflammation of the blood vessels damages the surrounding tissue. Still other children have central nervous system problems because they have taken too much corticosteroid over the years. Each of these types of damage has its own peculiarities, but all three may occur in the same child at the same time. Central nervous system damage may also occur due to high blood pressure, which was the result of renal disease.

A number of tests are used to evaluate a child with SLE who is showing neurologic abnormalities:

- An MRI will show structural changes in the central nervous system. It will also show increased water content that can occur with inflammation, bleeding, or other problems.

- A CAT scan will show structural problems and may also demonstrate bleeding, among other problems. When these test results are normal, there may still be significant findings on lumbar puncture.

- The cerebrospinal fluid (CSF) cell count, protein level, glucose level, or immunoglobulins all may be abnormal if SLE is affecting the central nervous system. They also may all be normal. **The most important reason to look at the CSF in this situation is to make sure that there is no infection or other unsuspected problem**.

- Nuclear isotope central nervous system scans called single photon emission computed tomography (SPECT) scans are utilized by some centers to evaluate central nervous system function, but these are generally considered unreliable in the setting of SLE. Positron emission tomography (PET) scans and functional MRIs may provide useful information if they are available.

Central nervous system damage due to strokes is usually very dramatic. It can result in sudden inability to use a hand, leg, or whole side of the body. Sometimes the stroke may affect a speech center, making it impossible for the child to talk, or the balance centers, making the child unable to walk normally. Whenever there is a sudden change in the ability of a child with SLE to function normally, the central nervous system should be carefully evaluated.

One of my patients was a teenage boy with SLE who loved to participate in sports. His disease was under control, and he was doing everything right. One day, the ward team called to tell me that he was in the hospital. No one had called me initially because he had hit his head on the goalpost playing football and had a simple concussion. When I went to see him, he could not move his head without the whole world spinning and was not talking. The neurologists said that he must have hit his head hard to cause the concussion. We waited for him to get better, but things did not improve. When an MRI was done, it showed inflammation and damage in the cerebellum. Once we treated the problem, he was able to tell us that while on the football field, he was suddenly unable to walk, and he fell down. He never hit his head on the goalpost; people just assumed that was what had happened when they found him on the field. The whole problem was a stroke caused by his SLE. The wrong story caused a two-day delay in proper treatment.

Central nervous system damage due to inflammation of the blood vessels by SLE is often much more subtle. Margaret, whose story opens this chapter, became withdrawn and did poorly in school because she was suffering from central nervous system involvement. Careful studies have shown that many children with SLE do not do as well as they should in school. In addition, they frequently use bad judgment. People often assume that they are just bad kids. Many years ago I cared for Susan, a teenage girl who was sent to me because of SLE. The physician who sent her told me that she was trouble. She had been arrested for joyriding and hung out with the wrong crowd. She had a reputation for being nasty to her doctors, talking back, and often refusing to take her medications.

In addition to her other problems, Susan had developed ballism. Patients with ballism have trouble controlling their movements. This is the result of irritation of the basal ganglia that control motor coordination. When the ballism was active, Susan could not control the movements of her left arm. It would wave around wildly. When she took enough corticosteroids this condition was well controlled, but during uncooperative periods, Susan would not take her medicine. When the left arm began to wave around and she could not control it, Susan would become very annoyed. She would come to the hospital for medication. I would give her a high dose of corticosteroids, and the arm would come under control. We went through several of these episodes before I realized that at the end of each treatment for her ballism, Susan was polite and respectful. Her misbehavior and refusal to take medications were also the result of her central nervous system involvement, just like the ballism. When I put Susan on intravenous cyclophosphamide and brought her SLE under good long-term control, she turned out to be a nice person all the time.

Cardiac Involvement

Recognizing Potential Problems

Mild cardiac involvement is common in children with SLE but does not usually become significant. Careful studies often find mild changes, but they are rarely symptomatic.

Pericarditis may cause chest pain, which may worsen with deep breaths or changing positions (such as leaning forward). This can be detected easily if an echocardiogram is performed. Children with chest pain must also be evaluated for pulmonary emboli. Small amounts of pericardial thickening are often found in children with SLE who do not report chest pain, but if a child reports chest pain and there is thickening of the pericardium, an NSAID may help. Another common problem is an increase in the amount of pericardial fluid.

When the inflammation of the pericardium causes thickening, pain is the most common symptom, but it rarely interferes with cardiac function. **Pericardial effusion** should be suspected if the heart looks enlarged on chest X-ray. Large pericardial effusions may ultimately interfere with cardiac output and produce shortness of breath, swollen feet, and other signs of cardiac failure. This is easily diagnosed with an echocardiogram.

It is rare for cardiac muscle to become significantly inflamed in children with SLE. If myocarditis is present, there may be chest pain and there will be an increase in the level of CK. This enzyme is found in other muscles as well and may be increased in many conditions. The laboratory can fractionate the CK to tell whether it is coming from the cardiac muscle, other muscles, the central nervous system, or elsewhere. Myocarditis may cause abnormalities in the cardiac rhythm that will show up on an electrocardiogram (EKG). It may also produce signs and symptoms of cardiac failure. Like the other cardiac findings, it is best evaluated by a cardiologist using an EKG and an echocardiogram.

Buildup of abnormal material on the surface of the cardiac valves is another common cause of problems in children with SLE. These children often develop accumulations of fibrous material on the surface of the valves termed

Libman-Sacks endocarditis. This endocarditis is a worrisome problem for two reasons. First, the vegetations may become big enough to interfere with the proper opening and closing of the valves. Second, vegetations on the valves often result in bacterial endocariditis. If a piece of vegetation breaks off from the valve and lands in the central nervous system, it can cause a stroke. If the piece that breaks off is infected, it can cause **septic embolization**. To minimize the risk of developing infected cardiac valves, children and adults with any type of cardiac valve involvement must take antibiotics before they go to the dentist. This is called *subacute bacterial endocarditis (SBE)* prophylaxis. Many rheumatologists give antibiotics before dental visits to all the children they treat with serious SLE, even if they do not have definite cardiac valve involvement. This decision is up to the individual physician.

Another problem for children with SLE is the development of **arteriosclerosis**. Chronic use of corticosteroids promotes the development of this condition, so children who have received a lot of corticosteroids may develop arteriosclerosis in their teens or twenties. High cholesterol levels (like those seen in children with nephrotic syndrome) also lead to arteriosclerosis. High blood pressure may be a consequence of corticosteroids and/or renal disease. Inflammation in the blood vessels promotes high blood pressure and arteriosclerosis, too. Some children with SLE have all of these factors. As a result, some children with SLE that has been treated with moderate doses of corticosteroids for many years will have myocardial infarctions in their twenties or thirties. This is one of the best reasons for using strong immunosuppressive drugs early in SLE.

Treatment of Cardiac Complications

Treatment of cardiac involvement varies with the type and severity of the condition. Mild pericarditis may be treated with NSAIDs. More severe pericarditis is often treated with corticosteroids. In rare cases, the problem recurs frequently or is very severe. When that happens, it may be necessary to perform a pericardiectomy to relieve the pressure. The treatment of Libman-Sacks endocarditis is more complicated. If the vegetations on the valves are small, the cardiologist may choose to leave them alone. If they are breaking off and causing problems, anticoagulation may be necessary. If the vegetations are infected, a long-term course of antibiotics is required. If too much damage has occurred, it may be necessary to replace the valve. With modern aggressive therapy this problem is becoming rare.

Pulmonary Involvement

Recognizing Potential Problems

Pulmonary involvement in children with SLE may take several different forms. Most children with SLE never experience pulmonary symptoms. However, weakening of the diaphragm is a common problem. This makes it more difficult for children with SLE to take a deep breath and to cough deeply. This poor air movement combined with medications that interfere with the immune response makes children with SLE more vulnerable to **pneumonia**.

Some children with SLE are found to have areas of fibrosis. Small areas of fibrosis are not important and usually disappear with treatment of the SLE. Occasionally, children develop more severe pulmonary fibrosis. If this progresses over time, it can be quite serious. In rare cases, children with areas of pulmonary involvement may form pockets of nonfunctional air cells, or *blebs*. If an area of fibrosis or a bleb breaks, it can lead to a **pneumothorax**. When this happens, the child will experience severe chest pain and difficulty breathing.

Pulmonary emboli may occur. Symptoms in children are sudden onset of chest pain and shortness of breath. Although children with clotting problems and anticardiolipin antibodies are at greater risk of developing pulmonary emboli (see the section on hematologic abnormalities in this chapter), children without these findings may also have pulmonary emboli. Any child with a sudden onset of pain and shortness of breath or severe chest pain must be promptly evaluated. Emboli may be diagnosed on the basis of X-rays, CAT scans, MRIs, or ventilation perfusion (VQ) scans. Newer tests such as D-dimer assays may be helpful.

Some children with SLE develop **serositis**. When this occurs in the chest, it causes pain and difficulty in breathing. The symptoms are very similar to those of pericarditis, and the two conditions can be reliably distinguished only by carefully evaluating the pericardium on an echocardiogram. The symptoms may also mimic those of a pulmonary embolus.

Pulmonary hemorrhage is a very serious complication of SLE. The body can handle a very small amount of pulmonary bleeding, but significant bleeding may fill the lungs with blood, preventing air exchange. A child who is coughing up blood should be investigated immediately. A little blood can come from irritation of the airway or from blood swallowed because of a cut in the nose or mouth. True pulmonary hemorrhage may be a fatal complication.

Treatment of Pulmonary Complications

In children with SLE, pneumonia needs to be treated aggressively. Children with pulmonary emboli should be anticoagulated.

Hematologic Involvement

Recognizing Potential Problems

Hematologic involvement refers to involvement of the bone marrow or a problem in the mechanism of blood clotting. The most common hematologic involvement is anemia. Mild anemia is common in children who are chronically ill for any reason. Children with SLE may also have anemia because of excessive bleeding: from an ulcer, the kidneys, heavy menses, or one of many other sources.

Red blood cell involvement is most often anemia of chronic disease. Some children with SLE develop **hemolytic anemia**. Anemia of chronic disease results in a low hemoglobin level and a low reticulocyte count. Bleeding results in a high reticulocyte count if the body has enough iron stores. Hemolytic anemia is suggested by a finding of low hemoglobin with a very high reticulocyte count without bleeding. It can be confirmed by Coombs' test. Epogen and similar drugs may be used to stimulate RBC formation.

White blood cell involvement is most often **leukopenia**. In children with SLE, there may be anti-WBC antibodies. Another possibility is that not enough WBCs are being made in the bone marrow. This may be due to drugs, infections, or SLE. Children with SLE often have low or normal WBC counts. High WBC counts can occur but may be evidence of infection.

Severe leukopenia is worrisome. If there are fewer than 1000 WBCs/mm3 the hematologist may recommend drugs to stimulate WBC growth. Any child with a low WBC count and a fever should be promptly checked for evidence of infection. Children who develop large scabs on their lips without having been injured may be getting an infection from the normal bacteria in the mouth. This is often a sign of a dangerously low WBC count.

Platelets are the third major type of cell made in the bone marrow that circulates in the blood. If the number drops too low, the child will start to bruise easily. With very low numbers, the child may start to bruise without doing anything. All of the hematologic abnormalities that occur in children with SLE need to be carefully investigated.

Treatment of Hematologic Complications

Increasing the dose of corticosteroids treats most hematologic abnormalities satisfactorily. Surprisingly, cyclophosphamide has proven useful for these conditions even though the blood cell counts may decrease after it is given. A variety of newer therapies are being used for these problems when they don't respond appropriately to corticosteroids. Rituximab has proven very effective for many children with low platelet counts.

Involvement of the Clotting System: Antiphospholipid Syndrome

Recognizing Potential Problems

Some children with SLE bleed too much, and girls with SLE are sometimes recognized because of excessive bleeding with their periods (**menorrhagia**). Bleeding due to the lupus anticoagulant is not like the bleeding in a child with hemophilia. If a child has hemophilia, you can mix his or her blood with a normal person's blood in a test tube and it will clot normally. This is because the child with hemophilia is missing a factor that the normal blood supplies. However, when you add normal blood to the blood of a child who is bleeding too much because of a lupus anticoagulant, it still won't clot. Most often, children with SLE are not missing a factor. Instead, there is something in their blood that prevents clotting.

There is no single lupus anticoagulant. Instead, children with SLE may make a variety of antibodies that react with a class of molecules called *phospholipids* or *cardiolipins*, hence the terms *antiphospholipid (APL) antibodies* and *anticardiolipin (ACL) antibodies*. These terms mean almost, but not exactly, the same thing. The antibodies that interfere with clotting in children with SLE may be very different from each other. In addition, over time they may change slightly. This is important because people with these antibodies sometimes bleed too much, but sometimes they clot too easily. Children with ACL or APL antibodies need to be monitored for problems both from clotting and from not clotting. They may even have both problems at the same time. The key is to stop the body from making the antibodies. Corticosteroids can do this, and so can other immunosuppressive drugs. Early studies suggest that rituximab may be helpful.

Treatment of Clotting System Complications

There is a lot of controversy over what to do with children who have ACL or APL antibodies. A child who has had a clot must be treated with anticoagulants.

However, many children test positive for ACL or APL antibodies but have never had a problem. It might seem obvious to treat them with anticoagulants, but then if they get cut or fall, they may bleed too much. It does not seem worth the risk for a child who has never had a problem. Some physicians feel it is best to just watch; others believe in treating with a baby aspirin every day to try to decrease the risk. This seems safe, but so far it has not been proven to be effective. There is no certain answer. I treat my children with SLE who have ACL or APL antibodies with a baby aspirin every day if they have never had an abnormal blood clot. Children who have had blood clots must be treated with anticoagulants (e.g., heparin and warfarin).

Gastrointestinal System Involvement

Recognizing Potential Problems

Irritation of the gastrointestinal system occurs frequently in children with SLE. It may play a large role in the initial malaise that many children with SLE experience. The resulting pain and loss of appetite often lead to depression and weight loss. These are common problems in the period before diagnosis (note that this can happen in many other conditions as well). The most common gastrointestinal complaint of children with SLE is **nonspecific stomachache**. It may or may not be associated with eating. Often the first thought of the family and physician is that it is the result of irritation from the medications the child is taking. If it persists, everyone becomes worried about ulcers. Although many of the medications used to treat SLE can cause ulcers, children with SLE do not often get ulcers. Ulcers usually occur in the setting of very severe active disease. (When a child is very sick in the intensive care unit, the stomach's protective barrier seems to fail and *stress ulcers* are common.) The typical stomach irritation associated with medications is **gastritis**.

Chronic abdominal pain that is not resolved by changing medications needs to be carefully investigated. Some children have sensitive stomachs, but more serious problems can also begin with these complaints. One of the key aspects of SLE is inflammation of the blood vessels. If the blood vessels lining the intestines are inflamed, it may cause vague nonspecific pain. In some children this results in damage to the intestinal tract. This may take the form of **pneumatosis cystoides intestinalis** or small areas of infracted bowel. Both of these conditions may start with only vague abdominal complaints. Fortunately, they are rare in children whose SLE is well controlled. However, they must be looked for in children whose complaints continue.

Serositis is another cause of chronic pain in children with SLE. The function of the serous membrane is to keep everything moist and to remove any foreign material. Mild serositis causes diffuse pain. In severe serositis, the pain may be quite marked and associated with *rebound tenderness.* There are many possible causes, including infections.

Irritation of the pancreas is another cause of chronic abdominal pain in children with SLE. The levels of amylase and lipase can be measured in the blood and will be elevated if the child has pancreatitis. Sometimes the pancreas is irritated by inflammation due to SLE. At other times it is irritated by medications (e.g., corticosteroids, azathioprine, mycophenolate mofetil) used to treat SLE. This situation can be complicated, as inflammation due to SLE requires more corticosteroids, but these may be the cause of the problem.

Gallbladder disease is particularly common in children with hemolytic anemia. This is easily detected on abdominal ultrasound. Usually, it can be followed conservatively, but if the gallbladder is very involved or has many stones, it may need to be removed. Children with liver involvement often have an enlarged liver that can be felt on careful examination and may be tender. Elevation of the liver enzyme levels on the blood tests will confirm this (see Chapter 25).

The spleen may also be enlarged in children with SLE. An enlarged spleen may cause pain on the left side of the abdomen. Children with continuing abdominal pain without an adequate explanation should be carefully examined. Thorough evaluation may require blood tests, X-rays, abdominal ultrasound, and either an MRI or a CAT scan of the abdomen. Consultation with a gastroenterologist and endoscopy may be necessary.

Treatment of Gastrointestinal System Complications

Whenever a child with SLE complains of abdominal pain, there is a desire to stop the medicines (note that this is not possible for steroids, which cannot be stopped abruptly; see Chapter 23) and see whether the pain goes away. However, if the pain seems to be that of typical gastritis and the medicines are important, it is often better to treat the irritation using an H-2 acid blocker or sucralfate. If these steps do not work, consider stopping the medicine, if possible, and see whether the pain goes away. If it does, restart the medicine. If the pain promptly returns, that's a strong indication that the medicine is the cause.

If, after careful investigation, SLE is determined to be the cause of serositis, treat with more corticosteroids or immunosuppressive drugs to better control the SLE.

CHILDREN WITH SYSTEMIC LUPUS ERYTHEMATOSUS AND JOINT PROBLEMS

Although the family may not be aware of it, arthritis is often present when a child with SLE first presents. It is usually very responsive to treatment with steroids or NSAIDs. As a result, arthritis is rarely a significant long-term problem. The exception is an unusual condition termed **Jaccoud's arthropathy**, a painless swelling, primarily in the fingers and wrists, that develops slowly during the course of SLE. It does not usually cause damage to the bones, but it may be painful and interfere with use of the hands. The cause of this problem is unclear. Unfortunately, it does not respond well to medication.

Other bone and joint problems may develop during the treatment of children with SLE. The most common, worrisome problem is **avascular necrosis**. Although the mechanism by which this occurs is not fully understood, it appears to be the result of decreased blood flow to the ends of the bones. This can occur in children who do not have SLE. It can happen to children with SLE who are not being treated with steroids, and it can happen to people being treated with steroids who do not have SLE. However, it is most common in children with SLE who are being treated with steroids. The problem often begins with vague complaints of pain in the involved bone without any findings on examination.

Early in the development of avascular necrosis, the X-rays will be normal. Sometimes avascular necrosis is suspected because on bone scans there is decreased uptake of the radionuclide by the involved bone (see Chapter 25). The MRI is the most sensitive test for this condition. It will detect it very early. Sometimes children with suggested avascular necrosis on MRI recover; we do not know whether this means that the MRI reading was false or that early avascular necrosis can be reversed. However, if a child has definite avascular necrosis on MRI, it does not disappear.

Unfortunately, the normal course of avascular necrosis is for the bone to crumble slowly under the continued stress of bearing weight. If this happens, the joint must be replaced (see Chapter 26). In children with SLE, the hip is the joint most commonly affected, but the shoulders, elbows, knees, ankles, and other joints also may be involved. The identical problem may occur in children with JA or JRA who have been treated with corticosteroids. There is no safe dose of corticosteroids with regard to this problem. Avascular necrosis has occurred in children who never took corticosteroids. However, the more corticosteroids the child takes and the longer he or she takes them, the greater the risk. Children taking a significant amount of corticosteroids for more six months have a steadily increasing risk of developing avascular necrosis. In addition, a child who has had avascular necrosis in one joint is at greater risk of developing it in another joint. Reducing the risk of avascular necrosis is one of the reasons it is important to minimize the dose of corticosteroids for children with SLE.

LABORATORY TESTING AND TYPICAL PATTERNS OF DISEASE IN CHILDREN WITH SYSTEMIC LUPUS ERYTHEMATOSUS

Imagine that you are driving down the highway late at night. There is very little traffic, and perhaps you are exceeding the speed limit. At the side of the road you see a large sign that says "Warning: construction ahead." There might be a big construction project, where workers might be working late at night, and you might have to come to a sudden stop. On the other hand, workers might be there only during the day, and there might be no problem or only a need to change lanes. There's no way to be sure. However, a wise person would let up on the gas pedal, look around carefully, and be sure to keep attention focused on the road until he or she was sure about what was happening. That's how both parents and doctors should respond to changes in predictive laboratory test values. There might not be trouble, but everyone should be paying careful attention.

Physicians who take care of many children with SLE are struck by the great variability of this illness. Approximately one-third of children have mild disease that never causes major problems; many children have moderate disease that may be severe at times but responds well to treatment. Many fewer children have obvious severe SLE from the start. Different patterns of abnormalities may help to distinguish children with severe disease from the others.

Virtually all children with SLE are ANA-positive. However, many children test positive for ANA but do not have SLE (see Chapter 25). Antibodies to DNA tend to be associated with more severe SLE and are infrequently found in children who do not have SLE. Antibodies to dsDNA are the important ones. Antibodies to single-stranded or crude DNA extracts can be found in many different conditions and are not very meaningful. However, a child may have very severe SLE and yet have no antibodies to DNA.

Further evaluation of patients with SLE led to the discovery of extractable nuclear antigens (ENA). These are Ro, La, Sm, and RNP (see Chapter 25). They do seem to be associated with different patterns of disease, but again, there is not enough certainty to make definitive predictions. The clearest associations are with Ro and Sm. Often Ro antibodies are found in children with more rashes, more frequent than average complaints of arthritis, and relatively less renal disease. A high titer of Ro and RNP, and low or absent Sm, has been described as typical of mixed connective tissue disease (MCTD; see Chapter 12). Over the years, a variety of studies have suggested that adults with SLE who are Ro-positive have milder disease, but this generalization does not always hold true. Ro antibodies are also associated with neonatal SLE and congenital cardiac block, discussed at the end of this chapter.

The other antibody that seems to be important is Sm. This antibody is not found in everyone with SLE. If it is present, it is associated with a greater frequency of severe disease. However, just as the association of Ro with mild disease is only approximate, so is the association of Sm with severe disease. Indeed, some children have antibodies to both Ro and Sm. Children with worrisome antibodies may do well, and children with protective antibodies may not.

The key laboratory findings in evaluating a child with SLE are generally similar to those in evaluating children with other chronic illnesses. If a child is doing well, he or she should have a good hemoglobin level, a normal ESR, and a normal urine analysis. If all of these results are good, it is highly probable that the child is doing well (though neurologic problems may still occur). The additional laboratory tests that are useful in evaluating a child with SLE are the levels of serum complement C3 and C4.

Antinuclear antibody levels and anti-DNA levels rise and fall in children with SLE without a reliable association with disease activity. Sometimes it is helpful to think of the 10 percent analogy. If the ANA goes up, that's a 10 percent risk. If the ESR goes up, that's a 10 percent risk. If the hemoglobin falls, that's a 10 percent risk. If the anti-DNA goes up, that's a 10 percent risk, and so on. A change in any one test does not mean much, but if they all start going the wrong way, be sure to pay attention.

The complement system plays an important role. We know that much of the damage in SLE is caused by the activation of complement following the deposition of immune complexes in the tissues. As a general rule, lower complement levels indicate ongoing damage. This is an imperfect correlation because doctors recognize that the complement levels in the blood are determined as much by how rapidly more complement is being made as by how rapidly it is being used up. There are very sophisticated tests to measure what are called *complement breakdown products*, but these tests are not routinely done.

All the laboratory findings in children with SLE are individual pieces of the puzzle. C3 and C4 are easily measured, and the results are well standardized. Some children have chronically low C3 levels but do very well. Others have normal C3 levels but develop more problems. While physicians would be unwise to disregard C3 levels, they are not the whole answer.

Another way to think about the evaluation of laboratory parameters in children with SLE is to understand that there are two types of tests. The routine tests that evaluate hemoglobin, renal function, liver function, and so on indicate what is happening to those organs right now. Tests such as the ANA titer, the anti-DNA level, and the C3 and C4 levels are more useful as predictors of the future. Nothing is a perfect predictor.

DRUG-INDUCED SYSTEMIC LUPUS ERYTHEMATOSUS

Drug-induced SLE refers to the development of a positive ANA and SLE-like symptoms in association with certain drugs. Among the drugs that can cause this are commonly used drugs such as tetracyclines, including doxycycline, used in the treatment of teenagers with acne. However, this can also occur with many of the drugs used to treat children with seizures and some of the antibiotics, including isoniazid, which is used to treat tuberculosis. In the past, a wide variety of drugs were suspected of causing drug-induced SLE. For some drugs the association with drug-induced SLE is well known, but for many others it is only suspected. The fact that a drug has been associated with drug-induced SLE does not mean that it should be avoided. This is a rare complication. However, when evaluating a child with the new onset of SLE-like symptoms, these drugs should always be considered as a possible cause.

Children with drug-induced SLE can be significantly ill with fever, rash, and inflammation. However, a key to the diagnosis of drug-induced SLE is that it disappears quickly if the drug is discontinued. If symptoms of SLE begin after a child has started taking a drug but do not disappear when the drug is stopped, the condition is not drug-induced SLE even if the drug is known to cause drug-induced SLE. While it bothers me a little, this is the official position of the American College of Rheumatology.

I am often asked whether a child who has SLE can use a drug that is known to cause drug-induced SLE. There was a lot of concern about this at one time. Some of the most important drugs for treating hypertension in the past were also known to cause drug-induced SLE. Nevertheless, physicians often found it necessary to use them. There is no evidence that they caused additional problems. Using drugs known to be associated with drug-induced SLE in a child with SLE does not seem to cause trouble, but everyone should pay attention to the possibility of side effects arising over time.

OTHER COMPLICATIONS OF SYSTEMIC LUPUS ERYTHEMATOSUS

Complications of SLE in childhood may be complications of the disease, of the therapy, or both. It is very important to understand that half of the children diagnosed with SLE in the 1950s (before the routine use of corticosteroids) died within two years. Although this happened in part because only severe cases were properly diagnosed, it remains true that untreated SLE may be a rapidly fatal disease. Everyone must be concerned about the possible side effects of treatment. However, it is obviously foolish to die from the disease because you are afraid of developing a side effect of the medications.

Severe complications of SLE, such as pulmonary hemorrhage, renal failure, and strokes, have all become less frequent with proper therapy. Infections remain a major concern for children with SLE, and these children are subject to all the usual infections of childhood. In addition, children with active SLE often have poorly functioning WBCs and reduced levels of complement. Since these are key elements in the defense against infection, children with active SLE are more vulnerable to infection than normal children.

Another problem that leads to an increased frequency of infections is that children with active SLE often have a poorly functioning spleen. Removing bacteria and other infectious agents from the blood is a major function of the spleen. Children who do not have a spleen (because of surgical removal due to injury, etc.) are well known to have more frequent **pneumococcal infections**. Systemic pneumococcal infections and pneumococcal pneumonia also occur more often in children with SLE. **Meningococcal meningitis** is another infection that occurs more often than expected in children with SLE.

Normally, the spleen, WBCs, and complement play an important role in preventing infections. One key to recognizing that the spleen is not functioning well in a child with SLE is the presence of Howell-Jolly bodies on the CBC. These bodies are leftover nuclear material in RBCs. A normally functioning spleen removes this material, and normal children do not have Howell-Jolly bodies. If they are reported as being seen on the CBC smear, it means that the spleen is not doing its job. Any patient with Howell-Jolly bodies is at increased risk for infection. (Note: the person whose spleen has been removed will always have Howell-Jolly bodies and will always be at increased risk of infection.) Finding Howell-Jolly bodies is very important in children whose spleen has not been removed. It is a warning that these children are at greater risk of infection. If a child with SLE is brought to my office or the emergency room with a significant fever and has Howell-Jolly bodies, I will often admit that child to the hospital for observation even if he or she doesn't look very sick.

When considering the possibility of infection, parents and physicians must remember that both active disease and the medications used to treat SLE decrease the child's ability to fight infection. Children with SLE can rapidly develop overwhelming infections requiring urgent care. In some cases, a child with SLE will be brought to the hospital looking extremely ill. It may not be clear whether the problem is an infection or a flare-up of the SLE. Physicians who do not have a lot of experience with SLE will be very confused: For an infection they will want to use an antibiotic, but for a flare-up of the SLE they will want to use more corticosteroids. The best answer is to give both antibiotics and corticosteroids in this situation. Often the infection makes the SLE flare up, and this interferes with the ability of the WBCs to fight the infection. At other times, the child develops an infection because the SLE is flaring and, again, the WBCs are unable to fight the infection. In either situation, using both corticosteroids and antibiotics is appropriate.

COMPLICATIONS OF TREATMENT

Corticosteroids have been a key element in the treatment of SLE since their discovery in the 1950s. They are effective in treating and preventing many of the complications of untreated SLE. However, they increase the incidence of infection, weaken bones, cause stretch marks, promote diabetes, and hasten arteriosclerosis and cardiac disease (see Chapter 23 for more detail). For the approximately one-third of children with mild disease, it should be possible to keep the dosage of corticosteroids at an acceptable level, and the likelihood of significant toxicity should be minimal.

Unfortunately, the remaining two-thirds of children with SLE may face a recurrent need to raise the corticosteroid dosage. This brings with it an increased risk of corticosteroid-related toxicity. Surprisingly, this is a greater problem for children with moderate disease than for those with severe disease. In experienced centers, children with severe disease are rapidly recognized and given more aggressive immunosuppressive therapy. This normally allows a dramatic reduction in the dosage of corticosteroids. As a result, corticosteroid-related complications are often less frequent in this group. After recognizing this, many physicians have begun to advocate advancing children with more difficult moderate SLE to immunosuppressive therapy early in their disease course in order to minimize corticosteroid-related toxicity, as discussed in the following section.

TREATMENT OF SYSTEMIC LUPUS
ERYTHEMATOSUS

The key to proper treatment of SLE involves balancing the risks of the disease against the risks of the treatment. Systemic lupus erythematosus is extremely diverse, and many children have only mild disease that is easily treated with low doses of corticosteroids. Other children have severe, life-threatening SLE that requires aggressive therapy. There are no absolute guidelines for recognizing when a child needs to be treated with immunosuppressive drugs. However, it is clear that prolonged treatment with even moderate doses of corticosteroids will lead to significant side effects. Immunosuppressive drugs often seem frightening to parents and physicians who do not work with them all the time. Although immunosuppressive drugs may be associated with serious side effects, those side effects are very rare when given by experienced physicians.

Many parents worry that their child will develop all the side effects of immunosuppressive drugs. Virtually every child who takes a significant amount of corticosteroids does develop corticosteroid-related side effects. In contrast, serious side effects of immunosuppressive drugs are rare. I've seen far more children do poorly and suffer permanent damage (even die) because their families were afraid to treat their SLE aggressively than I have seen children with serious side effects of immunosuppressive drugs. This does not mean that every child should be on immunosuppressive drugs.

For children with rash, malaise, and arthritis, but no evidence of significant renal or other internal organ involvement, initial therapy should involve a low dose of corticosteroids. Often this is combined with an NSAID to provide additional symptomatic relief. Over the longer term, the antimalarial drug hydroxychloroquine (see Chapter 23) has been shown to be very beneficial for this group. At the time of diagnosis, some physicians follow a cookbook approach of prescribing 1 or 2 mg/kg/day of corticosteroids (prednisone or its equivalent), but this is often excessive for these children. The physician should monitor to determine that the child feels better and the laboratory abnormalities improve over a period of four to six weeks. As soon as it is clear that this has happened, the physician should try to begin slowly reducing the dose of the corticosteroid.

Some physicians like to use a very high dose of a corticosteroid at the beginning and then dramatically reduce the dose when the child's condition improves. This is like putting the immune system on a roller coaster ride. In a sick child, a high dose of a corticosteroid may be necessary, but then a slow, gradual progressive reduction in the dose is much better. Even when physicians go very slowly, it is impossible to predict how much the corticosteroid dosage can be decreased before there is new evidence of disease activity (e.g., increased ESR, decreased hemoglobin,, or decreased C3 or C4; see Chapter 25). If it is possible to reduce the corticosteroid (prednisone or its equivalent) to 0.2 mg/kg/day or less without causing recurrent disease, the child should be carefully followed on a low dose.

Many parents are anxious to have their children discontinue steroids, but completely stopping them is rarely advisable for children with SLE. Many years ago, a very experienced rheumatologist described that last bit of corticosteroid therapy as "cheap insurance." Every physician who takes care of many patients with SLE has seen someone who was doing wonderfully on just 5 mg prednisone daily and who suddenly got very sick when he or she tried to discontinue it. It is not impossible to discontinue corticosteroids, but if the patient is doing well on a small dose, it is probably unwise to try to stop completely. Even when there has been no evidence of disease for more than six months, stopping completely is not the best idea.

Children who do not have internal organ involvement but develop more symptoms when the dose of corticosteroids is reduced are a difficult problem. Hydroxychloroquine often helps to bring the disease under adequate control. Some physicians have tried using low-dose methotrexate in this group, but the results are highly variable. Without evidence of internal organ involvement, physicians hesitate to recommend more aggressive therapy, but that may leave a child on too much corticosteroid use for too long. In my experience, children in this group who do not tolerate appropriate reduction of their corticosteroid dose usually develop internal organ involvement later on. It is important for physicians to monitor them carefully. Frequently, the first signs of internal organ involvement are changes in the urine analysis. Often these changes are minimal at first and might be dismissed. However, over time, it becomes clear that there is significant renal or other internal organ involvement.

Children who have internal organ involvement need to be treated aggressively. Although doctors tend to agree on the importance of treating renal involvement, there is less uniform agreement about when to treat other organ involvement aggressively. For children with internal organ involvement, it is often not possible to reduce the corticosteroid dose to an acceptable level (again, I consider this to be 0.2 mg/kg/day of prednisone or its equivalent). A variety of "steroid- sparing" regimens have been recommended. Mycophenolate mofetil is one of the most commonly recommended immunosuppressive medications at present (see Chapter 25). It is helpful for some children. Other physicians may recommend low-dose methotrexate or azathioprine. Each of these regimens has its advocates; none of them is always effective. I often use two courses of therapy with rituximab and cyclophosphamide in these children with good results (each course consists of two treatments separated by two weeks, and the courses are separated by six months).

Children with moderate internal organ involvement represent one of the greatest challenges for physicians who specialize in the care of children with SLE. They often do not appear sick enough to warrant significant immunosuppressive therapy, but over the years they receive too much corticosteroid treatment for too long. In the end, these children often have significant corticosteroid side effects, continued smoldering disease, and a generally unsatisfactory outcome.

It is hard for parents to accept a recommendation for aggressive treatment for children with continued moderate internal organ involvement because the disease is not that bad. Even many physicians do not believe that these children should be treated aggressively. However, when you watch what happens to these children over a five- to ten-year period, it is very discouraging. Ten years later, if they have not been treated aggressively, these children often have both significant corticosteroid side effects and significant damage from the disease, with no end in sight.

The reasons cited by many physicians to avoid cyclophosphamide include the risk of infection, the risk of sterility, and the risk of cancer later in life. However, chronic use of corticosteroids and azathioprine or methotrexate also carries significant risks of infection, sterility, and cancer later in life. Many physicians assume that these risks are greater for the children receiving cyclophosphamide, but after a very thorough review of the literature, I've determined that there are no clear data to support this conclusion. The physicians who are opposed to cyclophosphamide refer to data on children treated for cancer. Those children often received multiple drugs and radiation. The radiation greatly increases the risk of cancer and sterility. We do not give radiation to children with SLE.

The most compelling reason to use cyclophosphamide for children with moderately severe SLE comes from our experience in using it for the children with severe disease. Five or six years after receiving cyclophosphamide, most of the children with severe SLE are taking less than 0.2 mg/kg/day (prednisone or its equivalent) of corticosteroids and have no signs of steroid side effects. They have discontinued cyclophosphamide and all the other drugs except for the low dose of prednisone. They feel well and often tell me, "I don't remember that I have SLE except when I have to come to see you." In contrast, the children who did not receive cyclophosphamide because their disease was not that bad are still taking too much prednisone, have multiple prednisone side effects including weight gain and bone damage, and still have active disease. The children who had more severe disease at the beginning and were treated aggressively are doing far better both mentally and physically.

A physician who says that cyclophosphamide might have fatal side effects and that prednisone does not has never seen a child stop taking medications because he or she refused to go on "looking so ugly." Some children admit that they are not taking their prednisone; others just stop taking it and may suddenly die. It is very important for the physicians and parents who deal with these children on a day-to-day basis to be aware of the emotional toll of acne, obesity, and stretch marks related to chronic corticosteroid therapy. In addition, corticosteroids may have significant negative effects on bone structure and cardiac function. Recently, one of my patients, a young adult who had been treated at another institution with azathioprine and steroids for many years, seemed to be doing fine. For twelve years his steroid doses went up and down, but they were never really high (maximum, 40 mg/day of prednisone). He had mild renal disease but always did acceptably with azathioprine and was never treated aggressively. However, he had a massive myocardial infarction at the age of twenty-eight and needed coronary artery surgery. Prolonged use of corticosteroids was his only known risk factor for cardiac disease.

There is no perfect answer for children with SLE at present. Years of experience and seeing what happens to children over time have made me very aggressive in trying to prevent the side effects of long-term corticosteroid usage. Some physicians hesitate to use cyclophosphamide for fear of central nervous system involvement, pulmonary involvement, or mild renal involvement. However, in my experience, children who have disease in any internal organ system that is not well controlled by an acceptable dose of corticosteroids do best if aggressively treated. Not every physician agrees. The parents must always make the final decision. My goal is to make sure that physicians have enough information to clearly understand the risks and benefits of the alternatives. Cyclophosphamide does not help every child every time. It does have potential side effects, but these are rare when it is administered by experienced physicians. Corticosteroids and azathioprine appear to be safer in the short term, but I do not believe the results are as good in the long term.

For children with severe internal organ involvement, especially renal involvement, the majority of physicians now agree that cyclophosphamide is the best answer. In carefully controlled studies, it has been clearly demonstrated that cyclophosphamide prevents continued scarring of the kidney, while prednisone does not. No one has studied azathioprine in this regard. The academic answer is, "We know that cyclophosphamide works. Why should we subject patients to a different therapy that might not work?" The systematic use of monthly intravenous cyclophosphamide in seven doses, followed by cyclophosphamide every three months for an additional two to two and a half years, has been shown to produce the best long-term outcome for SLE patients (both adults and children) with renal disease. Many studies combining newer drugs such as rituximab, abatacept, and mycophenolate mofetil in varying combinations, with and without cyclophosphamide, are now underway. The goal is to find a combination that promptly puts the disease into remission and keeps it there with the least likelihood of either medication toxicity or recurrent SLE. No one has determined the best answer yet. Fortunately, there are relatively few children who fail standard therapy.

ADJUNCTIVE THERAPIES FOR CHILDREN WITH SYSTEMIC LUPUS ERYTHEMATOSUS

Nonsteroidal anti-inflammatory drugs are often helpful in controlling the minor aches and pains associated with SLE. Children with SLE usually tolerate these drugs without difficulty. Lupus may make these children more vulnerable to the effects of NSAIDs on liver or renal function, so, like children with other forms of arthritis who are on these medications, children with SLE should have liver function and renal function monitored. There are also reports of NSAIDs causing unusual reactions such as aseptic meningitis in SLE patients. If something unusual happens when a child with SLE starts taking an NSAID (or any other new drug), it should be stopped. While these reports are a cause for concern, most children with SLE take NSAIDs without significant problems.

Bolus methylprednisolone refers to the use of very large doses of this corticosteroid to control severe manifestations of SLE. In general, this is considered to be 30 mg/kg up to a maximum of 1 gm of methylprednisolone. These large doses can be very effective in controlling sudden severe flares of SLE. Some physicians are tempted to use this therapy over and over again. In certain situations, such as severe renal disease, it is often advisable to combine cyclophosphamide with bolus methylprednisolone each month until the disease comes under better control. However, bolus methylprednisolone also has side effects. I've seen children develop serious infections, serious irritation of the pancreas, and avascular necrosis of bone after these treatments. It is best to treat bolus methylprednisolone as a "fire extinguisher next to the stove." It's very handy to have in case of emergency, but if you find yourself using it over and over again, you'd better change the way you cook.

Mycophenolate mofetil and azathioprine are immunosuppressive drugs that work in a similar fashion. There is much more experience with azathioprine, but mycophenolate mofetil is believed to have similar effects and perhaps fewer side effects. These drugs do increase the risk of infection. In addition, there are good data demonstrating that azathioprine increases the risk of cancer and causes sterility in some children. Mycophenolate will probably be found to have the same effects once it has been around long enough. It blocks the same pathways that azathioprine does, just at a different point. Nonetheless, these drugs may be useful for children who cannot receive cyclophosphamide. I also use them in children who have received cyclophosphamide but who have some continuing or new disease activity that I do not want to treat with too much corticosteroid.

Methotrexate has been very useful in the treatment of arthritis. It is generally used in a low dose (less than 25 mg/week). Low doses of oral methotrexate have also been used as a steroid-sparing agent in children with SLE. In general, the response has not been dramatic. Physicians using methotrexate must be sure that the children are taking folic acid because children with SLE who have chronic anemia may be deficient in folic acid.

Cyclosporine is a strong immunosuppressive drug that often interferes with renal function (Chapter 23). It is known to cause renal problems, and this has kept most physicians from using it for the treatment of SLE. However, there are occasional reports of its successful use. It seems especially useful in children with membranous glomerulonephritis (class V renal disease) and excessive proteinuria. Cyclosporine should be given only by physicians experienced in its use. Like all immunosuppressive drugs, it is associated with an increased risk of infection and an increased risk of cancer.

New biologic agents and other experimental therapies are being tested for SLE. Some centers are also testing the use of autologous bone marrow transplants. However, at present, this is restricted to specialized centers and is used only for children in whom normal therapy has failed. Fortunately, such children are rare.

PROGNOSIS

With early and aggressive treatment, the vast majority of children with SLE do fine. There are some children who die from SLE. However, the survival rate is above 90 percent at five years in every experienced center. In many centers the survival rate is much higher. **Obviously, five-year survival for a fourteen-, fifteen-, or sixteen-year-old child certainly is not good enough.** The main reason for advocating early aggressive therapy is that we want to achieve excellent forty-, fifty-, and sixty-year survival. Proof? Not yet. Someone will have to follow these children for fifty years to prove that we've done the right thing. But we cannot continue doing what we know does not work while we wait forty or fifty years for proof of the right long-term answers. I will be very disappointed if in fifty years we haven't developed completely different methods for treating children with SLE over the long term. With current state-of-the-art therapy, the majority of children will do very well.Children with severe disease should be referred to the most advanced centers, where they have the greatest likelihood of achieving a good outcome.

ANTI-Ro ANTIBODIES AND NEONATAL SYSTEMIC LUPUS ERYTHEMATOSUS

It was surprising to find that babies born with a problem called *neonatal cardiac block* or *complete congenital cardiac block* often had mothers with SLE. This does not happen to most mothers with SLE, but it may happen if the mother tests positive for antibody to Ro. Most children with congenital cardiac block had healthy mothers who reported no medical problems. But when doctors began testing them, it was found that almost all of the normal, healthy mothers who gave birth to children with congenital cardiac block tested positive for antibodies to Ro. A few of these mothers had unrecognized SLE when examined carefully, and some of these mothers developed SLE or Sjögren's syndrome years later. There is a registry collecting information on all these mothers and their children (see the Appendix for resources).

At first, doctors were very worried that women who had SLE and were Ro-positive would be at high risk of having children with congenital cardiac block. This seems not to be the case. Most Ro-positive mothers have normal children. Even Ro-positive mothers who have had one child with cardiac block most often have a normal child the next time. If a woman who is known to be Ro-positive becomes pregnant, she should be monitored carefully.

Evidence of congenital cardiac block can be detected before birth, and experienced doctors should be standing by to take care of these babies when they are born. Most often, congenital cardiac block is not life-threatening and can be treated with a pacemaker when the child is old enough to need it. In rare cases, children with cardiac block are extremely sick and may not survive. The problem is sufficiently uncommon that we encourage women with SLE and antibodies to Ro to have children when they are ready—but with careful monitoring during pregnancy.

Other complications that may occur in children of mothers with SLE include low levels of platelets, WBC, or RBCs. These are thought to be the result of antibodies that have been passed from the mother to the child. These antibodies are usually cleared out of the child's system in a few days, and the problems are rarely severe. Other children of mothers with SLE may develop a rash when they are first exposed to the light or develop mild inflammation of the liver. These are all well-recognized problems that normally resolve after a few days to a few weeks. Serious complications in the children of mothers with SLE are infrequent.

SHOULD A WOMAN WITH SYSTEMIC LUPUS ERYTHEMATOSUS HAVE CHILDREN?

We know that SLE occurs with varying frequency in people of different races. It also occurs more frequently among relatives of people with SLE. This is evidence that genetics plays a role in the development of SLE (see Chapter 22). However, the risk of a mother passing on SLE to her child is very small. Precise numbers are uncertain, but one in fifty is the best estimate. Thus, the child of a mother with SLE is more likely to develop the disease than a random child is, but not frequently enough to discourage mothers with SLE from having children. If you are the physician of a woman with SLE who is considering whether or not to have children, the major concern is *her* health, not the risk of the child having SLE. A pregnant woman with SLE should discuss the subject with her doctor and be evaluated for any risk factors, such as antibodies to Ro or anticardiolipin antibodies, so that appropriate steps can be taken to minimize problems.

12

Mixed Connective Tissue Disease

At one time, mixed connective tissue disease (MCTD) was thought to be a milder version of SLE. To understand this disease, it is necessary to understand that it was defined "backward." A physician named Gordon Sharp noted an unusual laboratory finding in some patients who were ANA-positive. When he examined these patients, he discovered that they were most often atypical SLE patients. These patients differed from typical SLE patients in having more arthritis, more rash, more lung disease, and less kidney disease. Since many of these patients were also positive for RF (see Chapter 25) and had more arthritis than typical SLE patients, they were thought of as having "mixed" disease. Thus, the name of the disease was chosen to reflect this condition. It took only a short time, once the disease was described in adults, to realize that there were children with the same pattern of findings. Children with MCTD are ANA-positive, like children with SLE, but typically have high titers of antibodies to ribonucleoprotein (RNP) as well.

The precise relationship of MCTD to SLE and the other rheumatic diseases remains unclear. There are only three diseases that commonly cause nail fold capillary abnormalities (see Fig. 14–1): dermatomyositis, scleroderma, and MCTD. Indeed, it is now well known that some children with MCTD will go on to develop scleroderma, but most do not. Obviously, these diseases are somehow interrelated, but there is no clear explanation yet. At some future time we may understand how MCTD, SLE, dermatomyositis, and scleroderma are related to each other. Although MCTD was originally described as a subtype of SLE, it is probably more closely related to scleroderma and dermatomyositis. Children with MCTD often have mild muscle inflammation and may develop poor lung function.

Children with MCTD typically are brought to doctors because of cold, blue hands (Raynaud's phenomenon), joint pains, and a positive ANA. They often have elevated muscle enzyme levels and rashes over the outer surfaces of their knees and elbows, just like those seen in dermatomyositis, but they rarely are significantly weak. Often they have mild to moderate arthritis, but they may not have complained about it. Children with MCTD usually do not have serious kidney involvement, but they may have some and it may become serious.

DIFFERENTIAL DIAGNOSIS AND LABORATORY FINDINGS

For most diseases, these are two separate discussions. However, the clinical manifestations of MCTD overlap with those of dermatomyositis, SLE, JRA, and early scleroderma. In addition, over time, children initially thought to have MCTD may develop a clear case of one of these other diseases. As a result, physicians must rely more heavily on the laboratory findings to confirm this diagnosis. Much of the confusion in diagnosing MCTD results from the unclear nature of the disease itself. Indeed, it is quite possible that we will ultimately realize that at least two different diseases have been grouped together as MCTD.

A high-titer, speckled-pattern ANA is characteristic of MCTD. When the ANA subtypes are checked (see Chapter 25), children with MCTD are usually found to be Ro-positive, RNP-positive, and Sm-negative (some have low-titer Sm). Because these children are often RF-positive, they may be referred for JRA. Another finding is that these children may have very marked elevation of their quantitative immunoglobulins, especially IgG (again, see Chapter 25).

At one time, most children with MCTD were considered atypical cases of SLE. Children with MCTD can be mistakenly diagnosed with SLE because of the strongly positive ANA. Findings that help in making the distinction between SLE and MCTD include the speckled pattern of the ANA, a positive test for RF, and usually normal serum complement levels. Antibodies to dsDNA are sometimes found in children with MCTD.

As noted earlier, children with MCTD often have many findings that are also seen in dermatomyositis and scleroderma. In more severe cases, children with MCTD often have Gottren's papules and nail fold capillary abnormalities. They may initially have been labeled with one of these diagnoses. Although children with MCTD have the elevated muscle enzyme levels and a rash, they do not tend to develop dermatomyositis. However, MCTD may evolve into scleroderma over a period of years. The presence of antibodies to Scl-70, or anticentromere antibodies, strongly suggests the diagnosis of scleroderma. These antibodies may not be present initially, but they may appear years later.

COMPLICATIONS

The complications of MCTD are highly dependent on the evolution of the disease. The arthritis, rash, malaise, and Raynaud's phenomenon are usually easily treated with NSAIDs, low-dose prednisone, a calcium-channel blocker for Raynaud's phenomen, and hydroxychloroquine. Inadequately treated children may have recurrent problems with Raynaud's phenomenon, and may have distal fingertip ulcers and even infarction of parts of digits in the cold. Physicians must emphasize to families the importance of treating Raynaud's phenomenon and seeking care if a digit does not warm up appropriately with return to a warm environment. The elevated muscle enzyme levels and the markedly elevated IgG level will usually respond to a moderate or low dose of prednisone.

Children with fever and distress should be presumed to have poor spleen function, and should be hospitalized and given intravenous antibiotics until it is certain that they do not have an infection. If the laboratory reports the presence of Howell-Jolly bodies on the peripheral smear, this is evidence that the spleen is not functioning properly and that there is an increased risk of infection. Some children with MCTD have poor blood circulation in their hands and feet. If the circulation to a finger or toe has stopped and it is numb and discolored, this is also a reason for immediate hospitalization. In most cases, a numb and discolored finger or toe (impending digital infarction) responds to intravenous bolus methylprednisolone. A variety of regimens, including prostacyclin inhibitors, may be considered if this is not effective in restoring circulation.

Some children with MCTD will develop obvious scleroderma over time, and they should be treated appropriately for that diagnosis. Other children will not develop the typical skin changes of scleroderma but may develop shortness of breath and pulmonary function abnormalities. Pulmonary fibrosis may occur; I have seen children who developed pneumothorax as a result. In other children, pulmonary fibrosis may result in pulmonary hypertension, with resultant cardiac problems and an increased risk of infection.

Sudden overwhelming infection remains the most commonly reported cause of death for children with MCTD. This may be related to frequent problems with the spleen (functional asplenia), as discussed for children with SLE. Parents of children with MCTD should promptly seek medical care at the first suspicion of a serious infection. Whenever possible, children with MCTD should receive vaccination against pneumococcal infections.

MEDICAL TREATMENT

The standard treatment for MCTD is a low dose of corticosteroids combined with hydroxychloroquine and an NSAID for relief of the arthritis. The corticosteroid dosage should be adjusted as necessary to correct the elevated IgG level, the ESR, the anemia, and the clinical symptoms. Significant Raynaud's syndrome should be treated with an appropriate calcium-channel blocker. Although stronger agents are available if these do not provide relief, most children with MCTD will do well on this combination.

For some children with MCTD, it is not possible to reduce the corticosteroid dosage to a satisfactory level. Methotrexate seems to be an effective steroid-sparing agent for these children. Most often it is necessary to treat them with higher doses of methotrexate, such as those used in dermatomyositis and scleroderma (i.e., up to 1 mg/kg/week, 50 mg maximum). The key to successful treatment of MCTD is early identification of the children who are at high risk for progressive disease. This group must be treated vigorously with the goal of bringing the disease under control. Children treated aggressively generally do well.

Stronger immunosuppressive agents are rarely necessary for the treatment of children with MCTD unless the condition is evolving toward scleroderma. For children who do not respond to or tolerate methotrexate, azathioprine or mycophenolate mofetil may be considered. In the small subset of children who develop nephrotic syndrome, treatment with intravenous cyclophosphamide may be necessary and is often helpful. Children who progress to scleroderma are difficult to treat and should be treated as appropriate for scleroderma (see Chapter 15).

PROGNOSIS

The long-term prognosis for children with MCTD depends on the evolution of the disease. Most children do well with the treatment I have described. In many children, the disease seems to resolve slowly over time and they are able to discontinue all medications. Most of my initial teenage patients are now young adults. Ten years after diagnosis, they are doing well on no medication and have no significant problems. However, children who develop significant lung involvement or other evidence of progression toward scleroderma are much more worrisome. These children need to be treated aggressively, but even so the prognosis is guarded, as it is for all children with scleroderma.

13

Sjögren's Syndrome

Children with Dry Eyes and Dry Mouth

Children with Sjögren's syndrome are often sent to the rheumatologist by a dentist who has noted that they have unusually severe cavities or by an ophthalmologist who has noted that their complaints of eye discomfort are due to chronically dry eyes and poor tear production. Other children with Sjögren's syndrome are sent to the rheumatologist because of Raynaud's syndrome and a positive ANA or RF.

The combination of dry eyes and dry mouth may be the result of inflammation of the lacrimal glands and the parotid and submandibular glands that produce tears and saliva. These children may present with complaints of dry eyes, recurrent mouth sores, or tender and protuberant parotid glands. In the pediatrician's office, chronic eye allergies with dryness and itching are frequent complaints. The majority of children with Sjögren's syndrome test positive for antibodies to Ro. Most of these children are ANA-positive.

Sjögren's syndrome should be considered in the differential diagnosis of any child with recurrent corneal abrasions, unusually severe dental problems, or recurrent parotid gland swelling. Although there are viruses other than mumps (for which most children have received appropriate immunizations) that can cause recurrent parotitis, all children with recurrent parotid gland swelling should be evaluated for Sjögren's syndrome.

When they are fully evaluated, some children with Sjögren's syndrome are found to have SLE; these children are said to have *secondary* Sjögren's syndrome. Sjögren's syndrome is also a known complication of rheumatoid arthritis in adults, but it rarely occurs in children with JA. I have seen children with sarcoidosis who had Sjögren's syndrome and arthritis. Children who have dry eyes and dry mouth but lack other findings suggestive of connective tissue disease have primary Sjögren's syndrome. However, over time, some children with what was thought to be primary Sjögren's syndrome ultimately develop more symptoms and are diagnosed with SLE. The only way to deal with this is to treat the Sjögren's syndrome appropriately (usually with hydroxychloroquine and low-dose steroids) and to monitor carefully.

One source of confusion in caring for children with Sjögren's syndrome is the involvement of the acinar glands. The acinar glands include not only the salivary glands, but also the pancreas. All of the acinar glands are part of the digestive process, and if they are inflamed, the amylase level will be elevated. Although an elevated amylase level may indicate pancreatitis, in children with Sjögren's syndrome it may reflect inflammation of the parotid gland without pancreatitis. Sometimes children with Sjögren's syndrome have simultaneous inflammation in the pancreas and the parotid glands. It is important to recognize that there are several possible explanations for the elevated amylase level; evaluate the child carefully for each of them.

Children with Sjögren's syndrome may be referred because they have developed arthritis. Recently, a child was referred to me for knee pain. The mother was quite surprised when I asked whether he had sores in his mouth or difficulty swallowing. When she told me about his dry mouth and his treatment for three episodes of epidemic parotitis, we promptly did the appropriate tests and confirmed the diagnosis of Sjögren's syndrome.

Kidney involvement with Sjögren's syndrome may take the form of hematuria or proteinuria. There is also an association between Sjögren's syndrome and **renal tubular acidosis**. Children with this complication should be under the care of an experienced nephrologist.

COMPLICATIONS

The most common complications of Sjögren's syndrome are the direct result of the dry eyes. Dry eyes are easily scratched, and corneal abrasions are both painful and ultimately damaging to the lens. These children need frequent monitoring by an ophthalmologist. The dry mouth causes poor dental hygiene and the development of many cavities. These complications can become quite serious, and it is important to make sure that children use artificial tears and artificial saliva if necessary. Special toothpastes and medicines to increase saliva production also help.

Most of the other complications of Sjögren's syndrome respond well to treatment. The kidney involvement usually is responsive to appropriate treatment by nephrologists. Sometimes children with Sjögren's syndrome develop abdominal pain and a rash over the front of their legs. If they did not have the other symptoms, this would be considered **Henoch-Schönlein purpura**. It is thought to result from deposition of large immune complexes in the skin and intestines. Children with this complication may also develop a flare of their arthritis and other problems and should be evaluated carefully. Long-term follow-up of children with Sjögren's syndrome suggests that chronic inflammation of the acinar glands may result in significant glandular destruction and disability. It is important to keep the inflammation suppressed. This condition may be best monitored by following the immunoglobulin and amylase levels, not the ESR.

MEDICAL TREATMENT

Artificial tears and artificial saliva are very important parts of the treatment of children with Sjögren's syndrome. Some teenagers are reluctant to use them at school for fear of seeming different. However, dry eyes and dry mouth can do so much damage that it is very important to encourage routine use of artificial tears and saliva even at school. Hydroxychloroquine is often helpful in slowing the progression of the disease. Corticosteroids are useful if the symptoms are more severe or progress despite the use of hydroxychloroquine. In severe cases, methotrexate or another immunosuppressive agent may be necessary. Rituximab has shown promise in very severe adult cases and may be used in children with Sjögren's syndrome as well.

Children who develop ocular, dental, or renal problems need to be treated appropriately; in most cases, these problems are not difficult to treat. There is an association between Sjögren's syndrome and lymphomas and Waldenström's macroglobulinemia in adults. This is not generally true in childhood. Most children with primary Sjögren's syndrome do well.

PROGNOSIS

The long-term prognosis for children with primary Sjögren's syndrome is unclear. Some children develop other rheumatic diseases over time. In that case, the underlying rheumatic disease determines the prognosis. Failure to properly treat recurrent ocular or dental problems may produce significant problems over time. Serious complications related to kidney disease and vasculitis are infrequent. Because Sjögren's syndrome is rare in childhood, there are no good reports describing the extended follow-up of children with this diagnosis.

14

Raynaud's Phenomenon

Maurice Raynaud (1834–1881) was a French medical student in the 1860s who was required to write a thesis to fulfill the requirements for graduation from medical school. He described the color changes he noticed in the hands of some women while standing outside in the cold waiting for the streetcar during the winter in Paris.

- **Raynaud's phenomenon** refers to the typical hand changes Raynaud described.
- **Raynaud's disease** (primary Raynaud's phenomenon) refers to the typical hand changes occurring in the absence of any other rheumatic disease.
- **Raynaud's syndrome** (secondary Raynaud's phenomenon) refers to the typical changes occurring in the setting of an underlying rheumatic disease.

Many people have cold hands whenever it is cool outside—this is not Raynaud's phenomenon. Raynaud's phenomenon results from spasm of the blood vessels. This may occur as a result of exposure to the cold, embarrassment, or other stresses. Many of my patients with significant Raynaud's syndrome describe their worst problems as occurring in the summer when they walk into air-conditioned buildings from the heat outside. The fundamental abnormality is the hyperreactivity of the blood vessels. Raynaud's phenomenon may be the result of being thin (it is common for tall, thin women to have the condition) or of the blood vessels being sensitized by immune complexes or by inflammatory mediators (see Chapter 25) because the individual has an underlying rheumatic disease.

To have true Raynaud's phenomenon, there must be a three-phase color change. Initially, the tips of one or more fingers turn white as the blood flow is cut off by spasm of the blood vessels. Once the spasm passes, there is increased reactive blood flow and the fingers turn red, then slowly revert to their normal state of bluish discoloration, with sluggish blood flow. **Cold red hands or cold blue hands without the spasmodic white phase do not constitute Raynaud's phenomenon.**

The importance of Raynaud's phenomenon lies in its association with a variety of rheumatic diseases. While Raynaud's phenomenon is common in thin young women, it is often the first manifestation noticed in children with progressive systemic sclerosis (see Chapter 15). Raynaud's phenomenon is also found frequently in children with other vasculitic diseases, such as SLE, dermatomyositis, and anticardiolipin antibody syndrome. It may also occur in children with many other rheumatic conditions.

Since most young women with Raynaud's phenomenon are healthy, it is important to understand how to recognize children in whom it is a warning of an underlying condition. There are a number of simple steps for doing this. Every child with Raynaud's phenomenon should undergo routine testing, but boys with this condition are more worrisome than girls, and children less than twelve years of age are more worrisome than older children. Tall, thin girls with a family history of Raynaud's disease are less worrisome than those without a family history.

As in every evaluation, a good history, careful physical examination, and appropriate laboratory tests are key. When evaluating a child with Raynaud's phenomenon, it is important to note what provokes the attacks, how often they occur, their duration, and any associated symptoms. Attacks on entering an air-conditioned space in the summer suggest more serious disease. Long-lasting episodes, frequent episodes, coincident shortness of breath or chest pain, and morning stiffness (particularly in the fingers) all increase the probability of an underlying disease.

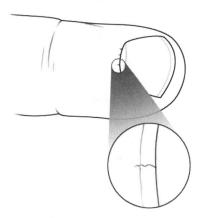

Figure 14-1 *Dilated nail fold capillaries may be easy to see with a small magnifying glass.*

When examining the child, look carefully for nail fold capillary abnormalities (see Fig. 14-1) or distal fingertip pitting. Either of these findings substantially increases the probability that an underlying disease is present.

Many physicians are concerned about lacking the proper equipment for nail fold capillary microscopy, but this examination can be easily done with an otoscope (the small hand-held magnifier used for looking in ears). In a normal individual, nail fold capillaries cannot be seen, even with an otoscope. Red streaks seen in the nail folds suggest the presence of nail fold capillary abnormalities, and the child should be referred to an experienced physician for further evaluation. All ten fingers should be examined, as the presence of these abnormalities on any finger is significant.

Distal fingertip pitting is another important finding that is also easily detected on routine examination. These pits are little areas where the small blood vessels have infarcted and the skin and underlying tissues have atrophied. As a result, these areas often feel callused to the examiner. The child will describe decreased feeling in the fingertips, as one would expect with calluses. If you look carefully, you may be able to see the areas of thickened skin, often with little central depressions or scars. However, it is easiest to screen for these abnormalities by feeling the tips of the fingers. The areas that are scarred feel like little bumps and are harder than the normal skin. **The presence of either nail fold capillary abnormalities or distal fingertip lesions strongly suggests the presence of an underlying rheumatic disease.**

LABORATORY TESTING

Laboratory evaluation of a child with Raynaud's phenomenon should include a CBC, ESR, ANA, RF, anticardiolipin antibodies, PT, PTT, and thyroid function tests. If there are no suggestive findings on the history or physical examination and all of these tests are normal, there is little likelihood of an underlying rheumatic disease. However, the presence of a positive ANA, positive RF, anticardiolipin antibodies, or an elevated ESR should all prompt more complete investigation, as should any suggestive findings on the history or physical examination.

COMPLICATIONS

If a child is known to have an underlying rheumatic disease, the presence of Raynaud's phenomenon does not necessarily indicate more serious disease. However, there are several complications related to Raynaud's phenomenon that must be considered. In more severe cases, children with this condition may have problems not only in their fingers, but also in their toes, ear lobes, and tip of the nose. All of these areas should be protected if the child is to be exposed to significant cold stress.

It is also important to recognize that children with increased vascular reactivity and Raynaud's phenomenon may have instability in other vascular beds. This is a rare complication, but I have cared for children with scleroderma who had chest pain and cardiac abnormalities owing to documented constriction of their coronary arteries that occurred whenever their fingers blanched because of Raynaud's phenomenon. If the internal organs are being deprived of blood flow, the Raynaud's phenomenon must be treated aggressively.

Any child who has distal fingertip pitting or a history of severe Raynaud's phenomenon should not be unnecessarily exposed to cold stress. Digital gangrene with loss of parts of fingers or toes can occur. Whenever a child has prolonged loss of circulation to a finger or toe, he or she should be taken to a local emergency room. I tell my patients that if a finger is white and numb for more than ten minutes, they should be indoors making every effort to warm it up. If it is not clearly back to normal after half an hour, they should be on their way to a medical facility. High-dose intravenous corticosteroids and prostacycline inhibitors have both been used, with good results, in this setting.

MEDICAL TREATMENT

For children with Raynaud's phenomenon without an associated disease, the most important aspect of treatment is common sense. The vast majority of children do well simply by dressing warmly and wearing gloves. If these measures are not enough, children may benefit from the use of calcium-channel blockers (Chapter 23). Most children tolerate the mild reduction in blood pressure associated with these drugs without difficulty, but some experience mild side effects. Many of my patients use these drugs only in the coldest weather. In addition to the calcium-channel blockers, it is possible to use drugs such as pentoxyfyline. Some rheumatologists use aspirin and other agents with varying success.

For children with an underlying rheumatic disease, the key to relieving Raynaud's phenomenon is treating the underlying condition. **In some children with an underlying rheumatic disease, Raynaud's phenomenon may remain a problem when the majority of the symptoms have resolved. Symptomatic** therapy with warm clothing and calcium-channel blockers may be helpful in these cases. Complete loss of blood flow for a prolonged period is extremely rare. However, prolonged vasoconstriction can result in loss of the affected finger or toe. For this reason, it is important that any child who has a cold, white finger or toe that has not returned to normal within a reasonable time period promptly seek appropriate medical care.

15

Scleroderma

Scleroderma is a broad term that simply means "hard skin." A variety of different diseases are grouped together under this diagnosis. The focal (or localized) forms of scleroderma are often mild and may not require treatment. In contrast, **progressive systemic sclerosis** (also called **diffuse scleroderma**) is a life-threatening disease typically involving the heart, lungs, and other organs. Fortunately, the mild forms of scleroderma are far more common than the severe ones.

Because the forms of scleroderma are so different from each other, it is necessary to discuss them separately. Typically, each form looks very different from the others, but confusing conditions that seem to overlap do exist.

Box 15-1 Forms of scleroderma

Local or focal forms of scleroderma
Morphea

Linear scleroderma

Linear scleroderma en coup de sabre

Parry Romberg syndrome (the relationship of this syndrome to scleroderma is uncertain)

Sclerodermatomyositis

Other overlapping syndromes

Systemic forms of scleroderma
Progressive systemic sclerosis

CREST syndrome

Diseases that can evolve into scleroderma
Eosinophilic fasciitis

Mixed connective tissue disease (see Chapter 12)

Box 15-1   Continued

Laboratory tests for scleroderma

Local or focal forms of scleroderma

ANA occasionally positive

RF usually negative

Creatinine phosphokinase (CPK) mildly elevated in linear scleroderma and sclerodermatomyositis but not in morphea or linear scleroderma en coup de sabre

    Anticentromere antibody negative

    Anti-Scl-70 negative

    Other blood tests usually normal

Systemic forms of scleroderma

Progressive systemic sclerosis

ANA often positive

RF often positive

Anti-Scl-70 sometimes positive (less frequent in childhood)

CREST syndrome

ANA often positive

RF sometimes positive

Anticentromere antibody usually positive

Eosinophilic fasciitis

ANA often positive

Eosinophilia

Mixed connective tissue disease

ANA positive

RF most often positive; Anti-Scl-70 negative

LOCALIZED FORMS OF SCLERODERMA

Morphea

Jill was an eight-year-old girl who developed a pink spot on her back. At first no one noticed, but it was obvious in the summer when she put on her bathing suit. It looked like a big pink circle with a whitish central area. Her mother thought first of Lyme disease, but two weeks of antibiotics had no effect. The lesion was treated with topical ointments for dry skin, then for ringworm, all without improvement. After six weeks, Jill's mother took her to a dermatologist. He examined the lesion and did a biopsy. The report was "consistent with scleroderma." By the time I saw Jill, the lesion had stopped growing and had developed a thick white center that was firm to the touch. Jill never developed any other lesions. She was treated with over-the-counter topical agents to soften the skin. Over a period of several years, the lesion softened. Now it is evident only because she has an area of darker skin where it occurred. The skin is soft and feels normal. She's never had another problem related to morphea.

Overview and diagnosis

Morphea is the most common form of scleroderma in childhood. It consists of areas of thickened skin commonly on the trunk but sometimes on the extremities. Families usually notice a patch of pink irritated skin that looks like many common skin conditions. If the patch is due to morphea, it typically does not itch or hurt. Often the area of reddened skin does not attract attention until it has persisted for several weeks. It will not improve with treatment for skin infections, but it might briefly look better if it is treated with corticosteroid creams.

Commonly, the family becomes concerned when either a second area of skin becomes involved or the area begins to enlarge. When areas of morphea are active, they slowly increase in size. The rim remains pink, but the center turns whitish and becomes hard. Dermatologists usually make the diagnosis of morphea on the basis of either a skin biopsy or clinical experience.

Laboratory abnormalities are rare in children with morphea. Although some children have positive tests for ANA, tests for anti-dsDNA, RF, Scl-70, anticentromere antibody, and routine blood tests including CBC, ESR, and muscle enzymes should all be normal. If they are not, a complete evaluation by an experienced rheumatologist is in order.

Some lesions of morphea are very small (nickel- or dime-sized), while others are several inches across. Over a period of years, they usually evolve from hard white areas to soft darkened skin. (*Note*: In dark-skinned people the areas of morphea may remain lighter than the surrounding skin.) If the morphea is not interfering with function and there are only a few lesions, it may be best to treat it with topical creams such as vitamin E cream or cocoa butter. Chronic use of corticosteroid creams can damage the skin and should be avoided.

Medical treatment

Children with rapidly developing morphea lesions that are disfiguring may need aggressive therapy. In my experience, methotrexate therapy has been very successful in stopping the progression of morphea. Low doses of methotrexate given as pills are rarely effective, but moderate doses (1 mg/kg/week [maximum 50 mg]) given as subcutaneous injections are very effective. However, the lesions must be significant enough to warrant the risks, as well as the time, effort, and expense of therapy. Borderline cases may benefit from treatment with hydroxychloroquine.

Complications

Morphea has two main complications. First, the lesions are unattractive. If they are in a location that is covered by clothing, the problem may be minimal. If they are in a location that is easily seen by others, it is necessary to address the psychological issues associated with the curious questions (see the section on dealing with friends and neighbors in Chapter 27). Second, the skin in the lesions will not heal well if it is cut or abraded. In rare cases, isolated lesions of morphea may be associated with mild arthritis or other rheumatic disease manifestations. These overlap conditions are of uncertain significance. However, any child with atypical lesions or unexpected problems should be carefully evaluated by an experienced rheumatologist.

Many parents worry that morphea lesions may be the first indications of systemic scleroderma. This is rarely, if ever, true. Children with new-onset morphea should be carefully evaluated by a physician who is experienced in dealing with children with scleroderma. An experienced physician may recognize indications that the child has a systemic disease. If there are no such indications, I recommend only periodic monitoring after the initial evaluation.

Prognosis

The cause of morphea remains entirely unknown. Many ideas have been proposed over the years, but none has withstood the test of time. The key facts to know about morphea are as follows:

- It usually disappears after a period of years and leaves only darkened skin behind. Sometimes this darkened skin is sunken due to subcutaneous atrophy.

- If there are many lesions, or if they occur in disfiguring locations, they can be treated.
- The earlier in its evolution morphea is treated, the better the outcome.
- Children with morphea should be carefully evaluated for other evidence of rheumatic disease. If nothing is found on careful examination at the beginning, the risk of other rheumatic diseases appearing later is small.

The long-term outlook for children with morphea is excellent. There should be no need for surgery or other aggressive interventions. Children with morphea should expect to grow up to lead normal, healthy, productive lives.

Linear Scleroderma

Kathleen was nine years old when her mother noted a patch of unusual skin on the top of her left foot. Over the next six months the area was always irritated and red, despite a number of treatments for athlete's foot and other minor conditions offered by her physician. No one was very concerned until new lesions appeared on Kathleen's calf. These were red at first and looked like an allergic reaction. Over time more lesions developed, and they began to appear above the knee. Gradually, these lesions began to turn white; then they darkened and hardened.

When Kathleen was eleven, a neighbor pointed out to her mother that Kathleen was limping. When Kathleen was undressed in the doctor's office, mixed white, dark, and pink lesions were found up and down her leg; there was even one on her stomach. The left leg was smaller than the right both in length and width. In addition, she could not straighten her left leg completely. There was a tight band of skin behind the knee that prevented the leg from straightening.

By the time Kathleen came to my office, the linear scleroderma on her leg was well advanced and causing significant problems. It required a year of treatment with methotrexate injections and physical therapy before the skin was soft and she could fully straighten her leg. We did not discontinue the therapy until she had been stable for another year. Unfortunately, she lost a lot of muscle bulk during the time before she was diagnosed and began treatment with methotrexate. As a result, the left leg is still thinner than the right. However, she is now able to function normally.

Overview and diagnosis

Linear scleroderma differs from morphea in that the areas of involved skin form linear bands instead of irregular ovals. These bands are often described as following the distribution of dermatomes, but this is not true. Nonetheless, linear scleroderma usually does not cross from one side of the body to the other. The idea that irritation of the nerves leads to the development of linear scleroderma received a lot of attention in the past. One group of researchers suggested that linear scleroderma was the result of herpes zoster infection involving the nerves. Another group thought that it was due to Lyme disease. These ideas have been disproved. The cause of linear scleroderma remains unknown.

A typical case of linear scleroderma is a child such as Kathleen, with a tight band of skin on the top of one foot extending up onto the leg. It may also begin on the hand and arm. These areas appear pinkish at first and don't hurt. Later, they become pale and harden. A small area of involvement may be of little concern, but if a large area is involved, tightening of the skin may cause the leg (or arm, toes, etc.) to develop a contracture.

We do not understand the patterns of linear scleroderma. Some children have one patch on one arm or leg. Others have several patches on one arm. Still others have involvement of both the arm and the leg on one side, and the lesions may extend onto the trunk. Less frequently, both sides of the body are involved. Involvement of both sides of the body is unusual and should prompt careful investigation. However, involvement of an arm and a leg on the same side is not uncommon.

Laboratory abnormalities in children with linear scleroderma are minimal. Although some children have positive tests for ANA, tests for anti-dsDNA, RF, Scl-70, anticentromere antibody, and routine blood tests including CBC and ESR all should be normal. Some children will have mildly elevated muscle enzyme levels. If a child has elevated muscle enzymes and the typical rash of dermatomyositis in conjunction with an area of linear scleroderma, the disease is termed **sclerodermatomyositis**, discussed later in this chapter.

Medical treatment

If the disease occurs while the child is still growing, it may interfere with the development of the underlying muscles, bones, and joints. This may result in stunting of the growth of an extremity and lead to permanent disability. For this reason, areas of linear scleroderma that cross a joint (e.g., an elbow, wrist, knee, ankle) require aggressive treatment. Studies have shown excellent success in treating linear scleroderma with methotrexate. Over a six-month period, weekly methotrexate injections (1 mg/kg/week up to 50 mg) are associated with dramatic softening of the skin and gradual reversal of contractures. Although this treatment cannot restore lost muscle or bone mass, it appears to stop progression of the condition and allow resumption of growth in young children. It should be started as soon as possible in children who are developing deformities.

Linear Scleroderma en Coup de Sabre and Parry Romberg Syndrome

Overview and diagnosis

Linear scleroderma en coup de sabre is a particular form of linear scleroderma that may not truly be related to the other forms. *En coup de sabre* is a French phrase once used to describe the injuries of foot soldiers struck on the head by the sword of a cavalry soldier riding a horse. If the foot soldier survived his injury, there was a scar and thickened skin involving one side of the forehead and extending along the scalp toward the back. Children with linear scleroderma en coup de sabre have an area of thickened abnormal skin that resembles this scar, but they usually do not have significant underlying problems. However, the distinction between linear scleroderma en coup de sabre and Parry Romberg syndrome is unclear. There are no clear criteria for a distinction at present.

Parry Romberg syndrome is a gradually progressive facial hemiatrophy. In a full-fledged case, there is significant deformity, with one entire side of the face smaller than the other. This is in sharp contrast to typical linear scleroderma en coup de sabre, where the abnormality is confined to the forehead. While the changes of linear scleroderma en coup de sabre are usually confined to the skin, in Parry Romberg syndrome there is an increased frequency of underlying changes in the brain.

The difference between linear scleroderma en coup de sabre and Parry Romberg syndrome is best exemplified by involvement of the tongue in Parry Romberg syndrome. Not only is one side of the face smaller, but so is one side of the tongue. Thus, Parry Romberg syndrome is clearly not a condition of the skin alone. However, both conditions may begin the same way, and there are children who have areas of atrophic facial skin that do not clearly fit either category.

These illnesses typically begin in the first or second year of life. Most often the family notices a pinkish lesion just to one side of the middle of the forehead. Since children in this age group fall frequently while learning to walk, most families assume that the child simply banged his or her head. Over a few weeks, the lesion does not disappear as expected. Instead, the veins may in the pink area become more noticeable.

The lesion on the forehead is often present for months before the family begins to notice indentation of the bone under the pink skin. On careful examination, there may be a continuation of the abnormal skin underneath the hairline. In other children, the area of pink skin extends farther down the face and along the side of the nose over time. Linear scleroderma en coup de sabre should not extend below the eyelid. True Parry Romberg syndrome involves the entire side of the face. Some children fall between these two conditions.

Because there are children with varying degrees of involvement, there is no agreement on where linear scleroderma en coup de sabre ends and Parry Romberg syndrome begins. If there the tongue is involved, it is Parry Romberg syndrome. I also believe that all children with involvement of the brain underneath the lesions have Parry Romberg syndrome and not linear scleroderma en coup de sabre, but the distinction between these diseases remains uncertain.

Laboratory abnormalities are minimal in children with both of these disorders. As with other forms of linear scleroderma, some children have positive tests for ANA, but tests for anti-dsDNA, RF, Scl-70, anticentromere antibody, and routine blood tests including CBC and ESR should be normal. These children should not have abnormal muscle enzyme levels or muscle weakness.

Medical treatment and prognosis

The treatment and prognosis for this group of children remain uncertain. If the lesions are confined to the scalp and forehead, as in typical linear scleroderma en coup de sabre, they are responsive to methotrexate. The long-term outlook for children with linear scleroderma en coup de sabre is generally excellent. In most cases, the cosmetic deformity is minimal and can be well concealed by the hair.

Some children with linear scleroderma en coup de sabre have been described as having underlying neurologic involvement. Again, I believe this is more likely a manifestation of Parry Romberg syndrome. Unfortunately, children with Parry

Romberg syndrome and facial hemiatrophy are rarely recognized before the atrophy becomes significant. In most cases, it does not appear appropriate to intervene medically at that point. However, with an experienced plastic surgeon who has worked with these children, cosmetic surgery is practical. Many special considerations are involved in this surgery, and it should be done only by a team experienced in dealing with such children.

A significant percentage of children with Parry Romberg syndrome also have underlying central nervous system lesions. These may vary from benign nonspecific findings on MRI to vascular malformations or neurologic abnormalities. Some children with Parry Romberg syndrome have learning disabilities. Children with this syndrome occasionally develop optic neuritis, which requires immediate treatment. I have also cared for children with linear scleroderma en coup de sabre who developed uveitis. **All children with these conditions should have periodic ophthalmologic evaluations**.

The combination of cosmetic and neurologic abnormalities in children with Parry Romberg syndrome makes the prognosis for these children more guarded. Most do well with corrective surgery, as needed, provided it is done by plastic surgeons experienced in dealing with this condition. A sympathetic family and physician are important. Special efforts must be made to help these children deal with the social stresses that result from their often abnormal appearance (see Chapter 27).

Sclerodermatomyositis

Overview and diagnosis

Sclerodermatomyositis is an overlap disorder that illustrates the foolishness of considering the rheumatic diseases to be completely separate entities. **Children with sclerodermatomyositis have a typical band of tight skin that appears to be linear scleroderma, but they also have muscle weakness, elevated muscle enzyme levels, and often a heliotropic rash** typical of dermatomyositis (see Chapter 16). The simultaneous occurrence of manifestations of two separate diseases in these children is unexplained. The muscle inflammation and heliotropic rash most often respond promptly to corticosteroid therapy and do not recur. The linear scleroderma lesion does not respond to corticosteroids, though it may become less pink in coloration. **Progressive systemic sclerosis with elevated muscle enzyme levels is not sclerodermatomyositis.**

Laboratory abnormalities found in children with sclerodermatomyositis include a positive test for ANA. Routine blood tests may show mild anemia, elevation of the ESR, and elevated muscle enzyme levels (CK and aldolase; see Chapter 25). Rheumatoid factor is rare, and anti-Scl-70 is normally absent. Although diffuse sclerodermatous changes, rash, and elevated muscle enzyme levels may occur in MCTD, children with MCTD do not have linear bands of tight skin. Children with sclerodermatomyositis do not have the typical pattern of laboratory findings seen in children with MCTD, and the two conditions are most likely distinct.

Medical treatment and prognosis

Complications of sclerodermatomyositis are rare. Usually, the muscle inflammation and rash are easily treated with corticosteroids. The area of linear scleroderma is rarely large enough to cause concern. If it is crossing a joint or causing significant deformity, methotrexate therapy may be necessary. Many children are treated with long-term hydroxychloroquine once corticosteroids are no longer necessary. Although a small percentage of children will develop further manifestations of rheumatic disease, in general the long-term prognosis is good.

Other Overlapping Conditions

As a physician caring for children with these diseases for many years, I am struck by the diversity of the diseases. Somehow, all of them, which look so different in their typical forms, are interrelated, but we do not understand the connections. Sometimes children simultaneously have skin lesions of morphea on their back and abdomen, indentations typical of linear scleroderma en coup de sabre on their forehead, ocular inflammation such as that seen in children with JA,, and areas of linear scleroderma on their legs.

Other overlapping conditions may also occur. The key element in caring for children who do not fit neatly into one category is to recognize each condition for what it is and treat it appropriately. At the same time, every atypical child must be carefully evaluated to make sure that an alternative diagnosis has not been overlooked. Some of these children are difficult to treat, and their long-term prognosis is uncertain. With the exception of neurologic and visual problems, no child with localized scleroderma has significant internal organ involvement.

SYSTEMIC FORMS OF SCLERODERMA

Progressive Systemic Sclerosis

Overview and diagnosis

The form of scleroderma called **progressive systemic sclerosis (PSS)**, also referred to as **diffuse scleroderma,** is the most severe form of the disease, with the subtle onset of skin tightening and, in many cases, shortness of breath. Children and families may be unaware of the disease until it becomes well advanced. However, careful questioning may reveal that the disease has been developing for a long period. Because the onset of disease is slow and gradual, families often are unaware of it until a dramatic event occurs. Sometimes this is a cold, numb finger. Sometimes it is the inability to participate in favorite sports when the season starts. In other cases, the family suddenly realizes that the child cannot open jars or perform other minor chores that he or she once did easily. These children have poor wound healing and may be brought to the physician because of painful sores that do not heal appropriately. These commonly occur on the ankles, elbows, or fingers.

The most common early symptom of PSS is Raynaud's phenomenon. However, it is important to be aware that most people who have Raynaud's phenomenon do not develop rheumatic disease (see Chapter 14). Other common early symptoms of PSS are gradually increasing tightness of the skin and progressive stiffening of the fingers. Unfortunately, the disease often progresses so slowly that the child and family may be unaware of changes that are striking to the outside observer. With time, children may notice that it is becoming more difficult to open their mouths fully to eat a large sandwich. Because the symptoms evolve slowly, none of them is likely to result in prompt referral. Typically, these children are ultimately brought to their physicians because of shortness of breath, difficulty swallowing, or weight loss.

An experienced physician easily diagnoses PSS when the skin involvement is prominent. The tight, shiny skin is often accompanied by sores over the knuckles (Gottren's papules), abnormalities in the nail fold capillaries, and distal fingertip lesions (see Chapter 14 for a full discussion). This combination of findings is diagnostic of PSS. Less often, children present with dysphagia. They may have difficulty swallowing foods in large chunks or those that have sharp edges, like potato chips.

Some children with scleroderma present initially with complaints of chest pain. These are usually the typical complaints of esophageal irritation. The distal esophagus is frequently involved in scleroderma, and the distal esophageal sphincter is often ineffective as a result. Occasional children present with chronic diarrhea and weight loss because of gastrointestinal involvement and malabsorption. In all of these cases, the key to the diagnosis is consideration of the possibility of scleroderma.

Other diseases may be associated with Raynaud's phenomenon or shortness of breath, but **the combination of chronic or recurrent shortness of breath and Raynaud's phenomenon is highly suggestive of PSS or CREST syndrome** (discussed later in the chapter). Mixed connective tissue disease, dermatomyositis, SLE, and, less frequently, other rheumatic diseases may also produce both symptoms. Typical cases of each can be easily differentiated. However, there is a broad spectrum of overlap among these diseases. While these diseases are clearly distinguished in textbooks, nature has not been so obliging. Over time, some children with obvious MCTD progress to PSS.

The diagnosis of PSS is based on the characteristic findings on examination of the skin. In some cases, it is necessary to biopsy the skin for confirmation. However, the diagnosis is often obvious to an experienced physician. If confirmatory findings are present on physical examination and in laboratory tests, a skin biopsy may be avoided. The skin of children with scleroderma often heals poorly, and the biopsy often leads to just one more scar.

There are several patterns of laboratory abnormality in children with scleroderma. No single test is abnormal in every child. Frequently, the routine tests (CBC, ESR, metabolic panel) are essentially normal. An increased number of eosinophils may be noted in the CBC. Very high levels of eosinophils may suggest **eosinophilic fasciitis** (discussed later in the chapter). Positive tests for ANA or RF are common but not necessary for the diagnosis. Levels of muscle enzymes (CK, aldolase) may be elevated. Antibodies to Scl-70 (antitopoisomerase antibodies) are less common in children with scleroderma than in adults but may occur. Anti-DNA antibodies are occasionally reported in low titer, but levels of serum complement (C3, C4) should be normal.

Except for the finding of anti-Scl-70, it may be impossible to differentiate MCTD and PSS on the basis of laboratory test results. Because some children with MCTD ultimately develop PSS, this may be a false distinction (see Chapter 12). CREST syndrome should be considered carefully in children with telangiectasias or high titers of anticentromere antibody.

Pulmonary complications

The most severe complications associated with scleroderma result from involvement of the internal organs. Lung involvement that leads to progressive shortness of breath may be quite severe. Children with PSS should have periodic pulmonary function tests (PFTs; see Chapter 25). High-resolution CAT scans of the chest are helpful if a child has abnormal PFTs and may be done in children with normal PFTs if there is clinical suspicion of lung disease. Areas of fibrosis or a honeycomb ground-glass appearance indicate significant lung involvement.

Children with significant lung involvement should be aggressively treated. Over time, the pulmonary fibrosis leads to right heart failure, with enlargement of the right ventricle, pulmonary insufficiency, and increased pulmonary artery pressure. Untreated pulmonary fibrosis often leads to heart failure, pneumonia, or both.

Cardiac complications

Heart problems in children with scleroderma are usually the result of lung involvement. However, some children develop **myocardial fibrosis**. This is easily recognized on an echocardiogram. It is a very difficult problem to treat. Normally, heart failure is treated with agents such as digitalis that increase the strength of the heart's contractions. However, these agents frequently are associated with arrhythmias in children with scleroderma.

The pericardium may also be involved in scleroderma. Pericarditis with or without significant pericardial effusion is well recognized. Typically, this can be treated with medications, but if it is very severe it may require pericardiocentesis.

Although myocardial infarction is rare in childhood, the coronary arteries may be involved in children with scleroderma. Gradual thickening of the coronary arteries is unlikely to cause problems until the children become adults. However, some children develop vasospasm in the coronary arteries. Most often, coronary artery involvement is discovered in children with scleroderma when they report chest pain occurring when they experience Raynaud's phenomenon. This should be aggressively treated, as it may result in myocardial infarction.

Renal complications

Involvement of the kidneys is another major concern. If the blood vessels supplying the kidneys become thickened and narrowed, there may be increased rennin production resulting in systemic hypertension. Rarely, children develop an acute rise in blood pressure called **scleroderma renal crisis.** This is an acute, life-threatening condition. Fortunately, ACE inhibitors are effective in treating this complication.

Gastrointestinal complications

Children with scleroderma frequently have involvement of the gastrointestinal system. Tightness of the skin around the mouth can make it difficult to open the mouth widely enough to eat normal foods. Thickening of the esophagus makes it difficult to swallow foods such as meat. In addition, it is common for these children to have significant **gastroesophageal reflux,** which causes severe irritation and often chest pain. Eventually, the gastroesophageal reflux may cause scarring leading to dysphagia. The pain and discomfort may lead to anorexia, and the child will begin to lose weight.

Involvement of the intestines by scleroderma also takes the form of diffuse thickening. Poor motility results in poor absorption of nutrients and chronic bloating. Some patients have constipation, others have diarrhea, and some have both problems. These problems frequently increase the child's weight loss. Liver involvement in children with scleroderma is rare. Some cases of **primary biliary cirrhosis** have been reported in childhood.

Medical treatment

Proper treatment of childhood scleroderma remains controversial. It is generally agreed that treatment with D-penicillamine (which was once the standard therapy) is ineffective. There is no clear agreement on the best treatment for mild cases. Some physicians feel that short courses of prednisone are helpful. I avoid them if possible. They are useful if the CK level is elevated, indicating muscle inflammation.

Most centers treat children with systemic scleroderma with mild agents such as hydroxychloroquine unless there is severe internal organ involvement. If significant internal organ involvement is present, they use intravenous cyclophosphamide.

I prefer to treat every child with definite PSS with injections of methotrexate and oral cyclosporine. While this is not proven therapy, I have found it to be very successful in preventing progression of scleroderma. Studies in adults show that low doses of methotrexate do not work. In my experience, the higher dose of 1 mg/kg is effective when given by injection every week.

Cyclosporine is another potent drug that provides additional benefit to these children. All of my PSS patients are treated with the combination of cyclosporine and high-dose methotrexate, and they do well. I do not wait for severe problems to develop; my goal is to prevent them. Not all physicians agree with this choice of therapy. Since no therapy for PSS has been proven effective, each center has its own preferences based on its own experience.

A variety of medications have been tried in adults with scleroderma. The use of agents that block TNF-α and agents that block B-cell activity, such as rituximab, is being considered. Additional new agents are in development. See Chapter 23 for a more complete discussion of these medications.

An assortment of medications is used to address specific problems. For example, ACE inhibitors are used to treat increased blood pressure. Calcium-channel blockers are used to treat Raynaud's phenomenon. A variety of medications that block acid secretion are used to minimize damage to the esophagus. In addition, prostaglandins such as inhaled iloprost, a stable analog of epoprostenol, have been used to treat pulmonary fibrosis and the resultant increase in stiffness of the blood vessels in the lungs. Imatinib mesylate (Gleevec) is also under investigation. There is no single best therapy.

Children with scleroderma should be followed by physicians who are familiar with the most current recommendations. Ideally, all children with significant PSS should be cared for at major medical centers with experienced rheumatologists, pulmonologists, cardiologists, nephrologists, and specialists in intensive care with extensive pediatric experience. The primary goal must be to prevent progression of the disease.

Prognosis

The prognosis for children with PSS is guarded. In the absence of significant internal organ involvement, these children may live for decades. Some children with only skin involvement may find that their skin eventually softens and will do well. Children with significant heart, lung, kidney, or gastrointestinal involvement did poorly in the past. However, with more aggressive therapy, the outlook is improving.

CREST Syndrome

CREST syndrome is a variation of systemic scleroderma that has several peculiar aspects. The acronym CREST comes from the findings of **calcinosis, Raynaud's phenomenon, esophageal problems, sclerodactyly,** and **telangiectasias**. The key findings that distinguish CREST syndrome from PSS are the presence of telangiectasias and anticentromere antibodies.

The general problems associated with CREST syndrome and their treatment do not differ from those of PSS. However, it is clear that these children are somehow different from the children with PSS. Often children with CREST syndrome have less skin and kidney involvement but more heart and lung involvement. Treatment is essentially the same for CREST and PSS. At one time, it was thought that the prognosis for CREST was better. In children this is uncertain.

EOSINOPHILIC FASCIITIS: A DISEASE THAT CAN EVOLVE INTO SCLERODERMA

Overview and diagnosis

Eosinophilic fasciitis is an unusual disorder characterized by the acute onset of pain and swelling of an extremity. Typically, the skin in the affected area is very red, tender, and swollen. This inflammation is followed by hardening of the skin and muscles in the area. Although the onset of eosinophilic fasciitis is commonly associated with extreme exercise or trauma, the cause is poorly understood. Evidence of inflammation, including an increased ESR and an increased eosinophil count, are common. Internal organ involvement does not occur.

Some cases of **eosinophilic myalgia** syndrome were initially thought to be eosinophilic fasciitis. This is a syndrome with muscle pain and redness but not fasciitis. An epidemic of eosinophilic myalgia was apparently caused by contaminated L-tryptophan purchased in health food stores. Children with eosinophilia and myalgias should be carefully questioned about their intake of vitamins, food supplements, and other agents. Most evidence points to a contaminated source of L-tryptophan as the cause of the problem, but these issues have never been fully resolved. I cared for one teenager with this syndrome who took many supplements but was sure that none of them contained L-tryptophan. Since there is no real supervision of the manufacturers, one never knows for sure what these supplements contain.

Medical treatment and prognosis

Eosinophilic fasciitis is usually very responsive to treatment with corticosteroids. However, the long-term course of the disease is highly varied. Sometimes it resolves entirely, but other cases persist, with varying levels of disease activity for years. A few children ultimately develop PSS after initially being diagnosed with eosinophilic fasciitis. However, most cases resolve completely over a period of months.

Children with eosinophilia and musculoskeletal complaints need to be evaluated very carefully. This combination of findings may occur in children with parasitic illnesses, eosinophilic vasculitis, and Churg-Strauss disease. These diseases are uncommon but may be life-threatening if not recognized and treated. Children with these diseases may have rashes, but these diseases are not associated with hardening of the skin.

16

Dermatomyositis and Polymyositis

Hillary was a delightful four-year-old. She had a younger sister who was just beginning to walk when the family noticed that Hillary was asking to be carried and was holding on much more often than she had previously. Her family thought this was a reaction to the increased attention given to her sister. But the next month, she became increasingly difficult. She often refused to walk and had tantrums if her parents would not carry her. Hillary's bedroom was on the second floor. Although she would come downstairs in the morning, she insisted on being carried up to bed every night. One morning she wanted a doll from her bedroom but refused to go upstairs to get it. Her parents could not understand why she was getting so lazy. Over the next few weeks, they noted that she was holding on to the stair rail with both hands when coming down the steps and seemed to be falling unexpectedly.

Concerned, her parents brought her to the pediatrician. On examination, she was weak and could hardly get up from the chair. She could not get up from the floor without assistance, and even when she was given help, she needed to push herself up, using the front of her legs, to rise to a standing position. Laboratory evaluation revealed an elevated ESR, CK, AST, and ALT.

In the office, Hillary could grab my fingers tightly with her hand but could not raise her arms over her head. She had red, irritated skin over the extensor surfaces of her elbows and knees. Her parents ascribed this condition to her frequent falling. They had not noticed the pinkish rash over her eyelids. The diagnosis of dermatomyositis was made. She was begun on a low dose of corticosteroids, and within one year she recovered completely.

Quick Summary

- Children with dermatomyositis do not have the increased risk of cancer described for adults with this disease.
- Polymyositis is rare in childhood. Any child with "dermatomyositis" without a rash should be evaluated very carefully.

- Children with the characteristic rash of dermatomyositis and elevated muscle enzyme levels should be treated even if they are not weak. It does not make sense to wait for their condition to get worse.
- If a child with dermatomyositis develops a nasal voice or begins to cough when eating, it may signal involvement of the pharyngeal muscles. This places the child at high risk of aspiration and is an indication for immediate aggressive treatment.

DERMATOMYOSITIS

Overview

Dermatomyositis in childhood is characterized by proximal muscle weakness and rash. In most cases the disease begins slowly, with the gradual onset of progressive weakness. However, a small percentage of cases begin with dramatic fever, rash, elevated muscle enzyme levels, and profound weakness. Dermatomyositis may begin in any age group, sometimes affecting very young children and at other times teenagers. The key to the diagnosis is recognition of progressive muscle weakness involving the proximal muscles to a much greater degree than distal muscles. Dermatomyositis is always associated with a rash, usually heliotropic, occurring over the upper eyelids and over the elbows and knees.

There are a number of other illnesses that may cause muscle weakness. In addition to dermatomyositis, the gradual onset of weakness in small children can come from botulinum spores (found in organic honey and possibly other unpasteurized or improperly processed foods), intrinsic muscle diseases, including muscular dystrophy, and a variety of metabolic diseases, such as lipid myopathies. The abrupt onset of muscle weakness may follow viral infections, exposure to insecticides and other poisons, certain venomous snakebites, and some medications. During flu epidemics, many children complain of pain in their calves and have elevated muscle enzyme levels. **The key findings that differentiate dermatomyositis from these conditions are the presence of rash and selective proximal muscle weakness.**

Diagnosis

In children with dermatomyositis, inability to raise the arms over the head (e.g., when brushing the hair) and difficulty raising the legs (e.g., when going upstairs) are often the first symptoms noted by the family. Any child of an appropriate age who cannot raise his or her arms over the head, get up easily from a chair, or get up from the floor without assistance requires thorough evaluation.

The diagnosis of dermatomyositis is made on the basis of the history and the physical examination findings plus appropriate blood tests. Either the CK level or the aldolase level will be abnormal in most children. They can also be abnormal following viral infections or intense physical activity (e.g., playing football, running track, lifting weights). Often these tests are not included in the routine metabolic panel and have to be specifically requested. All of the routine tests, including the ESR, may be normal, despite the presence of active dermatomyositis.

Absolute proof of dermatomyositis requires a muscle biopsy with the characteristic finding of muscle cell atrophy with perifascicular inflammatory cell infiltrates. The diagnosis can also be made if electromyography (EMG) demonstrates a characteristic "spike and wave" pattern. The muscle biopsy and EMG must be done on the inflamed muscle. Since dermatomyositis is primarily a disease of the proximal muscles, performing the biopsy on a distal muscle is not helpful. In addition, not all proximal muscles may be equally involved. Biopsy of an uninvolved muscle may lead to a false-negative report.

It is often useful to obtain an MRI of the thighs. Inflamed muscles are edematous and show up on the MRI. Thus, the MRI can show the surgeon which muscles are involved and where the biopsy is best done. However, once the MRI has demonstrated the presence of inflamed muscles in a weak child, unless another cause of muscle inflammation is suspected, the muscle biopsy is academic. Most often I will not do a muscle biopsy. The characteristic history and examination findings with confirmatory laboratory tests are quite sufficient. If the MRI shows the inflamed muscles, there can be little doubt of the diagnosis. Unfortunately, children with dermatomyositis have poor skin healing. As a result, the surgical site often breaks down and leaves a large scar where the biopsy was done.

Children who have a typical dermatomyositis-appearing rash with mildly elevated muscle enzyme levels but no evident weakness require particular attention. These children clearly have the disease. Although I have heard physicians argue that they do not require treatment, the elevated muscle enzyme levels and rash are evidence of ongoing inflammation and cell death. Rather than wait for the condition to get worse, I believe it is important to treat these children appropriately to bring the muscle inflammation under control. Often these children require only a short course of therapy.

Disease subtypes

Several subtypes of dermatomyositis have been recognized. The most common form is typically referred to as **unicyclic** (or *monocyclic*). This form of dermatomyositis most often occurs in small children, such as the girl described in the case history above. There is gradual onset of weakness and rash. On careful examination, these children are not found to have nail fold capillary abnormalities, poorly healing skin ulcers, or Gottren's papules.

Children with **polycyclic** disease usually have the same initial symptoms as those with unicyclic disease, but these children often do have nail fold capillary abnormalities and Gottren's papules. It is important to recognize that these children are different from the first group of children. They require more aggressive therapy for a longer period and remain at increased risk of relapse.

There is a group of patients with muscle disease and abnormal antibodies to transfer ribonucleic acid (tRNA) synthetase (Jo-1) and related molecules who have an increased frequency of lung involvement and other problems. Most of these patients are adults; these antibodies are rarely found in children. If they are present, more careful evaluation is required and more aggressive treatment may be necessary. It is not clear that this is the same disease.

Treatment

Unicyclic dermatomyositis responds well to corticosteroids and typically disappears within six months of beginning treatment. Treatment beyond a modest to moderate dose of corticosteroids is rarely necessary. Long-term complications of this form of dermatomyositis (including calcifications) are very rare.

Treatment for children with polycyclic disease is more complex. They more often require moderate doses of corticosteroids and seem to relapse more often. Methotrexate is often helpful, but these children may require therapy for six months or longer before they can be weaned off corticosteroids. Recurrences may occur, even years after the initial diagnosis. In some cases, children with poly-cyclic disease may require therapy with immunosuppressive medications such as rituximab or cyclosporine. Although some physicians like to use intravenous gamma globulin (IVIgG) in treating this group of children, I believe low-dose methotrexate is equally, if not more, effective, easier to administer, and far less costly. If they are treated aggressively, many of the children in this group do very well. Children with an extensive rash and skin ulcerations appear to have more severe disease and may follow a more protracted course.

Complications

Complications of properly treated unicyclic dermatomyositis are usually minor. In children with polycyclic disease vasculitis is characteristic. Its presence is strongly suggested by the occurrence of nail fold capillary abnormali-ties and Gottren's papules. There may be vasculitis of the intestines leading to abdominal pain and, rarely, perforation. Any child with dermatomyosi-tis who has chronic or recurrent abdominal pain must be investigated very carefully. Vasculitic complications can also occur in the central nervous sys-tem, lungs, and kidneys. Children with these complications require aggressive therapy.

Subcutaneous or intramuscular calcifications are the second major com-plication. These calcifications appear as the muscle inflammation is resolving and probably represent a scarring response. They may cause major problems. The calcifications may become infected. This occurs most often over the elbows or at other pressure points. They may spontaneously become swollen and ten-der and then drain to the outside. The initial drainage most often is not infected, but once leakage to the outside occurs, there is a significant risk that the lesion will become infected, with subsequent cellulitis and the risk of sepsis.

Large calcifications within the musculature may be a source of ongoing mus-cular irritation and also may become infected. Fine reticular calcification under the skin may also be seen on radiographs. There is little to be done for these com-plications. I have seen surgeons remove large calcifications, but this procedure may be associated with poor wound healing and significant long-term prob-lems. At one time, there were reports suggesting that these calcifications could be treated with warfarin, but this has proven unsatisfactory. There are reports describing substantial improvement after treatment with bisphosphonates. The best therapy for calcifications is to prevent their occurrence by providing prompt diagnosis and treatment for children with dermatomyositis.

Children with polycyclic disease may have several recurrences of muscle inflammation over a period of two or three years. They may be left with complications, but active muscle inflammation is less common beyond that point. Over time, many children with polycyclic disease slowly regain normal or near-normal strength and are able to function well as adults. The calcifications may also disappear over a period of years, though not always and not necessarily all of them.

A third group of children with dermatomyositis has **chronic recurrent disease**. The relationship of this form of the disease to the other forms is unclear. Children with chronic recurrent dermatomyositis often appear more sick during the acute phase of their illness. Their muscle enzyme levels are often very high and do not seem to respond significantly to therapy. Vasculitis is a common component of this form of the disease. Children with chronic recurrent dermatomyositis frequently require treatment with corticosteroids and methotrexate, but they may respond only incompletely. Fortunately, they are rarely as weak as their laboratory values suggest. The long-term prognosis for this group is uncertain.

POLYMYOSITIS

Sally was a six-year-old girl who was brought to me for a second opinion. Seven months previously, her mother had brought her to a local emergency room with a cough, cold, and fever. Blood work was done and an X-ray was taken. The child was sent home with cold medication. The next day, the emergency room physician called and insisted that the child return to the hospital. Sally was hospitalized and begun on corticosteroids because her muscle enzyme levels were significantly elevated. After a week Sally was discharged, and the corticosteroids were slowly withdrawn. Her mother had never noted Sally to be weak and noted only the changes caused by the steroids during the six months of therapy. At the end of six months, the corticosteroids were stopped completely. When her mother asked the doctors whether Sally was now well, she was told that nothing had changed. On evaluation, Sally was found to be a delightful young lady with no muscle weakness. Laboratory testing, however, revealed a markedly elevated CK level with no additional findings. Sally has remained well for five years with no treatment, but her muscle enzyme levels remain elevated.

Jenna was a five-year-old girl who became weak after an upper respiratory infection. Muscle enzyme testing revealed an elevated CK level, and the pediatrician was concerned that she might have muscular dystrophy. She was referred to the neurology clinic, where it was found that she had an inflammatory muscle condition but not muscular dystrophy (which is much more common in boys than girls and genetic in origin). She was treated with corticosteroids and slowly recovered.

Polymyositis is extremely rare in childhood. The absence of rash differentiates it from dermatomyositis. Children with polymyositis have the same pattern of proximal muscle weakness seen in children with dermatomyositis. This is a rare condition, and its natural history is unclear. Children such as Sally, who have markedly elevated muscle enzyme levels without rash or evident weakness, often have lipid myopathies or mitochondrial abnormalities—not polymyositis. Sally was not being evaluated for weakness or pain; her elevated muscle enzyme levels were discovered by accident. These levels did not normalize when she was initially treated, and since then she has done well without treatment. We are unsure of the significance of the prognosis for children like Sally. Such children do not benefit from corticosteroids In contrast, Jenna was weak, did have polymyositis, and did benefit from corticosteroids.

COMPLICATIONS OF DERMATOMYOSITIS AND POLYMYOSITIS

The common complications of dermatomyositis were discussed in the earlier sections on unicyclic, polycyclic, and chronic recurrent disease. In addition to these complications, there are rare complications related to **vasculitis of the central nervous system**. This can result in psychological disturbances, hallucinations, and even seizures. Children with these complications must be treated aggressively. The kidneys are also involved in some children with polycyclic or chronic recurrent disease.

Lipodystrophy is a more unusual complication seen in some children with dermatomyositis. This condition is associated with widespread loss of subcutaneous fat. Some children have lesser areas of involvement, a condition referred to as **localized** or **partial lipodystrophy**. Children with generalized lipodystrophy are very thin. Characteristic of the loss of subcutaneous fat is the ability to easily see the blood vessels through the skin. Even in its partial form, this condition may be associated with abnormal lipid metabolism and diabetes with insulin resistance. Although some centers report this in as many as one-quarter of their patients, in most centers lipodystrophy is a rare complication. Its relationship to the diagnosis of dermatomyositis is unclear. Children with lipodystrophy need to be under the care of a multidisciplinary team in an experienced center.

Medical treatment

The type of disease, the degree of weakness, and the nature of the complications determine the medical treatment of dermatomyositis. If a child is very weak, immediate intervention with high-dose intravenous steroids may be important. If a child has developed a nasal voice or has begun to cough when eating, immediate intervention is vital. These findings suggest weakness of the pharyngeal muscles and the risk of aspiration.

For children without evidence of vasculitis who are not profoundly weak, a low or moderate dose of corticosteroids is often sufficient. Some children with dermatomyositis have mild arthritis when they first present. This usually responds well to treatment with corticosteroids, but a brief course of NSAIDs may also be beneficial. Hydroxychloroquine is often useful as a steroid-sparing agent.

Children with evidence of vasculitis often respond well to a moderate dose of corticosteroids. Typically, as the corticosteroids are withdrawn, these children develop recurrent problems. The addition of methotrexate is often beneficial. Alternative regimens include cyclosporine, IVGIgA or—for severe methotrexate-resistant disease—rituximab and/or cyclophosphamide. These agents are rarely necessary for unicyclic disease but may be necessary for more severe polycyclic disease. Although preliminary reports suggested that TNF-α blocking agents, such as etanercept and adalimumab, may prove useful, in general they have not been satisfactory for dermatomyositis.

Optimal therapy for chronic recurrent dermatomyositis and polymyositis in childhood remains unclear. Most children are initially treated as if they had polycyclic disease, with subsequent therapy based on the severity of the symptoms and the experience of the physician. Children with the characteristic rash and elevated muscle enzyme levels require treatment even in the absence of evident weakness. They have ongoing inflammation, and there is no sense in waiting for enough muscle cells to die to make it obvious that they are weak before treating them.

Over the long term, persistent weakness and secondary calcifications remain the most distressing problems for children with dermatomyositis. Rapid diagnosis and appropriate treatment minimize cell death. Since calcifications in the skin and musculature are a healing response, early aggressive therapy is the best means of prevention. Bisphosphonates are helpful for children with extensive dystrophic calcification.

Physical therapy

Physical therapy to maintain range of motion and maximize the strength of the remaining musculature is a major component of care for children with dermatomyositis. During the period of active muscle inflammation, the therapists should concentrate on passive range of motion. Only after the muscle inflammation has been controlled should active range-of-motion exercises begin.

Surgical therapy

In general, surgical therapy is not a significant component of the care of children with dermatomyositis. Excision and drainage of infected calcifications may be necessary in some children. Poor wound healing limits the utility of surgical efforts to remove large calcifications. Children with intestinal vasculitis may require urgent intervention.

Prognosis

The prognosis for most children with dermatomyositis is very good. Unicyclic disease is the form most commonly seen, and these children should do well. With early diagnosis and prompt therapy, most children with polycyclic disease also have a good outcome, provided the patient's family seeks care promptly. Children with polycyclic disease have a more guarded prognosis. This is also true for children who have substantial muscle atrophy or suffer from multiple intramuscular calcifications. These conditions are often the result of delayed diagnosis or inadequate therapy. These children should be referred to specialized centers.

Repeated pulmonary infections resulting from excessive muscle loss leading to difficulty in coughing and clearing the respiratory tract occur in the most severe cases. Sepsis and right heart failure are major concerns. Fortunately, such cases have become rare, and with prompt diagnosis and treatment, the majority of children with dermatomyositis will do well.

17

Kawasaki Disease

Billy was a three-year-old boy who had always been in good health. Ten days before he was sent to my office, his mother noted that he appeared irritable. He had a low-grade fever, and the next day he was taken to the pediatrician to be checked for an ear infection. There was no otitis, but Billy was given antibiotic drops for his conjunctivitis. Over the next two days, Billy remained irritable. Although his eyes got better, his fever continued.

When his mother noted a tender lump under his chin, she brought him back to the pediatrician. Billy was started on antibiotics for a cervical adenitis. He developed a rash the next day, and the antibiotic was changed because he was possibly allergic. Three days later, his mother returned to the pediatrician because Billy was not getting better. He still had fever, and the tender lump under his chin was getting larger despite the antibiotics. Now his lips were dry and beginning to split. His tongue was red and irritated.

The WBC count, ESR, and platelet count were all very high. Billy was sent to me, and the diagnosis of Kawasaki disease was confirmed. He was treated with intravenous gamma globulin (IVIgG), and his symptoms disappeared promptly. We monitored his heart; there was no sign of heart involvement. Billy recovered completely.

Quick Summary

- Kawasaki disease (KD) most often affects young children (generally under the age of five years), and the diagnosis should be questioned in anyone over the age of ten.
- **"Atypical" KD is almost always typical something else!**
- Children with KD who do not respond promptly to treatment with IVIgG should be carefully evaluated to be sure that the diagnosis is correct, and corticosteroid treatment should be considered.

- It is not true that IVIgG is ineffective after the tenth day. Efficacy after the tenth day has never been studied! The original study was set up to determine whether IVIgG was effective in preventing aneurysms. Since most aneurysms are thought to begin at or soon after day ten, earlier treatment gave IVIgG the best chance of blocking the aneurysms. Children seen after the tenth day were excluded from the study.

- If a child who is being evaluated for KD has a low platelet count, something is definitely wrong. Kawasaki disease does not cause low platelet counts.

- Kawasaki disease is not the only disease that causes coronary artery aneurysms or thickening of the coronary arteries on echocardiograms. These findings alone do not establish the diagnosis.

- Kawasaki disease is not the only condition that causes peeling of the skin in the perineum or on the fingertips. Again, this finding does not establish the diagnosis.

- Anti-inflammatory therapy is important even after IVIgG has been given. Children should be given one aspirin daily (81 mg baby aspirin for small children) to reduce the risk of blood clot–related problems, but traditional NSAIDs, such as naproxen, are safer and easier to use as the main anti-inflammatory therapy. They can be given with the one aspirin daily. The NSAIDs should be continued until the ESR has been normal for several weeks. The duration of the aspirin therapy depends on the child's cardiac status.

Kawasaki disease usually begins in a young child as fever and irritability without apparent explanation. Otitis may be suspected. Within the first few days, some children develop a swollen lymph node below the jaw. Usually, this is thought to be cervical adenitis and is treated with antibiotics. Young children with high fevers who do not develop a swollen lymph node are frequently begun on antibiotics for presumed ear infections. Some children already have a rash at this point, but often the child will develop a rash the next day that may be confused with an allergy to the antibiotic.

Physicians usually do not begin to think about KD until the child continues to have fever and rash even after antibiotic therapy. In a typical case the child will continue to look worse, with nonpurulent conjunctivitis and dry, cracked red lips or an irritated tongue. These symptoms usually appear over the next few days of the illness. The hands and feet often become diffusely swollen at about the seventh day of the illness. Laboratory tests indicate a rising WBC count, ESR, and platelet count—sometimes to very high levels.

Early diagnosis of KD is difficult because many serious infections are identical to KD at the beginning. The diagnostic criteria require a fever for at least five days with no response to antibiotics. Children with measles and severe streptococcal infections may fulfill the criteria for KD. One interesting observation is the frequent occurrence of marked redness and swelling at the site of bacille Calmette-Guérin (BCG) vaccinations in children developing KD.

Box 17-1   Criteria for the diagnosis of Kawasaki disease

Fever of at least five days' duration plus four or more of the following:

- Nonspecific rash or polymorphic exanthem (any rash)
- Cracked (fissured), red lips or irritated tongue ("strawberry tongue")
- Diffuse swelling of the hands or feet with redness of the palms and soles
- Conjunctivitis without pus affecting both eyes
- Swelling of the cervical nodes (in the neck, usually just under the chin)

ETIOLOGY

The cause of KD is not well understood. The disease tends to occur in epidemics, which suggests that it is an infection. However, infections usually spread among children in the same household. For KD it is rare (about 3 percent) to find a second child in the same household or a playmate with the disease. However, there is evidence that KD is spread by exposure to some type of agent. It is more common in areas that have been recently flooded and in households where the carpets have recently been shampooed. These observations suggest that dampness must play a role. Careful investigations of viruses, fungi, and bacteria have not produced convincing findings. It is likely that KD is not a common result of an uncommon agent, but rather an uncommon result of a common agent. This would explain the disease's predilection for young children and its occurrence in epidemics.

MEDICAL TREATMENT

Once the diagnosis of KD is established, the antibiotics can be stopped and appropriate anti-inflammatory therapy started. Intravenous gamma globulin should be given as soon as possible after the diagnosis has been established because this often quickly stops the inflammation associated with KD. The early administration of IVIgG (within ten days of the onset of symptoms) has been shown to dramatically reduce the risk of developing coronary artery aneurysms. If physicians are unsure of the diagnosis but want to treat with IVIgG, they should save a tube of blood for later serologic testing. Intravenous gamma globulin contains pooled antibodies from many different people. Once it has been given, serologic tests to look for other explanations for the child's illness will be unreliable for many weeks.

Some physicians believe that IVIgG should be given only during the first ten days of illness. This is wrong. Even if the disease has been going on for more than ten days, it is safe to give IVIgG, and IVIgG is effective in treating the inflammation (see "Quick Summary" at the beginning of this chapter). The efficacy of IVIgG in preventing aneurysms when given after the tenth day has not been studied. However, it still does an excellent job of bringing the inflammation associated with KD under control in most patients.

Some children with KD have less common symptoms. One well-described pattern is severe abdominal pain with gallbladder involvement. This responds to therapy for the KD and in most cases does not require special treatment. Severe headaches and neck pain are also well-described but less common findings. Some children with KD develop aseptic meningitis. Arthritis with pain and swelling of the knees also occurs in some children with KD. Other uncommon but well-described findings include inflammation of the pancreas, the kidneys, and the urinary tract. All of these findings may cause confusion, but if they are due to KD, they respond quickly to IVIgG therapy.

Intravenous gamma globulin treatment is followed quickly by an end to the fever and prompt improvement in other symptoms in children with typical KD. Occasionally, children require a second dose of IVIgG. **Any child who is not better after two doses of IVIgG should be carefully reevaluated.** I have seen children with polyarteritis nodosa, systemic-onset JRA, and other rheumatic diseases and infections mistakenly diagnosed as having KD. They do not get better with IVIgG or they improve only briefly.

At one time, it was thought that treatment with corticosteroids might make a child with KD more likely to develop coronary artery aneurysms or make the aneurysms worse. This has now been disproven.If two doses of IVIgG have not improved the child's condition, the diagnosis of KD should be reconsidered. **In the absence of infection or any other contraindication, corticosteroids may be given to children who have not responded to IVIgG.** Although there are reported cases of children with KD improving significantly but relapsing a few days later, this is rare. There are also reports of children having had KD twice, with months to years separating the episodes. These recurrences are very infrequent.

COMPLICATIONS

Once the diagnosis of KD has been established, the major concern is whether the child has any cardiac involvement. Early in the illness, a small number of children develop pancarditis. There are also children who develop coronary artery aneurysms very early in their disease. Children with very large coronary artery aneurysms (greater than 8 mm) early in KD have frequent cardiac problems and should be cared for at an advanced center.

Fortunately, most children with KD have no aneurysms or only thickening of the coronary arteries on echocardiogram. This thickening is often not meaningful and can be seen in children who have other conditions. Children without coronary artery aneurysms have an excellent prognosis. Although IVIgG decreases the frequency of coronary artery aneurysms, it does not always prevent them.

Children who do develop coronary artery aneurysms need careful follow-up. There are two major concerns. The first is a myocardial infarction due to blockage of the artery. This may occur during the first weeks of illness. Fortunately, it is rare in children who are properly diagnosed and treated. The second is that the damaged coronary artery may ultimately scar, predisposing the child to heart problems years later. This is why it is important for children to have continued cardiologic follow-up, even if they look fine.

A small number of children with KD do develop aneurysms in other arteries; these aneurysms may cause problems either during the initial illness or later. A variety of other unusual complications of KD have been described. Their relationship to the disease is uncertain. The long-term prognosis for most children who have been properly treated for KD is believed to be excellent.

DIFFERENTIAL DIAGNOSIS

The most important aspect of the diagnosis and treatment of KD is prompt recognition of the disease. At the same time, it is necessary to remember that there are a variety of illnesses that may produce a similar appearance. It is very important to be sure that the child is not suffering from a significant infection. Measles, streptococcal infections, drug reactions, and many forms of vasculitis may result in a clinical picture that satisfies the criteria for a diagnosis of KD. Hemolytic uremic syndrome has also been confused with KD.

There is a significant concern that children diagnosed with atypical KD in fact have another illness. Such children should be carefully evaluated. Coronary artery aneurysms may occur in children with a number of rheumatic diseases, including polyarteritis nodosa and Takayasu's arteritis. Further, thickening of the coronary arteries on echocardiogram is a nonspecific finding and should not be used to establish a diagnosis of KD. It may occur in many other conditions.

Mucocutaneous lymph node syndrome is simply an old name for KD. This is the name it was originally given by Dr. Kawasaki, who first recognized the syndrome among his patients in Japan. The name was changed to honor him years after his initial description of the disease. There is also an illness called **infantile polyarteritis nodosa**. The clinical symptoms of this disease are different from the normal symptoms of KD. However, when specialists compare the pathologic material from children who died of KD with material from children who died of infantile polyarteritis, it is not possible to distinguish the diseases. Most likely, infantile polyarteritis is KD. It is now rare for anyone to make the diagnosis of infantile polyarteritis.

Laboratory findings in KD typically include a dramatically rising WBC count, ESR, and platelet count. Failure of any of these indices to rise appropriately by the seventh day of illness should raise suspicion. A falling platelet count is never consistent with the diagnosis of KD unless there are severe complicating factors. Although small amounts of RBCs and WBCs may appear in the urine, significant kidney involvement is not a normal manifestation of KD. These findings should cast doubt on the diagnosis of KD and prompt a thorough reevaluation of the child.

18

Benign Hypermobile Joint Syndrome and Ehlers-Danlos Syndrome

Benign hypermobile joint syndrome is not really a disease at all. Instead, **it is an inherited variation on normal.** Children with benign hypermobile joint syndrome are often referred to as being *double-jointed*. Many children have loose joints or joints that they can voluntarily subluxate. The diagnosis of benign hypermobile joint syndrome requires that a child be able to do each of the following:

- Bend the fingers back over the wrist so that they are parallel with the forearm (i.e., they point straight backward)
- Easily bend the thumb back to touch the forearm
- Extend the elbow beyond 180 degrees
- Extend the knee beyond 180 degrees
- Bend over and touch the palms to the floor with the knees straight

The ability to bend joints to a greater than normal degree does not usually seem to be a handicap. Indeed, many young girls with benign hypermobile joint syndrome are extremely good gymnasts. They can do splits and other gymnastic activities that other girls can only imagine doing. The problem becomes evident when they do too much gymnastics too early in life—as in Tania's story at the beginning of Chapter 5.

Imagine that you have two sets of small wooden trains to play with. In one set the train cars are connected by metal hooks that hold each car firmly attached to the car in front. This train may not be able to turn sharply, but all of the cars will always remain in the proper position. If you don't intentionally damage the set, the train will stay in perfect condition. Now imagine another set with the train cars attached to each other by rubber bands. These cars will be able to move about much more flexibly, and the train will be able to make very sharp turns without difficulty. However, when you pull the train forward, the second car may not begin to move right away. Instead, it waits for the rubber band to tighten before moving. The same thing happens with each of the remaining cars. Once they all start to move, the train will move well until the first car stops. Then the momentum of the second car is likely to cause it to crash into the back of the first car. Each of the remaining cars will also crash into the car in front of it. If you play with this train set very often, all of the cars will be damaged by the repeated crashes. Pretty soon, it won't look nearly as good as the first train set.

The role of the ligaments is to maintain the bones in proper position with respect to each other. If they are loose, they don't perform this function properly. In children with benign hypermobile joint syndrome, the ligaments are loose and the bones are not held tightly in alignment. Over time, this leads to damage to the bones and joints that may become quite severe. You can't surgically correct the ligaments that are loose because the collagen they are made from is structurally weaker. The key is to recognize the syndrome and allow the children to reduce their activity and minimize the damage.

Most often, the children I see with benign hypermobile joint syndrome are ten- or eleven-year-old girls who have been recognized to have a lot of talent in physical education class. They are taking extra gymnastics or ballet classes and are believed to have great potential. However, they are beginning to complain of pains in their knees or other joints after practice. This can result from overuse of normal joints, but the child with ligamentous laxity is likely to have both earlier problems and more severe problems. Often when I take the history, I find that the symptoms began at seven or eight years of age. If the activity has been continued despite the pain, there may be joint swelling and pain on compression. Sustained painful activity can lead to permanent damage to the bones and joints.

At present, the relationship of Ehlers-Danlos syndrome and benign hypermobile joint syndrome is complicated by a disagreement over nomenclature. Some physicians refer to benign hypermobile joint syndrome as Ehlers-Danlos syndrome type III. Since a search for Ehlers-Danlos syndrome on the Internet will reveal descriptions of major complications, this causes the children's parents to become very alarmed unnecessarily.

Classical Ehlers-Danlos syndrome is that of a child who is tall (and usually thin), with long arms, long legs, and long, thin fingers (children with Marfan's syndrome may also have some of these characteristics). These children have a severe collagen defect and are easily recognized because it is easy to stretch their skin. If these children have a cut, it will heal poorly and the scars often become unusually large and thin ("cigarette paper" scars). By the time they are ten or eleven years old, these children have often had multiple orthopedic problems because of their loose ligaments.

If you are evaluating a child for benign hypermobile joint syndrome, you should look carefully for any unusual scars. Ask their parents how well the child's skin heals. Any child with unusual scars, poor healing, or unusually loose joints should be referred to an experienced center where a complete evaluation for the possibility of Ehlers-Danlos syndrome can be done. Genetic testing will detect the most common forms of Ehlers-Danlos syndrome, but it does not detect every case.

The evaluation of children in whom Ehlers-Danlos syndrome is suspected should include an echocardiogram to evaluate the aortic root. This should be done when they are first brought to the physician's attention and periodically thereafter. However, it is unclear whether children with simple benign hypermobile joint syndrome ever have these problems. If you are in doubt, you should refer the child for further evaluation but avoid frightening the parents by calling the problem Ehlers-Danlos syndrome.

MEDICAL TREATMENT

The joint pains and irritation associated with benign hypermobile joint syndrome can be relieved with mild NSAIDs, but the key to proper treatment is minimizing the activities that cause pain until the body matures further. It is important for pediatricians to emphasize to families that continued activity will not promote the child's future ability; it will instead cause damage. "No pain, no gain" may apply to muscles, but it is completely wrong when applied to bones and joints. Joints are being damaged!

PROGNOSIS

Most children with benign hypermobile joint syndrome do very well. They may need to work with a physical therapist to strengthen the muscles around the joint. Surgery is necessary only if severe joint damage has occurred. I occasionally see children who have had repeated surgery in an effort to stop recurrent subluxation. Because the ligaments are structurally weak, this surgery often fails. It is best avoided if possible.

Significant complications of benign hypermobile joint syndrome are very rare. However, it is important to recognize that type II collagen utilized in ligaments is also used in structures such as the aortic root. Children with very significant ligamentous laxity should have an echocardiogram as a precaution. Some children with Ehlers-Danlos syndrome are mistakenly thought to have only benign hypermobile joint syndrome.

19

Fibromyalgia and Chronic Fatigue Syndrome

Sue Ellen was a sixteen-year-old who complained of fatigue and weakness. She was unable to go to school because she could not get out of bed in the morning and complained of hurting all over. Six months previously, she had developed a severe viral infection with fever, rash, and diffuse aches and pains. Although the fever and rash resolved within a week, she never regained her strength. She had been seen by several physicians and had been treated for Lyme disease—despite negative blood tests—with no response. A thorough physical examination and comprehensive laboratory testing found no abnormalities except for multiple trigger points. I explained to Sue Ellen and her family that we would all have to work together to help her get well. With the aid of her family, and friends, a program of steadily increasing activities and school attendance was devised. She often became discouraged because she tried to do too much and exhausted herself. It took several months for Sue Ellen to resume her normal activities. However, once she realized that she was the most important member of the team working to restore her health, she made steady progress to a full recovery.

Tracy was brought to me at the age of fourteen after being diagnosed with fibromyalgia. She was obese and came from a troubled family. Tracy was not very interested in physical activities, and complained that she hurt all over and tired easily. Pressure over the expected trigger points for fibromyalgia produced complaints, but so did pressure in many other places. Laboratory evaluation indicated a mild elevation of the ESR and a positive ANA but nothing specific. Tracy was started on therapy for fibromyalgia and followed carefully. After a few visits, she came to trust me and asked for help with her depression. She was referred to a psychologist.

Over the next six months, it was noted that Tracy was developing an increasing number of red spots on her hands and face. These were telangiectasias. Testing for anticentromere antibody revealed that she was

246

positive with an extremely high titer, and we began appropriate treatment for her CREST syndrome. Had she simply been dismissed as another teenager with fibromyalgia, therapy for her CREST syndrome would have been significantly delayed.

Mrs. Smith was the mother of a three-year-old girl who was referred to the neurology clinic for developmental delay. Mrs. Smith's daughter did not reach the milestones of sitting independently, crawling, or walking by herself at appropriate ages. Even after she was able to do these activities, the little girl never wanted to play as much as her friends did. She seemed very bright otherwise; she just tired too easily. During the evaluation of her daughter, Mrs. Smith asked if chronic fatigue syndrome could be inherited. All her life, Mrs. Smith had tired easily and had never been good at getting everything done. Even as an adult, she had been sent to a psychiatrist because she felt too worn out to complete all of her household chores every day. She had been told that she had a typical case of chronic fatigue syndrome.

As the evaluation of Mrs. Smith's daughter progressed, it became evident that she was abnormally weak. A muscle biopsy found that the little girl had nemaline myopathy—an inherited condition producing muscle weakness. While talking to Mrs. Smith, the neurologist who cared for her daughter realized that Mrs. Smith had all the symptoms of nemaline myopathy as well. A muscle biopsy confirmed the diagnosis. The diagnosis of chronic fatigue syndrome was wrong. Her case illustrates why it is important to make sure that a diagnosis of chronic fatigue syndrome is correct. However, it should be remembered that Mrs. Smith had been weak all her life. This is not the expected history in someone with chronic fatigue syndrome.

Quick Summary

The most important thing to remember in evaluating a child with fibromyalgia or chronic fatigue syndrome is to be sure that the diagnosis is correct. Although these are complex syndromes that may be difficult to treat, many of the children who come to me as complicated cases had not improved simply because they had been given incorrect diagnoses. Every child with chronic pain and fatigue deserves a complete diagnostic evaluation. There should be no significant laboratory abnormalities in children with either fibromyalgia or chronic fatigue.

WHAT IS FIBROMYALGIA?

Children with **fibromyalgia** complain of widespread pain and fatigue that interfere with normal activities. Often they have missed many days of school because of difficulty getting up in the morning. With increasing school absence, these children have often been to a variety of physicians without receiving a definitive diagnosis. The generally accepted criteria for a diagnosis of fibromyalgia require widespread pain (above and below the waist and on both the right and left sides) and the presence of at least eleven of eighteen defined trigger points.

Many different etiologies of fibromyalgia have been proposed, but none is uniformly accepted. It often follows a severe viral infection or an injury. In the majority of cases, it appears that the child never fully recovered from the injury or infection. Often the parents and physicians have become frustrated because "it should have gotten better a long time ago." Because of the long-term nature of their complaints and their poor response to medications, children with fibromyalgia have one of the most challenging illnesses.

Proposed explanations for the continuing pain and fatigue suffered by children with fibromyalgia emphasize increased sensitivity of the nervous system. This has been ascribed to damaged nerve conduction pathways, altered hormonal balance, persisting infectious agents, and many other possible causes. **None of the proposed explanations has provided the scientific basis for consistently useful therapy**. This has resulted in a large number of frustrated families and physicians.

The children and their families do not understand why the doctors cannot help the children. I often see children who have had a bad viral infection just like several of their friends, but unlike their friends, they never recovered. They continue to complain that they are tired and do not feel well. Often they do not go to school or miss as many days of school as they attend. Whenever they try to do what the doctors recommend to help them get better, it just makes them feel worse.

The first thing to do in such circumstances is to conduct a thorough evaluation to find out whether something has been missed. Often this will yield an unsuspected clue, and the child's regimen can be adjusted so that he or she recovers. However, in many cases, no explanation is found and the child remains disabled.

CHRONIC FATIGUE SYNDROME

Chronic fatigue syndrome differs from fibromyalgia because the patients lack the typical trigger points associated with fibromyalgia. Like fibromyalgia, chronic fatigue syndrome is not associated with laboratory abnormalities, a known cause, or a known cure. Physicians should be cautious in making this diagnosis. I have seen numerous children with rheumatic diseases who were initially dismissed as having chronic fatigue syndrome because nothing was found on routine examination and their blood tests were normal. Once the diagnosis of chronic fatigue syndrome has been established **and other significant medical problems have been excluded,** children with chronic fatigue syndrome should be rehabilitated using the method described for fibromyalgia in the next section.

HOW TO TREAT FIBROMYALGIA AND CHRONIC FATIGUE SYNDROME

In the absence of a well-accepted scientific explanation for fibromyalgia, many physicians and families feel frustrated. They are waiting for someone to discover the cause and the cure. They feel helpless and do not know what to do. Pediatricians must make it clear to families that simply tolerating the situation is unacceptable. Often, too much time and money have been wasted on promised "miracle cures," such as natural medicines, diets, or supplements. Instead, I ask the families to think of how they would respond if a truck had hit their child.

If you were hit by a truck, you could easily suffer serious damage to both femurs, which might require surgery and/or traction for many weeks. Then one day the orthopedist comes into the room, orders the traction removed, and announces that your femurs have healed. You won't just get out of bed and walk away "cured." While lying flat on your back, you suffered a major loss of muscle strength and endurance. It is very difficult to start walking again. Even sitting at the side of the bed may make you dizzy.

Relearning how to walk and rebuilding strength and endurance is a slow, painful process. People who have suffered major injuries go through a long and difficult period of gradual recovery. There is no magic pill that will speed up the process. They have to do the work. The physicians and physical therapists can provide guidance and encouragement, but only the patients can make themselves better. Emotionally, however, it's relatively easy if a truck hit you. There are many witnesses to what happened, and no one thinks that it is your fault.

Children with fibromyalgia suffer a similar degree of disability and have an equally difficult path to recovery. But it's much harder for the child when no one understands what hit him or what's wrong with him. However, there is still only one person who can start the recovery process, and that person is the patient. There is no magic pill for fibromyalgia any more than there is a magic pill for recovery after being hit by a truck.

My approach to caring for children with fibromyalgia is to emphasize reha-bilitation and return to activities of daily living. If one views recovery from fibromyalgia as one would view recovery from a major physical injury, the appro-priate steps become self-evident. At every step, the child, family, and physicians must recognize that there will not be a sudden, miraculous recovery. Progress is made through a rigorous program of slow and steadily increasing level of activities, just as if both legs had been broken. It is equally important for every member of the team to acknowledge the reality of the initial injury and the psychological difficulty of dealing with it, just as they would acknowledge the difficulty of recovering if the child had been hit by a truck.

The absence of a uniformly effective therapy for fibromyalgia places a signif-icant burden on the parents and physicians caring for these children. Several key points must be remembered:

- This is not a self-induced illness. The children definitely want to get better.
- Children with this illness suffer from disordered sleep, and often complain of difficulty sleeping at night and being tired all day.
- Opiate pain medications do not relieve any symptoms other than pain. They frequently cause nausea, worsen sleep patterns, increase the child's sense of ill health, and interfere with school attendance and normal life.
- Depression probably does not cause fibromyalgia, but fibromyalgia defi-nitely does cause depression.

Injured children often recover faster than children with fibromyalgia because everyone understands the injury and what needs to be done to promote healing. Injured children are treated sympathetically but firmly. We need to treat children with fibromyalgia the same way.

Some children recover well with time, reassurance, medications, and support from their family and doctors. For more difficult cases, a hospital-based team approach is often beneficial. The team in a large children's rehabilitation center consists of nurses, physical and occupational therapists, social workers, psychologists, and pediatricians. Most often, even children with difficult-to-treat fibromyalgia can be managed on an outpatient basis, but that does not eliminate the need for all team members to participate in their care. Once the diagnosis of fibromyalgia has been confirmed, it is important for the family to meet with all the appropriate members of the team. While this is being done, the family can take the first steps toward recovery.

STEPS TO RECOVERY

Getting Back on Schedule

Anyone who has traveled overseas and suffered jet lag understands the impact of disordered sleep patterns. Although a variety of remedies may be useful, the key to all of them is to promptly begin to set your body's wake/sleep cycle on the appropriate schedule for the time zone you are in. Similarly, families can start to put their children back on a regular schedule of getting up at an appropriate time in the morning (the same time as if they were going to school). This should be accompanied by a policy on lights, computers, televisions, video games, and so on that must be turned off at the appropriate time for a school night. **Do not expect instant success.** Inexperienced travelers often report two to three weeks of difficulty in adjusting to a new time zone. However, if they get up at the appropriate time in the morning, it becomes easier and easier to fall asleep at the appropriate time and sleep through the night.

Increasing Physical Activity

Even as the child is adjusting to getting up at the appropriate time each morning, it is important to begin a program of gradually increasing physical activity. For children in the rehabilitation center, this is done under the supervision of a physical therapist. For children attending school and receiving outpatient treatment, this may not be necessary. Children who are not attending school will need regularly scheduled physical therapy at least three days a week with parent-supervised physical activity on the other days. Too often, families overreach in this initial physical therapy. (There are special supervised programs that "jump-start" therapy for children with severe disease under carefully supervised conditions. Intense therapy is appropriate for the children selected to participate in these programs.)

A child who has been incapacitated for a prolonged period will need to start exercising slowly. At first, three or four fifteen-minute sessions may be all the child is capable of in a given day. Significant muscular discomfort normally accompanies the resumption of activities in a child who has been disabled for a prolonged period. This discomfort may be treated with NSAIDs, topical creams for sore muscles, and massage. The key to the success of this program is that it be continued despite the muscle soreness and related complaints—just as it would be for someone hit by a truck.

Physical and Occupational Therapy

Physical and occupational therapy play a vital role in the care of children with severe fibromyalgia. Just as a child severely injured by a truck would never be expected to recover without physical therapy, a child with severe fibromyalgia should not be expected to do it alone. The key is to find a therapist who understands that the injury in fibromyalgia is every bit as real as the injury to the child who was hit by a truck. The program of slowly increasing physical activities to improve strength and endurance must be tailored to the disability level of the child. However, it must have the ultimate goal of achieving complete recovery. If a truck had hit the child, everyone would understand that complete recovery might require months of therapy and that, even a year later, the child might not be fully recovered. Fibromyalgia is no different.

Psychological and Emotional Support

During the initial weeks of establishing a program of normal wake/sleep hours and exercise, **it is normal for the child to increase his or her complaints and the parents to become discouraged.**Psychological and emotional support from the family and the psychologist treating the child is critical at this point. Antidepressant medications may be necessary for some children during this stage. Over a period of three months, it should be possible to gradually increase the level of physical activity to the point where the child feels capable of returning to school. In a rehabilitation setting, this corresponds to three or more thirty-minute periods of sustained exercise each day.

It is normal for children to experience significant discomfort and resist the program of rehabilitation at several key points in time. Despite the best intentions, at the beginning they will have difficulty adjusting their sleep schedule and resuming physical activity. There is frequently another period of difficulty and resistance six to eight weeks into the program. Children frequently decide that "This is not working, and I'm tired of it." **Just as we would never allow a child to give up on recovering after being hit by a truck, we cannot let these children give up.** These periods of stress and frustration are a normal part of every recovery. Parents and children should be told to expect them before they occur. Continuing physical, emotional, and psychological support is key to working through these episodes.

The major long-term disability associated with fibromyalgia results from the loss of strength and endurance and the accompanying loss of self-confidence and self-esteem. If the child hit by a truck had bad dreams or was afraid to return to school, no one would be embarrassed to ask for psychological help. Unfortunately, because we do not understand what happened to them, children with fibromyalgia often do not get the sympathetic support given to children with obvious injuries. From a psychological point of view, this makes the situation much worse for children with fibromyalgia. A sympathetic family, a sympathetic physician, and a sympathetic psychologist or psychiatrist are all very important.

Just as we would force a child with an obvious physical injury to do the work necessary to recover, we must push the child with fibromyalgia to recover. Psychological support is critical for both the child and the family when the inevitable resistance occurs. The physical and emotional pain of going a little further and trying a little harder every day is often best dealt with by solid emotional support. A psychologist or psychiatrist can play a vital role in helping the child and family to deal with these issues.

Expect a Relapse

Some children will relapse within four to six weeks of returning to school and having a normal schedule. The rehabilitation team routinely anticipates this setback. Children are so anxious to succeed that they often push themselves beyond their limits during their first days back. Depending on the situation, the rehabilitation team may choose initially to have the child restart school on a part-time basis in order to avoid this problem. This is a decision that should be made by the entire team working together.

Periodic relapse or fear of relapse in association with viral infections and other stresses may occur. The key to successful management of these episodes is for the child and family to pull together and keep things on track. While it may be necessary to spend twenty-four to forty-eight hours in bed with the flu, it is essential that children with a history of fibromyalgia promptly get back on their feet and resume their normal activity. The attitude of the rehabilitation team and the family must be one of steady reassurance and support for the child.

Equally important in the care of children with fibromyalgia is recognition of the needs of other family members (see Chapter 27). Children who are recovering from a severe illness suffer significant additional stress when the stress of their illness is visibly upsetting other family members. Given the difficult nature of the gradual recovery process following any major injury, this additional stress may cause a significant psychological setback. This is why it is important that the entire family, including parents and siblings, be involved in the educational activities and psychological counseling that are part of the rehabilitation process. Too often other family members view the sensitivity of the child with fibromyalgia as manipulative behavior. These complex dynamics can be properly dealt with only if the entire family is willing to participate in the process.

Treatment in the Home

Children with mild fibromyalgia often do not require hospitalization. Their treatment at home should be based on the same principles described in the previous sections. It may be slower and more difficult because it is harder to provide a consistent wake/sleep schedule and physical therapy in the home environment. Willing participation by all family members will lead to a greater chance of success. Everyone needs to help the affected child recover. Many school districts have nurses and psychologists who can coordinate their efforts with the treating physician. Central to this process is education of those caring for the child. Physicians, nurses, teachers, or others who convey a negative attitude toward children with fibromyalgia need to be properly educated.

Resentment and resistance are just as likely to occur in children treated at home as in those treated in the hospital. Parents must be instructed both to expect these episodes and to deal with them in an understanding manner. However, understanding does not mean giving in. The program of exercises and activities necessary to regain strength and confidence can succeed only if it is carried out. Families that find themselves unable to handle the ups and downs of managing a child with fibromyalgia at home will need to consider inpatient therapy. With appropriate support from the physician and other care providers, most families can succeed.

Medical Treatment

Medications are a key component of therapy for adults with fibromyalgia. They are less important in children. However, NSAIDs, including tramadol, may be helpful in controlling the aches and pains associated with activity. Pregabalin is a medication that has been approved for the treatment of fibromyalgia. It reduces the transmission of nervous impulses carrying the sensation of pain. However, although it is certainly helpful, it is not magic. Amitriptyline is an antidepressant that has been found to benefit children and adults with fibromyalgia. While some of the benefit may be from the antidepressant effect, amitriptyline appears to have additional effects that help fibromyalgia sufferers. Children who are greatly troubled by muscle spasm often benefit from the addition of cyclobenzaprine or a similar agent (all of these drugs are discussed in Chapter 23).

What I have described in this chapter is not a cure for fibromyalgia. None exists. Nor is there a cure for having been hit by a truck. Our goal must be to help children overcome the symptoms of fibromyalgia and regain useful lives. Children with fibromyalgia must be educated to understand their illness and how to cope with it. With the benefit of this knowledge, they can deal with symptoms that might recur and continue their lives in a normal fashion.

PROGNOSIS

The prognosis for children with fibromyalgia or chronic fatigue syndrome who get proper care is excellent. However, just as a child left to languish in bed after an injury will do poorly, so will a child with these illnesses. A child with fibromyalgia or chronic fatigue syndrome should be able to be rehabilitated and to resume a fully productive life.

20

Reflex Sympathetic Dystrophy, Reflex Neurovascular Dystrophy, and Complex Regional Pain Syndromes

Fourteen-year-old Cindy was the ultimate figure skater. Her parents had met while skating in college. Briefly after college, her father had skated professionally, but her mother stopped skating shortly after graduating from college so that they could start a family. Cindy's father was now a successful businessman, and Cindy's mother stayed home to promote Cindy's development as a figure skater. Cindy had been skating as long as she could remember. But for the past six months, Cindy had been unable to skate because of ankle pain. There was no doubt about how Cindy's ankle was injured. Hundreds of spectators witnessed her fall at the regional skating championships. X-rays did not show a fracture, but her orthopedist immediately placed her foot in a cast to rest the ankle and make sure that it healed properly.

After three weeks of complete rest, the orthopedist expected Cindy to require only a few days of physical therapy before resuming full normal activity. However, when the cast was removed, Cindy continued to complain of pain and was unable to bear weight on her foot. Over the past few months, every study has been performed to evaluate the ankle and find out why Cindy cannot walk or skate on it. Her laboratory tests are normal, the MRI is normal, and X-rays show only mild osteoporosis. Her bone scan shows patchy uptake that does not suggest a specific diagnosis. Since it has been six months from the time of her injury, Cindy's parents and the orthopedist are very frustrated.

Cindy's foot and ankle are steadily getting worse. The entire foot is purplish in color and cool to the touch. Cindy cannot put a shoe or sock on her foot and often complains that even the weight of a sheet on her foot causes severe pain. Figure skating and Cindy's entire future have been put on hold. How can she go on to become a professional figure skater and fulfill her dreams? Her parents are willing to try anything.

Reflex sympathetic dystrophy (RSD), reflex neurovascular dystrophy, and **complex regional pain syndrome** are different names for the same condition. It is a cause of great frustration for parents and physicians, and it is far more common than you might think. Reflex sympathetic dystrophy can involve the upper or lower extremity. It rarely occurs in children under the age of eight, but it may occur at any age. Because there is usually a well-documented history of injury, families and physicians are often distraught over their inability to solve the problem. The child who has suffered the injury is invariably described as "my best child," "the hardest worker," "truly dedicated," and so on.

UNDERSTANDING AND DIAGNOSING REFLEX SYMPATHETIC DYSTROPHY

The key to understanding RSD is to recognize that the problem is no longer a simple physical injury. Children with RSD are overachievers who have been put under too much pressure to perform. At first, parents often refuse to believe this. Like Cindy's parents, they know their child loves the activities he or she is involved in. The parents are sure that they are not driving the child; the child is pushing to achieve. Any suggestion that there may be a psychological aspect to the problem is immediately rejected.

It took many months before Cindy's family agreed to psychological intervention. When they finally did agree to seek help, Cindy's symptoms began to slowly disappear. Over a further six months of physical and psychological therapy, Cindy recovered completely. She did not go on to become a professional figure skater. One of the first things the psychologist discovered was that Cindy had dreams of being a fashion designer, not a figure skater. However, when all was said and done, the whole family could enjoy skating and everyone ultimately accepted that Cindy needed to grow up to be what Cindy wanted to be, not what her parents wanted her to be.

Extensive experience with children with RSD has allowed physicians to understand that it is invariably a "cry for help." The problem may be as obvious as Cindy's or much more complex. The key to solving the problem is careful investigation and recognition that it is not simply a physical injury. Once this is done, the child and family can concentrate on dealing with the related issues and working with their physicians and psychologists to fully resolve the problem. Physical therapy is often still necessary because of the long period of disuse.

The first step in treating a child with RSD is to make sure that the diagnosis is correct. As often as I have seen physicians fail to make this diagnosis, I have had children with undiagnosed arthritis referred as having RSD. The laboratory tests are usually normal. In long-standing cases, X-rays may show mild osteoporosis due to disuse. An MRI may show patchy marrow edema, and the bone scan may show increased uptake, decreased uptake, or patchy increased and decreased uptake.

On physical exam, the involved hand or foot is often markedly discolored. It may feel warm to the touch, but far more often it is cold. The child is often very tense when the involved limb is examined and may cry out with pain. However, it is often possible to distract or calmly reassure the child and proceed to examine the limb fully. Often a child will cry out when I first take the involved foot in my hand, but then calm down quickly as I rub the foot gently and continue to talk to him or her about a favorite activity. Most often, this will not work if there is a fracture, infection, tumor, or other significant injury.

Making the diagnosis of RSD is usually far easier than explaining it to the family and getting them to accept it. Affected children are almost invariably overachievers who are very anxious to please their parents. In many cases, the combination of an abnormal bone scan and the obvious initial injury makes it very difficult for the parents to accept the idea that there is a psychological issue.

Reflex sympathetic dystrophy is a true somatization disorder. The child really feels the pain, and the pain is real. **The child is not making up a complaint of pain to manipulate the parents.** Since the child is in pain and the injured extremity is discolored, parents ask, "How can this be psychological?" It takes a lot of explaining to make the family realize that you do not think this is something the child is making up. Reflex sympathetic dystrophy is not a voluntary illness. The child does not think to himself, "If I say my foot hurts, I will not have to skate anymore." **Whatever goes on in somatization disorders happens at a subconscious level that the child is no more aware of than the parents.**

TREATMENT

Once the correct diagnosis has been made, physical therapy and psychological therapy become equally important. Physical therapy should concentrate on desensitization. The key is to persistently massage the tender extremity and gradually reassure the child that it is safe to put on a sock, to walk on the foot, or to use the hand. This is a process that may require weeks to months to accomplish. It should be accompanied by ongoing family psychological therapy to help the family and child understand the origins of the problem. (I have seen families refuse the psychological aspects of care and insist on only physical therapy. Although physical therapy may help even in the absence of psychological therapy, it fails to address the fact that this illness is a cry for help. In several cases, children whose parents refused psychological intervention recovered from their "injuries" but ultimately required psychiatric hospitalization.)

MEDICAL TREATMENT

Pain specialists often believe that drug therapy is appropriate for these children. Corticosteroids, regional sympathetic blocks, and narcotic analgesics all may provide temporary relief, but they fail to address the primary underlying problem. In several studies of large groups of children, it has been shown that the long-term outcome is far better for children treated with physical and psychological therapy than for children treated with medications and injections.

PSYCHOLOGICAL CONSIDERATIONS

The complex nature of the medical and psychological issues makes RSD a very difficult illness for pediatricians, but they are the front-line professionals who will see these families and be relied on for advice. Establishing rapport with the family is essential. Most families will not accept consideration of possible underlying psychological issues until a very thorough medical evaluation has been completed. Often psychological evaluation is accepted better if it is initially proposed as an aid to coping with the pain and disability.

21

Osteoporosis and Osteopenia

Charlotte was twenty-one years old when I first met her. She had been cared for by another rheumatologist for many years but was referred to me because of her need for joint replacement surgery. She was diagnosed with JA at the age of twelve years and treated with corticosteroids when her disease did not respond to NSAIDs. She felt much better with the corticosteroids and was able to attend school and go on to college. During the college years, Charlotte was away from home and managed her own medications. Although she was officially on a low dose of corticosteroids, she freely admitted that when she felt stiff or sore she took extra doses. Charlotte completed college with honors and planned to go on to graduate school. However, she had fallen and fractured her femur. X-rays revealed that she had severe diffuse osteoporosis. Over the next few years, she suffered multiple fractures. She has never been able to attend graduate school.

Osteoporosis and osteopenia are conditions involving decreased bone mass and hence a decrease in the strength of the bones with an increased risk of fractures. An individual has **osteopenia** if his or her bone mass is more than one standard deviation below the normal level and **osteoporosis** if the bone mass is more than two and a half standard deviations below the normal level. These definitions have been difficult to apply to children because the normal levels have not been well defined for children of different ages and races. Children who do not get enough calcium in their diet, children with chronic arthritis, children who take corticosteroids or other drugs (especially diuretics such as furosemide), and children with a variety of hormonal disorders are all at risk of developing osteopenia and osteoporosis.

Decreased bone mass in children is particularly disturbing because bone mass normally increases during childhood and then begins to decrease during adult life. If a child never reaches his or her expected peak bone mass level as a young adult, the risk of having significant problems later in life is greatly increased.

AT RISK

Anticonvulsants, diuretics, and corticosteroids are the most commonly used drugs causing osteopenia and osteoporosis in children. Children receiving drugs that are known to cause osteoporosis should be monitored carefully. If a child is discovered to have osteoporosis or osteopenia and is not known to have arthritis or to be taking medicines that cause the problem, he or she should be carefully evaluated to determine the cause. It is very rare for a child to have a low serum calcium level if he or she is consuming a normal diet. Most children with osteoporosis have normal serum calcium levels. In this day and age of dietary fads, pediatricians must be aware that many teenage girls are on vegan diets or participate in other dietary fads that may severely impact their health. **Young female athletes who train extensively while eating poorly are at particular risk for osteoporosis and stress fractures.** Teenagers should be specifically counseled that both alcohol and smoking increase the risk of osteoporosis.

DIAGNOSIS

There are no laboratory tests that are regularly useful in detecting osteopenia or osteoporosis. While osteoporosis may be suspected on the basis of routine X-rays, bone density studies should be done to confirm the diagnosis using DEXA (dual-energy X-ray absorptiometry) or a similar technique. It is important to use a method of measuring bone density that will provide quantitative results so that changes in bone density can be followed over time.

COMPLICATIONS

The major complications of osteoporosis are fractures. These may be stress fractures in the limbs of athletes or vertebral fractures in children with chronic disease. Stress fractures become evident as pain at the site of the fracture. Vertebral fractures cause severe back pain. Occasionally, children are recognized to have osteoporosis only when they fracture an arm or leg after a minor fall. Because childhood is a time when bone mass normally increases, the most important complications of childhood osteoporosis may not occur until many years later. Everyone starts to lose bone mass gradually shortly before the age of thirty. Even if the loss of bone mass occurs at a normal rate, a person starting with a low bone mass because of childhood osteoporosis will reach a critical level much sooner than a normal individual.

For children with an underlying rheumatic disease, the key to prevention of osteoporosis is control of the inflammatory process. However, while corticosteroids are effective anti-inflammatory agents, they promote osteoporosis. Their use should be restricted, but you do not want to risk serious damage from uncontrolled rheumatic disease because of the future risk of osteoporosis due to corticosteroids. **If a child or young adult requires corticosteroids, it is very important that he or she understands the importance of not taking extra doses when he or she feels bad.** The doctor may feel the need to increase the dose to improve disease control, but the doctor is also well aware of the need to reduce the dose as soon as possible. At one time, it was thought that deflazacort might cause less bone loss than other corticosteroids, but this turned out not to be true when the dose was adjusted for an equal anti-inflammatory effect.

MEDICAL TREATMENT

The most important element of treatment for childhood osteoporosis is prevention. Adequate calcium intake should be assured for every child. If extra calcium is given, it must be accompanied by vitamin D, but avoid giving excessive amounts. **Excessive vitamin D consumption is dangerous and can be fatal.** Excessive intake of calcium should be avoided because it often causes constipation and stomach upset. This is not a situation where "some is good, so more must be better."

For children with mild osteopenia, attention to diet and appropriate supplementation should be adequate treatment. Children with fractures or DEXA-documented osteoporosis may require more aggressive therapy. However, appropriate treatment for children with osteoporosis remains controversial. Bisphosphorates such as alendronate and other drugs used in adults may be required. They have been proven to reverse osteoporosis to some extent in children. However, their long-term safety for use in childhood is not established. Bisphosphonates are stored in the bones for many years. We do not know whether taking bisphosphonates earlier in life will cause problems for a woman if she becomes pregnant; this has limited our ability to use these drugs.

Calcitonin, a hormone that is normally made by the body to promote bone formation, is an alternative therapy that deserves serious consideration. Calcitonin isolated from fish is now available for prescription use.

PROGNOSIS

The prognosis for a child with osteopenia is very good. Identification of any underlying problem, correction of the diet, and appropriate medical therapy should lead to improvement.

The prognosis for children with osteoporosis is more guarded. Pediatricians caring for children with osteoporosis must consider whether these children should be treated with bisphosphonates. At the time of this writing, the long-term safety of bisphosphonates in children is unproven. There are also no clear data regarding their effect on future pregnancies. However, they have been shown to improve bone density. Children with severe osteoporosis should be referred to large centers with experienced staff where they can be offered the best possible therapy.

22

Genetic Conditions

Jennifer was a thirteen-year-old girl who puzzled her physician. Routine blood tests were normal, but she complained of feeling stiff all the time. She had had frequent upper respiratory infections as a young child, and they continued as she got older. On exam she was found to have limitation in her elbows without swelling. The pediatrician thought she might have JA. The pediatrician had also noticed a heart murmur and Jennifer was scheduled to be seen by a cardiologist, but she had gotten an appointment with me first. She was pleasant and normal in both appearance and intelligence. However, on complete examination I noted that while she had slightly cloudy corneas, she had never complained to her family of visual difficulties. The heart murmur was evident, as was mild hepatosplenomegaly. X-rays of her arms revealed a curved radius with a tilted radial epiphysis, and the radiologist was uncertain what that meant. Putting the symptoms together, it was clear that Jennifer had Scheie syndrome, a milder variant of mucopolysaccharidosis (MPS) I that was likely to cause progressive difficulties over time if not treated.

There are a variety of genetic conditions with significant musculoskeletal manifestations. These range in severity from those that are obvious at or shortly after birth to those that only become evident in later childhood or in the early teenage years.

- More common syndromes like Ehlers-Danlos syndrome and HLA B27–associated conditions with musculoskeletal manifestations and a significant genetic component have been discussed in previous chapters, as have sickle cell disease and beta-thalassemia.

- A variety of conditions associated with fever, rash, and varying degrees of joint pain have recently been discovered to be caused by defects in the CIAS1 gene and production of pyrin, ranging from very rare syndromes like neonatal-onset multisystem inflammatory disease to more common conditions such as familial Mediterranean fever. Children with these diseases are helped by treatment with agents that block IL-1.

- The lysosomal storage diseases also may present with joint pain or stiffness and, in some cases, fever and rash. Many forms of lysosomal storage disease, such as Hurler syndrome, often become obvious in early childhood, but children with Scheie syndrome and Fabry disease may present with joint complaints (and, with Fabry disease patients, fever and rash) long before they are recognized as having a life-threatening condition. Often these complaints lead to a misdiagnosis of JA or another rheumatic disease.

While all of these conditions are rare, early recognition is essential to early treatment. Several of the lysosomal storage diseases that a rheumatologist may see can be alleviated by periodic intravenous infusion of exogenous enzymes made by recombinant DNA technology (e.g., laronidase [Aldurazyme] for MPS I, idursulfase [Elaprase] for MPS II, galsulfase [Naglazyme] for MPS VI, and agalsidase beta [Fabrazyme] for Fabry disease), which perform the function of the enzyme that is missing owing to the genetic defect. Early recognition and treatment are important because these conditions cause cumulative damage over time that appropriate treatment can slow or prevent. All of these children are seen initially by primary care providers, who must take the initiative in referring them to appropriate specialists.

LYSOSOMAL STORAGE DISEASES WITH PROMINENT JOINT PAIN OR STIFFNESS: MUCOPOLYSACCHARIDOSIS I (HURLER-SCHEIE SYNDROME) AND FABRY DISEASE

Mucopolysaccharidosis I (MPS I) is the prototype of MPS disorders. It is known as *Hurler syndrome* when it presents in its most severe form and *Scheie syndrome* when it presents in a milder form. It is an autosomal recessive disease that results from a variety of genetic mutations on chromosome 4, leading to defective production of the lysosomal enzyme alpha-L-iduronidase. Some mutations produce complete absence of the enzyme and very severe disease, while others produce defective enzyme with some residual function. Although the estimated incidence is only 1:100,000 newborns, the ability of enzyme replacement therapy with laronidase (Aldurazyme) to reverse or limit progressive organ damage makes early recognition and treatment of affected children vitally important.

While Hurler syndrome becomes obvious in children within the first two years of life, resulting in early diagnosis, children with Scheie syndrome lack the typical abnormal appearance and mental retardation found in Hurler syndrome patients. Children with Scheie syndrome often complain of joint stiffness, but there are no abnormal findings on routine testing and these children may be misdiagnosed as having JA. Children with untreated Scheie syndrome develop progressive problems over time and ultimately may develop cardiac failure, deafness, spinal deformity, and blindness if not treated. Thus, early recognition and early therapy are vitally important.

The key to the diagnosis of Scheie syndrome is suspicion of the diagnosis of "atypical JA." The occurrence of joint pain and stiffness without obvious synovitis should raise suspicion. Additional suspicious findings include valvular heart disease, frequent upper respiratory infections, or hepatosplenomegaly. Corneal clouding in a child with joint complaints should prompt immediate consideration of Scheie syndrome. While children with JA may have band keratopathy complicating their disease, this occurs in the setting of uveitis, which does not accompany the corneal clouding in children with MPS I.

Rheumatic or orthopedic disease may be suspected in children with Scheie syndrome when they present with carpal tunnel syndrome, genu valgus, or hip dysplasia. Characteristic abnormalities on radiographic examination include an abnormally curved radius and a tilted radial epiphysis. In more advanced cases, clavicular and rib abnormalities may be present, but these should not be relied on in considering the diagnosis of Scheie syndrome.

More severely affected children may have an intermediate form of MPS I, Hurler-Scheie syndrome, with coarser features including frontal bossing and more prominent hepatosplenomegaly as well as a history of umbilical hernia, but with normal intelligence with or without a learning disability.

Children can be screened for MPS I by sending urine for quantitative glycosaminoglycan measurement. This test is routinely available from commercial laboratories. Definitive testing requires measuring alpha-L-iduronidase levels in blood or tissues and is provided by specialized laboratories. Any child in whom MPS I is suspected should be seen in a center with appropriate specialists.

FABRY DISEASE

Fabry disease results from the decreased function of alpha-galactosidase. The resultant accumulation of globotriaosylceramide results in damage to multiple organs, with vascular damage and ultimate renal, cardiac, and central nervous system disease. Fabry disease in childhood typically presents with recurrent episodes of fever and joint pain. A distinguishing finding is acroparesthesia— burning or tingling of the extremities. In addition, these children develop hypohidrosis accompanied by fatigue and exercise intolerance. Key to the diagnosis is the recognition of angiokeratomas or otherwise unusual whorled corneal opacities. The presence of combined heat and cold intolerance is another unusual finding that should prompt consideration of the diagnosis.

Misdiagnosis of Fabry disease in childhood is common. Children with this syndrome have been mislabeled variously with growing pains, fibromyalgia, erythromelalgia, Raynaud's syndrome, rheumatic fever, and systemic-onset JA. The combination of fever, elevated ESR, and joint pains often leads to rheumatic disease referral. However, Fabry disease is a rare condition, and review of the records of diagnosed cases indicates that the proper diagnosis is often not made until patients are in their twenties. Some patients have been discovered only by retrospective screening of adults being treated for "unexplained" renal failure or cardiomyopathy.

Fabry disease is X-linked recessive and thus the majority of patients are male, although a growing number of female patients with variable symptomatology are being recognized. Screening of males for deficient enzyme activity is available from specialized laboratories. Since females with Fabry disease typically have levels of enzymatic activity that overlap with the normal range, their diagnosis can be made reliably only by genetic testing.

Fabry disease is a storage disease, and replacement enzyme therapy (with agalsidase beta [Fabrazyme]) is clinically beneficial. As with MPS I, early recognition and treatment can limit organ damage and provide an optimal outcome. While the disease is rare, most affected children appear to be undiagnosed, with severe consequences that could be prevented if it was properly recognized.

DISEASES ASSOCIATED WITH MUTATIONS IN THE CIAS1 (NALP3) GENE: NEONATAL-ONSET MULTISYSTEM INFLAMMATORY DISEASE, MUCKLE-WELLS SYNDROME, AND FAMILIAL COLD URTICARIA

Children with NOMID (also called *CINCA syndrome*: chronic, infantile, neuro-logic, cutaneous, and articular syndrome) are afflicted with fever, urticarial rash, deformed joints with abnormal bone growth, and meningitis. Nearly all of these children have obvious problems by three months of age. At first, many of them were thought to have a severe variant of systemic-onset JA, but it was quickly recognized that this was not the same disease. Fortunately, NOMID is a very rare condition.

In the 1960s, Muckle and Wells identified a family with several genera-tions affected by the autosomal dominant occurrence of early-onset recurrent urticaria followed over time by deafness and amyloidosis. Children with this syndrome often develop urticaria following exposure to cold. When the urticaria appears the children often have fever, joint pains, and other nonspecific symp-toms. Typical attacks last up to twenty-four hours, but there is a great degree of variability.

A separate syndrome of familial cold urticaria (FCAS) has been described with the onset of urticaria and fever within the first six months of life that is not associated with deafness and only rarely with amyloidosis. Children with FCAS seem different from those with Muckle-Wells syndrome in that the former have almost daily episodes and are significantly debilitated.

Each of these syndromes seems to be clinically distinct. However, investiga-tors soon recognized that there were children who overlapped the boundaries. When precise genetic testing became available, it was found that the majority of the children with all three diseases have mutations that result in defective CIAS1 (NALP3) gene expression.

The CIAS1 (NALP3) gene is critical to the formation of an inflammatory molecular complex, which processes IL-1 beta. Defects in this molecular com-plex result in overproduction of IL-1 beta in response to a variety of stimuli. This discovery led to the use of kineret (Anakinra) to block IL-1 in children and adults with NOMID, FCAS, and Muckle-Wells syndrome, with prompt relief of their symptoms. It is now proposed that these three diseases are varying phenotypes of a single disease, since all result from malfunction in the CIAS1 (NALP3) gene.

FAMILIAL MEDITERRANEAN FEVER

Familial Mediterranean fever (FMF) is an autosomal recessive disorder. More common than the other disorders discussed in this chapter, FMF occurs in approximately 1 in 500 persons of Mediterranean ancestry. It has long been recognized as a cause of recurrent abdominal pain and fever, which may be difficult to distinguish from acute appendicitis. Although the disease is more common in Mediterranean populations, it can also occur in other ethnic groups. Attacks of FMF typically begin with a sense of discomfort followed by rapidly worsening abdominal pain and fever. Peritonitis with rebound is typical. In some children there is significant pleuritis, with chest pain as well. Rash on the extremities (erysipeloid erythema) is less commonly seen. Episodes typically last for two to three days, with gradual resolution beginning at the end of the second day.

The diagnosis of FMF is often delayed unless there is a strong family history that is recognized by the parents and presented to the primary care physician. Often the diagnosis is suspected only after the appendix has been removed and the episodes of abdominal pain have continued or when the periodicity of the attacks has been recognized by the family or physicians. Mild FMF with rare attacks may not require therapy. However, certain ethnic groups appear to have an increased risk of amyloidosis, and all children with FMF should be periodically monitored for proteinuria as the earliest manifestation of amyloidosis.

Arthritis is an episodic problem in children with FMF, but it may become severe. There is a predilection for involvement of the sacroiliac joints and hips. Some children have severe disease necessitating hip replacement in their early twenties.

Colchicine has been an effective therapy for FMF since the 1960s. A variety of regimens have been proposed, but chronic use is most successful. However, if attacks are infrequent, some families prefer to simply tolerate them. In the absence of amyloidosis or inappropriate medical intervention, this may be the best course.

Careful evaluation of the genetics of FMF has shown it to be the result of mutations in the MEFV gene, which is important in the production of pyrin. Interestingly, pyrin interacts with CIAS1 (NALP3) in the control of inflammatory responses. This has led to speculation that Kineret may be effective in the treatment of FMF as well.

CONCLUSIONS

As physicians caring for children, pediatricians, family practitioners, and specialists in childhood diseases have an important role to play in educating the public and in identifying children with the early manifestations of progressive diseases. Only by early recognition of these diseases, which cause increasing damage over time, can we institute proper therapy and minimize their impact. These are all rare diseases, but every affected child is seen by a primary care physician before referral to the appropriate specialist. Heightened awareness on the part of physicians is the key to early diagnosis and early therapy for these children.

PART III

LIVING WITH A CHILD WHO HAS A CHRONIC CONDITION

23

Medications and Immunizations

I do not discuss every possible medication in this chapter. I discuss the medications I commonly use. There are many choices and many individual styles. At the right time and in the right place, there are a number of medications that I use that are not covered here. The omission of a medication indicates only that I do not use it routinely or that I don't think of it as a rheumatic disease drug (e.g., I don't discuss antibiotics here).

GENERAL CONCEPTS

The physician strode confidently into the room and offered the child a cup of liquid to relieve his distress. "But wait," cried the parents. "Does that have any possible side effects?" The physician paused thoughtfully for a minute and then said, "Well, if taken in excess, it can cause problems for anyone with heart or kidney disease. It may dramatically worsen the condition of children with heart or kidney failure. It can cause both nocturia and urinary urgency and frequency. If taken too rapidly, it may cause nausea. If too much is ingested and the body becomes overloaded, it may cause seizures. Excessive use is often associated with a bloated feeling, weight gain, and swollen feet. It should not be left on the skin for a prolonged period or it may result in maceration and skin breakdown. Further, you should always be careful where it comes from, because some sources are contaminated with bacteria or viruses capable of causing severe infections." With that, the parents immediately jumped up and discarded the cup of water the doctor had brought because the child was thirsty.

No one likes to have to take medicine, and no one wants to take even the slightest risk of getting a side effect. Pediatricians must understand that even children who start off willing and excited about taking medications will become bored with the need to take them over time. Furthermore, most parents are not happy to give their children chronic medication. **But children who do take their medicine**

273

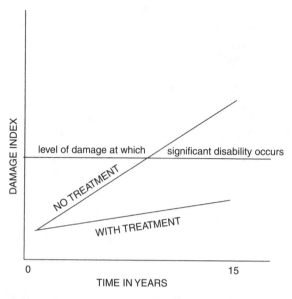

Figure 23-1 *Children who received treatment were able to continue functioning much longer after the children who did not receive treatment were significantly disabled, even though members of the treated group felt that they never really got better.*

routinely are the ones who get the best results, and that is what we want. Children often do poorly because their parents do not do what they are supposed to do. This is because the parents do not understand why the doctors are telling them to do certain things. It is our role as pediatricians to make sure that we properly educate families so that they recognize the importance of complying with the medication regimen (see Fig. 23-1).

There are two frequent responses from parents who want to avoid medication. The first group of parents does not want to give the child medication but wants the problem to disappear: *If only I could work miracles.* Parents in the second group realize that the child is much better off when he or she takes the medicine, but they do not want to do the blood tests and come to the physician to be monitored. It is ironic that the same parents who are very concerned about side effects are the ones who keep "forgetting" to do the appropriate monitoring tests.

When to Withhold Medication

If a child is sick with the flu or a virus and is vomiting, you should not prescribe NSAIDs or immunosuppressive medications. The only arthritis medications that should be given when the child is sick are corticosteroids. All other medications should be avoided. Children who are vomiting are at risk of becoming dehydrated and of developing Reye's syndrome.

Reye's syndrome usually follows a viral infection with symptoms of nausea, vomiting, and sleepiness. Aspirin and other drugs, including NSAIDs, may aggravate the condition. Nonsteroidal anti-inflammatory drugs should not be given to a child with nausea and vomiting who is at risk of becoming dehydrated. This includes aspirin and ibuprofen-containing products (e.g., Motrin and Advil).

CHILDREN WHO RESIST TAKING THEIR MEDICATION

There are a number of elements to consider in dealing with children who resist taking their medication. The easiest answer is to avoid getting into this situation. Finding a suitable compromise by converting the medication into a liquid or offering ice cream, candy, and so on is usually preferable to an all-out battle. For younger children, a reward system (or bribery) is often the easiest and most effective answer. As parents, we all believe that we should not have to bribe our children to get them to do what they should be doing anyway. However, with over twenty-five years of experience in watching parents deal with their children, it's become clear to me that whether it's called a reward system or bribery, giving children positive reinforcement for taking their medication works better than anything else.

If there are continuing problems in getting the child to take medication, it is important to deal with them openly. As children grow up, they become increasingly frustrated by their lack of control over what happens to them. Often a struggle over taking medication is really the declaration "I hate having my disease." If everyone can sit down and discuss what's going on, it may be possible to simply talk it out. If not, psychological intervention may be required. Often a child who refuses to take medication at home will respond quickly to being placed in a hospital environment where nurses instead of parents administer the medication. Awareness that the medication is a symbol of the disease and may become a focus of normal parent–child conflicts may help everyone bring the situation to a quick resolution.

PROPER MONITORING

It does not reflect everyone's standard of practice, but here is what I believe should be done to get the best possible results. Medicines tend to have two types of side effects. There are idiosyncratic reactions in which the patient responds in an unusual way. Some patients are unusually sensitive to certain medicines. Other side effects are related to the amount of the medicine: both the amount taken in each dose and the total amount taken over time. These two types of side effects require different forms of monitoring.

For medicines such as NSAIDs, which are generally safe, I want children to be tested within two or three weeks of starting the medicine to look for any unusual reactions, six weeks after starting the medicine to look for any cumulative reactions, three months after starting the medicine, and then every three months thereafter. This is very conservative, careful monitoring, but as a result, I have never had a serious medication side effect that was not resolved. Many physicians check much less frequently, and usually there are no major problems.

For medicines known to have an increased frequency or severity of side effects, such as methotrexate, I ask my patients to get their blood checked every week at the beginning and then every two weeks. Only when I am sure that they are tolerating the medicine in the full dose do I extend the frequency of blood testing to every month and eventually every three months. If parents add a new supplement to the child's diet, I start the monitoring tests again, because some supplements increase the risk of side effects. **I recommend that children on supplements be monitored just as carefully as children on prescription medicines.** There are numerous well-documented cases of children who became ill from dietary supplements.

WHY PRESCRIBE MEDICINES IF THEY ARE POTENTIALLY DANGEROUS?

Imagine that you are sitting in the library reading a book when six firemen come running in with axes and a fire hose, their boots clanking. "You cannot come in here with that hose!" the librarian shouts indignantly. "You're making too much noise, and my goodness, if you turn on that hose, you'll get water everywhere and damage the books! It will take forever to clean up the mess." That's all true, you think. But then one fireman points to the smoke coming out of a vent on the side wall and says, "Lady, if we don't start using this hose and get that fire under control, very soon there will be no library or books to worry about."

Medications for rheumatic diseases do have side effects, and their use must be carefully monitored. However, if the majority of children taking them did not do well and the benefits did not far outweigh the risks, no physician would recommend them.

Some parents will ask you why they should give their child medicine. It is important to make them realize that severe problems can occur if medicines are not taken. No sensible physician prescribes a medication unless he or she believes that the potential benefits outweigh the potential risks. I often hear parents say, "It's only a sore knee," or similar statements. But it's not. If a child's problem is interfering with his or her ability to keep up with friends and do normal things, it's damaging the child's self-concept and the feeling of self-worth. Failure to take care of these problems may have disastrous consequences in both the short and long terms (see Fig. 23-1).

WHY DOES MY CHILD HAVE TO KEEP TAKING MEDICATION AND GOING TO THE SPECIALIST EVEN AFTER HE OR SHE FEELS WELL?

The old zookeeper smiled quietly to himself as he listened to the children talking. "Look at the big kitty cat, Mommy! Why do they keep him locked up in that cage? Can't they let the big kitty cat out, Mommy? Why don't they let us get closer? I want to pet him, Mommy!" The mother stopped to explain that the big kitty cat was a lion—a fierce animal that looked very calm and quiet when resting but that could suddenly pounce on its prey with blinding speed and kill it mercilessly. The children were unconvinced. "It just looks like a big kitty cat to me, Mommy."

There are many times when, as a physician, I feel just like that mother in the zoo. Sometimes it's been several years since the child was brought to me with active disease that was causing serious problems. With the right medicines, hard work, and some good luck, the child's disease has been brought under control. At other times, it's a few months after the disease has come under control and I'm just beginning to be confident that things are going to go well. But the parents who never missed an appointment while their child was sick now don't want to come back so often and don't want to keep giving the child medicine. Like the children above, they see only a big kitty cat in the cage.

Many of the rheumatic diseases are chronic and recurrent. They can be controlled, but they can never be eliminated. When the disease is under control, the parents and the child would like to forget about it. They have forgotten that without the cage, the big kitty cat could again become a ferocious lion without warning. If you think this is a silly story, let me assure you that I've seen children suffer permanent damage because their parents thought the problem was gone and stopped giving the medicines. They stopped the medications because they ran out of them after forgetting to keep their appointments to have the blood work checked and the prescriptions renewed. After all, they saw no problems, and they did not want to continue taking time off from work or removing the child from school to keep "unnecessary" doctors' appointments.

"DISEASE-MODIFYING" DRUGS?

Parents are often concerned that they may be giving their child a drug that has possible side effects but is not disease-modifying. Why bother? If the drug is not going to cure my child's disease, why can't I just have him deal with the pain so that he does not have to risk the side effects of medicine?

Consider two construction workers who are working on a large project. I'll take a brick that weighs ten pounds and hold it six feet over each one's right big toe—no shoes or socks. When I drop the brick on their toes, they'll both scream in pain and will not be able to walk. I have dropped the same brick from the same height on both workers. Worker 1 is told that he's a tough guy. He can rest or go home if he wants to and come back when he feels he can work again—but he's not to take medications of any kind. Worker 2 is given NSAIDs that reduce the pain and inflammation. The NSAIDs do not change the fact that I dropped a brick on his toe. He, too, is told that he can rest or go home and come back when he feels he can work again. Who is likely to be back on the job first, earning money again first, feeling better about himself first, and more productive?

Taking NSAIDs may not change the fundamental nature of the disease, but it certainly will change the outcome by keeping the children in less pain, able to do more, and feeling better about themselves. The NSAIDs may not be disease-modifying, but they definitely modify the functional outcome, and that's what's most important.

In every discussion of drugs for children with chronic rheumatic disease, you will hear a debate about disease-modifying versus non-disease-modifying drugs. Sometimes the disease-modifying drugs are referred to as DMARDs (disease-modifying antirheumatic drugs) or SAARDs (slow-acting antirheumatic drugs). Ideally, there should be drugs that cure the rheumatic diseases. "Here, take these pills for ten days and the problem will be gone." Unfortunately, those pills do not exist. Instead, we have pills that reduce inflammation and both decrease pain and increase function.

With the development of newer drugs, there has been a lot of discussion about what constitutes a disease-modifying drug as opposed to what simply makes the patient feel better but does not fundamentally change the outcome of the disease. This is an important argument, but it has been misapplied and has caused a lot of confusion. The first thing to remember when dealing with children with arthritis is that we want the best possible outcome in terms of ability to function, not just from day to day but in later adult life as well. **If I decrease their pain and allow them to be more active and feel better about themselves, they will have a better outcome.**

In treating adults with rheumatoid arthritis, there has been an extensive discussion of how to define *disease-modifying*. To focus on objective measurements, the original plan was to concentrate on observing the changes in the bones on X-rays. So, for the original studies, two groups of patients on different medications were compared for the number of new erosions seen over a period of years. If patients on one drug developed fewer erosions, then the drug was disease-modifying. Most physicians now agree that this misses the point. What counts is whether the patient can go to work or school every day. That is determined more by how much pain and stiffness the patient has than by the number of erosions.

NONSTEROIDAL ANTI-INFLAMMATORY DRUGS

Nonsteroidal anti-inflammatory drugs are the mainstay of therapy for children with rheumatic disease. All of them interfere to varying degrees with the cyclooxygenase pathway. This pathway is responsible for the production of prostaglandins, which are important inflammatory mediators. By blocking the production of these inflammatory mediators, NSAIDs reduce the amount of pain, fever, and irritation that the child experiences.

Most NSAIDs interfere with cyclooxygenase-1 (COX-1) and cyclooxygenase-2 (COX-2). Choosing the proper NSAID for a given child involves balancing convenience, cost, effectiveness, and the probability of side effects. All of the NSAIDs can irritate the stomach, irritate the liver, interfere with kidney function, or result in a rash. However, all of them can be used safely with appropriate monitoring.

Side Effects of Nonsteroidal Anti-inflammatory Drugs

Allergic reactions can occur with any medications. Few children are allergic to NSAIDs, but if there is a history of allergy to aspirin or similar medications, one should be cautious. Some children who are allergic to aspirin are allergic to all NSAIDs, but others are not.

All NSAIDs may cause gastritis. This may manifest as indigestion or loss of appetite. It is important to make sure that the child takes the medicine on a full stomach. If stomachaches are common or persistent, you may need to change the medication or add a gastro-protective agent. Some children develop ulcers while taking NSAIDs, but this is uncommon. Remember, if every NSAID causes a child to have stomachaches, perhaps something else is going on.

Bruising is a common side effect of all NSAIDs. These drugs interfere with platelet stickiness and cause the patient to bleed or bruise more often than normal. Frequent bruises over the shins are common for children on NSAIDs, but if they are significant, make sure that there is no other explanation. It is also important to stop the NSAIDs before any elective surgery where there is a high risk of bleeding. Consult the physician doing the surgery. It may be necessary to stop the NSAIDs two weeks in advance.

Liver irritation may also occur with these medications. Most often the patient is not aware of the irritation, and it is detected only by blood work. With aspirin, liver irritation was very common and mild inflammation of the liver was tolerated. Given the variety of medications available today, we are less tolerant of liver irritation, but minimal amounts are acceptable.

Nonsteroidal anti-inflammatory drugs also affect the kidneys. They usually interfere with the glomerular filtration rate, causing the child to hold more water in the body. This causes a few pounds of weight gain and may be reflected in a slight drop in the hemoglobin value and a slight rise in the BUN level. These are normal effects of the medications.

Chronic NSAID use may lead to **interstitial nephritis**. This is a more serious condition that requires stopping the NSAID. It may have to be treated with steroids and could result in permanent damage. Routine urine tests are part of monitoring for side effects of NSAIDs in order to detect any signs of this problem. It may not occur until many months or years after starting the medication. This is why the monitoring must continue.

An unusual rash called a **pseudoporphyria reaction** has been described in some children on NSAIDs. This rash appears when the child is out in the sun. At first, it just looks like a number of tiny blisters, but the blisters leave a small scar when they heal. With continued medication and continued sun exposure, there will be more and more blisters and scars. The medication should be stopped and the sun avoided until the medicine is cleared from the body. This reaction has been noticed most often with naproxen, but that may be because so much naproxen is used. It has been reported with other NSAIDs, and all children on NSAIDs should be monitored for it.

Behavioral problems in children taking chronic medication can result from many different causes. In general, the NSAIDs do *not* cause misbehavior, changes in attitude, poor sleeping, difficulty studying, or similar side effects (though indomethacin is known to cause headaches, depression, and dizziness). If there is a significant behavioral problem in a child on an NSAID, I will observe at first and then stop or change the NSAID to see whether there is improvement. Other problems may occur. Almost anything can happen to a patient and possibly be the result of an NSAID he or she was taking. In large studies, there are always patients taking placebo who complain of headache, itching, sweating, constipation, diarrhea, difficulty concentrating, and so on. There are often a few more patients with these complaints in the group taking the real medication.

Important Points for Pediatricians to Remember

I have prescribed NSAIDs for thousands of children without ever seeing a side effect that did not disappear when the drug was stopped. Over thirty years, I have briefly stopped or changed the NSAIDs in many children with complaints of stomachache, but I have seen only four ulcers caused by NSAIDs. I would never prescribe these drugs if I did not think that the benefits far outweighed the risks. Nonetheless, I monitor very carefully with blood and urine tests. If a parent describes a change he or she thinks might be due to the NSAID and it continues, I always stop the NSAID to see whether it goes away, and then I carefully restart the NSAID to see whether it comes back. If it does come back, I stop the drug. Some physicians monitor less frequently. I like to play it safe.

As a physician, I want to give children with arthritis the NSAID that makes them better with the least likelihood of side effects and the greatest convenience. The probability of side effects is different for each NSAID. If one NSAID was more likely to make children better and less likely to cause side effects, all of the others would be discarded. The list of side effects is essentially the same for all NSAIDs; it is the probability of the side effects that changes.

One of the most common problems is for children to be treated with only one NSAID and told that there is no other choice. Despite their similar mechanisms of action, all NSAIDs are not the same. Some NSAIDs are far more effective for certain types of arthritis. Failure to recognize the different types of JA (see Chapter 7) means that many doctors have failed to understand that different NSAIDs are better for different diseases. Changing to the appropriate NSAID can often make a dramatic difference for a child. However, it may take some trial and error. You cannot predict which NSAID will be most effective for a given child just by looking at him.

Many physicians will not prescribe NSAIDs that have not been tested and approved by the Food and Drug Administration (FDA) for use in childhood. But testing costs a lot of money, and there are not many children with arthritis. As a result, many excellent drugs have never been specifically approved for children. This does not mean that they cannot or should not be used by physicians who are experienced with them, do appropriate monitoring, and are comfortable with their use. In some cases, newer drugs have been shown to be more effective and safer, but some physicians continue to use less effective and more toxic drugs because no one has told them that the safer drug is approved for children.

In the subsections that follow, I discuss the NSAIDs that are commonly used and the ones I prefer to use. This is not a complete list of all NSAIDs or of every NSAID I ever use. I have found a variety of NSAIDs that I am comfortable using in children and feel are effective. I have not tried them all, and the absence of an NSAID from this list simply means that I do not use it often. A few, like aspirin, are included because other physicians commonly use them, even though I rarely do. The FDA has not specifically approved all of these medications for use in children at this time. That means that they cannot be advertised "for use by children"; however, it does not mean that children cannot use them.

Aspirin

Aspirin, the original NSAID, was the mainstay of therapy when I began my career. Worldwide, aspirin remains one of the most widely used treatments for children with arthritis. However, its use in the United States is limited by the ready availability of other medications that are more convenient, equally effective, and less likely to cause side effects. Disadvantages of aspirin include the following:

- It must be given three or four times each day.
- It is available only as pills.
- It frequently causes gastric irritation.

Although aspirin is available without a prescription, regular use must be monitored, just like the use of prescription NSAIDs. Aspirin has all the side effects of other NSAIDs, and in many instances they occur more frequently with aspirin than with the prescription NSAIDs. Various forms of salicylate are available, including choline salicylate (which comes in liquid form), but these are infrequently used. The modern NSAIDs are more effective, more convenient, and less irritating to the stomach. An additional concern with the use of aspirin is that it has been linked to Reye's syndrome.

Naproxen and Ibuprofen: Propionic Acid Derivatives

Naproxen and ibuprofen are marketed under a variety of names (Alleve, Naprosyn, Motrin, Advil, Nuprin, Buprofen, and more). Both are available in liquid form and are used extensively in the treatment of children with arthritis. Naproxen has the advantage of being given only twice a day, while ibuprofen may need to be given as many as four times a day. Ibuprofen liquid and pills, and some forms of naproxen pills, are available without a prescription. The reason ibuprofen liquid, but not naproxen liquid, is available without prescription is unclear. **Both of these drugs require monitoring, just like all other NSAIDs, whether they are prescribed by a doctor or bought without a prescription**. Other than stomach upset, side effects of these medications are relatively infrequent. However, all of the side effects listed in the section on NSAID side effects may occur. These NSAIDs are effective for true pauciarticular-onset JA and helpful in many other conditions. For many children with more difficult forms of JA, more potent NSAIDs may be necessary.

All of the following drugs require a prescription in the United States.

Nabumetone

Nabumetone (marketed as Relafen) is an NSAID that is useful for pediatric rheumatologists. It seems to be very effective for arthritis while rarely causing stomach irritation. It's easy for parents because it has to be given only once each day. Although it does not come as a liquid, nabumetone dissolves in warm water with no apparent loss of efficacy. It can also be crushed. Since it has a long half-life, it can easily be given after dinner for a peak effect the next morning, when it helps to reduce morning stiffness.

Diclofenac and Tolmetin Sodium (Phenyl Acetic and Heteroaryl Acetic Acids)

Diclofenac and tolmetin sodium are marketed as Voltaren and Tolectin, respectively. They are effective for all onset types of JA and for spondyloarthropathies. Many children who are not doing well enough on naproxen or ibuprofen improve dramatically when switched to diclofenac. However, complaints of stomachache and increases in liver enzyme levels seem more common with these medications. Physicians must monitor the children for these problems. In general, I prefer diclofenac to tolmetin because there are fewer complaints of stomach irritation; also, most preparations of diclofenac are enteric-coated. A compounding pharmacist can provide diclofenac as a liquid for small children. The liquid cannot be enteric-coated, but that does not seem to cause problems.

Piroxicam (Enolic Acids)

Piroxicam (marketed as Feldene) is an NSAID that is very effective for many older children with spondyloarthropathies and the related types of arthritis. It has a very long half-life and slowly builds up to an effective level in the body. Often it takes two or three weeks to start having an effect. However, it is often very effective when other NSAIDs are not sufficient. Gastrointestinal and renal side effects may be more common with piroxicam and do not always occur at the beginning of therapy. I have seen interstitial nephritis as a complication of piroxicam more often than with other NSAIDs, but it can occur with any NSAID.

Indomethacin (Arylalkanoic Acids, or Indole Acetic Acids)

Indomethacin (marketed as Indocin) is generally agreed to be the most potent of the routinely used NSAIDs. It is an excellent inhibitor of inflammation. Indomethacin is also much more likely to cause side effects. In addition to the side effects listed for all NSAIDs, it commonly causes headaches. However, many of the children old enough to talk about it say that the trade-off in improved relief of arthritis is worthwhile. The headaches can be treated with acetaminophen, and decrease in frequency and severity over time. Some individuals become depressed when taking indomethacin, and the physician and family must watch out for this complication. In small children, it may cause inexplicable temper tantrums. Kidney and liver irritation are also well-recognized infrequent side effects.

Because indomethacin is very effective and is available as a liquid, it is valuable in the care of children with arthritis. In children with systemic-onset arthritis, it may relieve fever and other symptoms when no other NSAID is effective. Indomethacin is also very effective for some children with spondyloarthropathies who have not responded to other NSAIDs. Keep in mind that it requires careful monitoring.

Celecoxib (Celebrex)

Celecoxib (marketed as Celebrex) is a useful NSAID that provides good relief for some children. It is available as a liquid and has been specifically approved for children. It has less frequent side effects, but it does contain sulfa. **Children who are allergic to sulfa drugs may be allergic to celecoxib.**

There has been great concern about the incidence of heart attacks in people taking a variety of drugs. Some of the selective COX-2 inhibitors were pulled off the market for this reason, but no pediatric rheumatologist has ever reported a child with a heart attack while taking these drugs. Recently, a variety of drugs have been associated with an increased risk of heart attacks. It is important to remember that no drug is completely safe. All of these drugs are far less likely to cause heart attacks or cancer than smoking cigarettes or exposure to a parent who smokes.

SUCRALFATE (CARAFATE)

This drug is not an anti-inflammatory. Rather, **it is a drug that was developed to minimize stomach irritation secondary to the use of other medications**. It is frequently added by rheumatologists if a child complains of stomach irritation with an NSAID. Sucralfate is a surface active agent. It coats the inside of the stomach but lets the medicine be absorbed into the body. It dramatically reduces gastric irritation due to medications.

The most important thing to remember about sucralfate is that it takes time for the medication to dissolve in the stomach and spread over the surface to provide its protective action. Sucralfate should be taken at least half an hour before other medicines. If medicines are taken with meals, it is recommended that the child take the sucralfate, eat, and then take the other medications.

Side effects of sucralfate are rare. A few people are allergic to it. Others complain of bloating or constipation. Some of my patients say that it makes them feel full. It is available in liquid form for young children.

SULFASALAZINE (AZULFIDINE)

Sulfasalazine was developed in the 1930s, when it was still strongly believed that rheumatoid arthritis was caused by an infection. It turns out that sulfasalazine is very effective for spondyloarthropathies (enthesitis-associated arthritis), which are common in Northern European and Asian populations, but less effective for other forms of arthritis in childhood. **This illustrates why it is important to know exactly what condition you are talking about and not lump all children with arthritis together as having JRA.**

Often children with enthesitis-related arthritis who have not responded to other NSAIDs respond dramatically to this drug. The mechanism of action of sulfasalazine is unclear. It is metabolized into an aspirin-like molecule and an antibiotic. However, neither alone seems to be as effective. Sulfasalazine can be used in addition to other NSAIDs, so it can be added to the regimen of a child who is not doing well enough without stopping the medications the child is already taking.

The major disadvantage of this drug is that anyone who is allergic to sulfa drugs will be allergic to sulfasalazine. These allergies often take the form of rashes that can be quite dramatic. Other common side effects include liver enzyme elevation, gastritis, and leukopenia. Allergic reactions require discontinuation; other problems might respond to a change in the dose. Because of the allergic reactions, I usually start children on a small dose of sulfasalazine and monitor them carefully as I increase the dose.

For children who respond well to sulfasalazine, I will continue using the drug for years. Although there are no hard data, I have had a number of children who did well on sulfasalazine for years, stopped taking it, and then had problems again within a few months. These problems ultimately were controlled with sulfasalazine, but the children suffered much more joint damage in the interim.

Parents frequently ask me why they should use sulfasalazine if it often has side effects. The answer is that this drug is extremely effective for children who do not experience the side effects. If a child does not have an allergic reaction to the drug, he or she can often tolerate it without difficulty for years (if properly monitored). I have many patients who did not need to take potentially more toxic medications, such as methotrexate, because sulfasalazine was effective for them.

HYDROXYCHLOROQUINE (PLAQUENIL)

Hydroxychloroquine is an interesting drug that has been widely used in the treatment of rheumatic diseases since the 1950s. It is a derivative of quinine, which was originally used to fight malaria—hence, it is an antimalarial. Quinine was first reported to benefit patients with rheumatic disease in the 1890s. Hydroxychloroquine is a derivative that has fewer side effects. Its precise mechanism of action remains unknown. The drug's onset of action is very slow. Indeed, families often wonder whether their child just got better rather than improving with hydroxychloroquine. However, many controlled studies have shown that patients receiving hydroxychloroquine did better than the controls.

Hydroxychloroquine has been found to be helpful in children with most forms of arthritis, SLE, dermatomyositis, and scleroderma in both its localized and systemic forms. It is probably helpful for many other conditions as well. At one time, it was thought that hydroxychloroquine was uniquely effective for skin manifestations of dermatomyositis and SLE, but it is not clear that this is true.

One of the most interesting things about hydroxychloroquine is that evidence suggests that it truly is a disease-modifying drug. Hydroxychloroquine is probably the safest of all the medications that are thought to be disease-modifying. It is rarely associated with toxicity.

Unfortunately, there has been discussion of possible blindness as a side effect of hydroxychloroquine. It is important to know that this warning comes from a period in the late 1960s and early 1970s when the wrong dosage was used. Once the dosage was corrected, this problem essentially disappeared. It is recommended that children have an eye examination by an ophthalmologist before starting the drug and every six months thereafter while taking it.

Since hydroxychloroquine appears to be safe and effective but very slow-acting, children are often kept on it for years. Like all medications, hydroxychloroquine is associated with a wide variety of minor complaints or abnormalities on blood tests and therefore needs to be monitored appropriately. Fortunately, these problems are very infrequent. A compounding pharmacist can provide the drug in liquid form and add ingredients to hide the taste.

DOXYCYCLINE (VIBRAMYCIN)

Doxycycline is marketed under a wide variety of trade names around the world. It is a tetracycline antibiotic that has received a lot of publicity because it is used for Lyme disease. It is also useful for patients with arthritis. **The use of doxycycline and related tetracyclines in children is restricted by the fact that tetracyclines permanently stain growing bones and teeth.** Most physicians prefer not to use doxycycline before the age of ten, though some physicians use it earlier.

The discovery that doxycycline is effective for arthritis generated a lot of publicity. The physicians who initially proposed the use of doxycycline thought that it was effective in treating certain infections that caused arthritis. Instead, it has been shown that doxycycline works by blocking a group of enzymes called metalloproteinases. This effect is independent of its effect as an antibiotic.

In addition to staining teeth and bones in young children, doxycycline causes gastritis and photosensitivity. These complaints limit its use. It is also used in the treatment of acne in teenagers and in the treatment of Lyme disease. Some caution against using doxycycline for acne because it has been associated with rare cases of drug-induced SLE. There are a number of studies indicating that doxycycline is an effective adjunctive agent for arthritis, but the vast majority of teenagers I give it to discontinue its use because of stomachaches.

IMMUNOSUPPRESSIVE DRUGS

If a child with arthritis has failed to respond to NSAIDs, hydroxychloroquine, and sulfasalazine, the family will have to consider immunosuppressive medications or one of the newer biologics discussed below (although the biologics are classified separately, they are in fact immunosuppressive). **Fortunately, the majority of children with arthritis do not require immunosuppressive drugs. However, children with more severe arthritis will do much better if they are appropriately treated and their disease is brought under good control—the earlier the better!** Stronger immunosuppressive drugs are commonly used for children with illnesses such as SLE, dermatomyositis, scleroderma, polyarteritis nodosa, and Wegener's granulomatosis.

The majority of the poor outcomes result from families refusing aggressive therapy for severe disease or physicians failing to offer it. With careful monitoring, poor outcomes due to medications are extremely rare. Certain potential side effects have to be considered with every immunosuppressive medication. The two most important ones are the increased risk of infection and the possibly increased risk of a malignancy. **While the risk of potential side effects cannot be denied, the damage caused by uncontrolled disease is not a possible problem, but a real and immediate one that must be dealt with.**

Some immunosuppressive drugs, such as cyclophosphamide, azathioprine, and mycophenolate mofetil, work by inhibiting the rapid turnover of inflammatory cells. These drugs may increase the risk of infertility as well as the risks of infection and malignancy. Others, such as cyclosporine, tacrolimus, etanercept, infliximab, anakinra, and adalimumab, work by directly blocking the cytokines that promote tissue inflammation. Still other immunosuppressive drugs work by interfering with cytokine synthesis (thalidomide), eliminating the cells that are driving the response (rituximab), or blocking cell-to-cell messaging (abatacept). These drugs increase the risk of infection, and perhaps of malignancy, but are not thought to carry the risk of infertility.

> Prescribing medications is often like being the wise man in a mythical village. It is a wonderful place ruled by a good king. However, to keep evil at bay, the dragon must be fed fifty people each year. The king cannot make such a choice from among his subjects. Instead, a hundred people are chosen by lot and assigned to stand in a house with no roof where the dragon comes to

eat. The house has two rooms. One room has red walls and the other room has blue walls.

Since you are a wise man, some of the people who must stand in the house come to you and ask what to do. Experience has taught you that the dragon prefers to eat people in the red room. However, the dragon is nearsighted. Every year he eats forty people in the red room, but misses ten times and eats ten people in the blue room. Your advice is always to stand in the blue room. Every year there will be someone in the red room who lived and someone in the blue room who did not. There is no foolproof advice. But the blue room is clearly the better choice, even if the advice seeker's best friend survived in the red room the year before. With medications we aren't talking 40:10—it's more like 999:1.

Methotrexate

Methotrexate has significantly improved the outlook for children with arthritis. Before it became widely used for arthritis in the 1980s, children who did not respond to NSAIDs were treated with gold shots (discussed later in this chapter). If a child was allergic to the gold shots or had a toxic reaction, there were very few choices left. Methotrexate is now one of the mainstays for the treatment of children with significant arthritis. It can be used alone or in combination with anti-cytokine agents such as etanercept and adalimumab.

In the doses used in cancer therapy, methotrexate works by interfering with DNA synthesis and blocking the rapid reproduction of cells. In the dosage normally used for children with arthritis, methotrexate is believed to have a different mechanism of action. Nonetheless, it is very effective in reducing pain and swelling in children with most forms of arthritis. Careful studies in adults suggest that it may be a disease-modifying drug and may reduce the number of erosions. It is certainly a drug that improves function and controls arthritis symptoms for most children who take it.

Most often methotrexate is given as pills (or shots) that are taken just once each week. Some physicians start out at the full dose and monitor blood tests after a few weeks. However, there are children who are unexpectedly sensitive to methotrexate. I prefer to start out with a small dose and monitor the blood tests every week until I am sure that the child is tolerating the drug. Children on methotrexate should also take folic acid, which sharply reduces the frequency of side effects of the drug. There are many ways of administering folic acid; it doesn't matter how it is given as long as it is taken. My patients take 1 mg every day (even on the day when they take methotrexate) and do fine.

The onset of action of methotrexate is slow. It usually begins to show effects after a few weeks, but it may be six to twelve weeks before it has a significant effect on the arthritis. For many children, methotrexate is a very effective drug and provides excellent control of the arthritis. The normal dosage range for children with arthritis is 5 to 10 mg/m^2/week.

Many children who were having significant problems with arthritis do well after starting to use methotrexate. Although there is no uniform agreement, most physicians keep children on methotrexate until they have been well for at least six months. Some physicians then reduce the weekly dose, while others prefer to spread out the dose so that it is given every two weeks, then every three weeks, and so on, until it is slowly discontinued over a period of many months. Unfortunately, the arthritis flares in a substantial proportion of children as the methotrexate is withdrawn.

Common side effects of methotrexate include nausea, leukopenia, thrombo-cytopenia, and liver enzyme elevation. The nausea often responds to reassurance. However, methotrexate-induced nausea does not come from stomach irritation; it acts on the central nervous system. If the nausea is severe, it can be treated with ondansetron (Zofran). Changes in the blood counts and liver enzyme levels are monitored by blood tests. Sores in the mouth or an irritated tongue are rare in children taking folic acid. Children with warts often notice that their warts either return or get worse when the methotrexate reaches an effective level.

Children taking methotrexate also need to avoid going out in the sun. Although most children have no problem, some children taking methotrexate are photosensitive. In rare cases, methotrexate has been associated with renal or pulmonary problems. It should be very carefully monitored in children with pre-existing liver, kidney, or lung conditions. Methotrexate is normally excreted by the kidneys, but it is not removed by dialysis.

When methotrexate was first used for patients with arthritis, many of these patients underwent periodic liver biopsies to make sure that they were not developing cirrhosis of the liver. These routine biopsies were not found to be helpful. Children with persistent or recurrent liver enzyme abnormalities should be taken off methotrexate. Failure to do so could result in long-term liver damage. Occasional leukopenia or liver enzyme elevations may be the result of viral infections or other unrelated problems. These situations are best dealt with by withholding the methotrexate until the problem corrects itself and then restarting the methotrexate while monitoring carefully to make sure that the problem does not return. Everyone must remember that individuals using methotrexate must not drink alcoholic beverages. The use of alcohol greatly increases the risk of liver damage. While patients under the age of twenty-one will not be drinking legally, it remains necessary to caution them about the risks associated with the use of alcohol while taking medications.

BIOLOGICS

The biologics are a new class of medications that provide dramatic relief to children with severe arthritis. They are designed to target a specific molecule that plays an important role in the inflammatory process. Each of the biologics has strengths and weaknesses that I discuss later in this section. Because the biologics relieve arthritis by directly affecting the immune response, they are immunosuppressive. As a result, they carry the same risks of infection and possibly late development of cancer that are discussed in the section on immunosuppressive medications. Although in the past methotrexate was commonly prescribed before biologics, it has a slower onset of action, is often less effective, and has a higher frequency of side effects involving the bone marrow and liver. Therefore, many physicians are starting to use biologics before methotrexate. The biologics are more expensive, but in the long run their early use appears to be cost effective. It should be remembered that in the most severe cases the biologics and methotrexate have been shown to be synergistic, and it may be necessary to add methotrexate after starting a biologic if it has not been used before.

Parents often worry that because the biologics are new medications, we do not know what will happen to someone who takes them for ten years or more. Of course, until a medication has been in use for ten years, it is impossible to know what effects it will have. However, you would not go out and buy a ten-year-old model television or computer. You'd want the latest version.

It is always difficult for parents and physicians to balance the potential risks and benefits of new therapies, and often the list of potential side effects seems terrifying. But think about travel. Most of us would gladly accept two free round-trip airline tickets to Paris, but this doesn't mean that we are unaware of the risks of airplane travel, the hassles at airports, or the possibility of being mugged on the street in Paris. We accept them as part of traveling. There are a few people who are afraid to travel, but most agree that the benefits far outweigh the remote possibility of something truly unfortunate happening. The same is true of taking medications. The difference is that the government requires pharmaceutical companies and physicians to explain the risks; no one requires airlines or travel agencies to do so. Further, the cost of not taking a vacation in Paris is minimal compared to accepting a lifetime of discomfort resulting from inadequately treated disease. There are remote risks of undiscovered long-term side effects with every medication, but there are many uncontrollable risks in everyday life. **We recommend these medicines because we know for sure that ten years of uncontrolled arthritis will cause significant disability.**

It is recommended that any child at risk for tuberculosis be appropriately screened before beginning to take any biologic agent.

Agents That Decrease the Function of Tumor Necrosis Factor-α

A variety of biologic agents interfere with the activity of TNF-α, and several more are in early clinical testing. When large amounts of TNF-α are in the circulation, people tend to feel very ill. The effects of blocking TNF-α are often very impressive. Parents frequently report striking improvement within hours of taking the first dose. In most cases, the improvement continues as long as the child remains on the TNF blocking agent. By blocking TNF-α activity, these agents not only prevent agents not only prevent symptoms of the disease, but also allow healing of the bone and joint damage to begin.

Common side effects of TNF-blocking agents include rhinorrhea, injection site reactions, and headaches. Few parents or children feel that these are significant when measured against the dramatic relief of arthritis symptoms. Periodic monitoring of blood tests is required, as with every medication, but significant problems are few.

There are several important considerations regarding uncommon side effects in children on TNF-blocking agents. The most important one is the increased risk of infection. Fortunately, serious infections are rare. **Because of the risk of severe infection, if a child receiving TNF-blocking agents looks sick, he or she should be seen by a physician sooner, not later.** In this situation, I err on the side of antibiotic coverage.

Tumor necrosis factor–blocking agents and other biologics should not be given to children with fever unless the fever is part of the disease for which they are being treated (and then only with care). Skin and lung infections may be the most important ones to watch for. Infection is a risk with all of the immunosuppressive medications used for children with severe arthritis.

Another concern is that all of the drugs that affect the immune system are associated with altered immune regulation, which may lead to the development or worsening of other diseases. Some children receiving TNF-blocking agents have developed minor serologic abnormalities related to SLE, and this needs to be monitored. However, medically significant problems appear to be extremely rare. The TNF-blocking agents can prevent serious damage from arthritis. For the majority of children, allowing the arthritis to continue is far more worrisome and dangerous than the remote risk of a serious side effect from TNF-blocking agents.

Parents often ask how long their child will need to continue taking TNF-blocking agents. This is a very difficult question to answer. Although TNF-blocking agents often do an excellent job of controlling disease, they do not cure it. I have had two experiences with children who were "miraculously cured" by TNF-blocking agents, so that the family thought there was no reason to continue the shots or return for their appointments. After six or eight weeks off medication, the disease came back and was much worse than before.

Parents often become so worried after hearing about all the potential side effects that they hesitate to accept TNF-blocking agents. Everyone should remember that the most common thing I hear from parents after they start children on TNF-blocking agents is "She's doing wonderfully. Why did you let me wait so long?"

At present, a child who is doing well on a TNF-blocking agent should continue to use it. After the child does well for a year, it is often possible to decrease the frequency of injections. The proper means of discontinuing TNF-blocking agents remains to be determined. In the few children for whom these agents have not been beneficial, there have been no problems with discontinuation. All parents worry about giving their child a medication without a clear indication of how and when they will be able to stop using it. But seeing a child with significant arthritis suddenly and dramatically improve provides an immediate reminder of how much trouble the child was having. **It is true that parents and physicians should be worried about giving a child a medication without a clear indication of how and when to stop using it. But they should be far**

**more worried about allowing a child to have active uncontrolled arthritis
and all of its complications without a clear indication of how and when the
arthritis will stop.**

Etanercept (Enbrel)

Etanercept was the first widely available biologic. The etanercept molecule
consists of two artificial receptors for TNF-α attached to an Fc receptor that
allows the etanercept to which TNF has been bound to be cleared from the
body. It has made a dramatic difference in the care of children with JA. Many
pediatric rheumatologists feel that it is the most significant advance in many
years. It is effective for most children with polyarticular-onset arthritis, spondyloarthropathies, and psoriasis-associated arthritis and for some children with
systemic-onset arthritis. It may prove to be effective for many other forms of
childhood rheumatic disease, but this has not been fully investigated. Although
etanercept is also effective for children with severe pauciarticular-onset arthritis,
it is infrequently necessary for that disease.

Etanercept was initially studied in children with severe disease who were
not responding adequately to methotrexate. All of the published data indicate
that methotrexate plus etanercept is better than methotrexate alone. However,
etanercept is now commonly used alone because of its lower frequency of side
effects. Many physicians add methotrexate only in more difficult cases that have
not responded to etanercept or another biologic.

Etanercept works by binding to TNF-α. The major disadvantage of this drug
is that it must be given by subcutaneous injection weekly. That means that parents or the child will need to learn how to give the shots. Alternatively, the shots
can be given in the physician's office, by a visiting nurse, or by another individual. However, since subcutaneous injections are easy to administer, most parents
learn to give them without difficulty.

Common side effects of etanercept include rhinorrhea, injection site reactions, and headaches. Few parents or children feel that these are significant when
measured against the dramatic relief of arthritis symptoms. Periodic monitoring
of blood tests is required, as with every medication, but significant problems
are few. There are several uncommon side effects to consider for children on
etanercept and all the other TNF-blocking agents described above. Etanercept is
now approved for use in children with JA and psoriasis. It is being evaluated for
gastrointestinal and other diseases as well.

Adalimumab (Humira)

This is another new biologic. It is an antibody to TNF-α that can be given as a subcutaneous injection either every week or every other week. It attacks TNF-α not only in the circulation circulation but also on the surface of cells, destroying both the TNF-α and the cells. It is a very effective treatment for severe arthritis. It is effective for most children with polyarticular-onset arthritis, spondyloarthropathies, and psoriasis-associated arthritis, as well as for some children with systemic-onset arthritis. It may also prove to be effective for many other forms of childhood arthritis.

Adalimumab has been effective in some children who have not responded to etanercept. In addition, it has been extremely effective in children with uveitis associated with arthritis. Because adalimumab is a "fully humanized" antibody, there appear to be fewer side effects and less development of human antichimeric antibodies (HACAs) with adalimumab than with infliximab. Adalimumab has also proven effective in the treatment of Crohn's disease and seems particularly effective in children with psoriatic arthritis. Although adalimumab acts by directly binding to TNF-α rather than being a "fake receptor," because it also blocks the activity of TNF-α it shares with etanercept the increased risk of risk of infection and the possible future development of malignancy.

Adalimumab and etanercept have a similar frequency of side effects, but adalimumab requires less frequent injections. Children receiving adalimumab should be cautioned that the injections sting; those who expect this seem to tolerate the injections without difficulty. The efficacy of adalimumab in children who have conditions that do not respond well to etanercept is sufficient to offset the discomfort of its use.

It should be noted that the official product literature for adalimumab suggests that the injections be given every other week and increased to a weekly schedule only if the drug proves to be ineffective. I often find it more effective to give adalimumab weekly for the first six to twelve weeks, establish good control of the inflammation, and then decrease the frequency of injections. For children with uveitis, weekly injections often need to be continued indefinitely.

Infliximab (Remicade)

Infliximab is another useful biologic for the treatment of children with arthritis. It too is an antibody directed against TNF-α. The published information states that infliximab is used in conjunction with methotrexate. This is because the antibody molecule that is the active part of infliximab sometimes stimulates an immune response in which the body produces HACAs. These HACAs attack the infliximab molecule and block its effect. There is reason to believe that methotrexate reduces the incidence of allergic reactions and other complications that may interfere with the way infliximab works. It is also believed that methotrexate slows the formation of HACAs. If a child cannot tolerate methotrexate and requires infliximab, one of the other immunosuppressive drugs may be useful.

The major difficulties associated with infliximab relate to its administration. Infliximab is given as a periodic intravenous infusion. It can be given in a physician's office, in a hospital infusion unit, or by a visiting nurse. The dosage regimen is variable. After the initial doses, which are given more frequently, infliximab may be given monthly or every other month. The optimal dosage regimen and frequency are different for every patient. Allergic reactions seem to be more common with infliximab than with other biologics, and some patients need to be medicated for them. As a result, the first dose of infliximab is normally given under a doctor's supervision. Even after the first dose, any side effects during administration should be promptly reported to the physician for evaluation.

Infection is a concern with infliximab, just as it is with other immunosuppressive and biologic agents. Tuberculosis is a particular concern, and children should be screened for tuberculosis and tuberculosis exposure before infliximab is begun. The use of very high doses of infliximab is associated with a marked increase in the risk of infection.

If a child has fever or there are other reasons to suspect that there might be an infection, infliximab should not be given. Significant side effects of infliximab, except for mild allergic reactions and infections, are very rare. All of the concerns related to altering the immune system with immunosuppressive medications should be considered. As with etanercept and adalimumab, the ultimate duration of infliximab therapy is unclear.

Anakinra (Kineret)

Anakinra is a novel biologic agent that works by blocking a messenger called IL-1, preventing its attachment to the IL-1 receptor. The experience with kineret in children is limited. However, it has proven uniquely effective for many (but not all) children with systemic-onset JA. Unlike infliximab, adalimumab, and etanercept, which are given less frequently, anakinra needs to be administered as a daily subcutaneous injection. It may be associated with abnormalities on routine blood tests and local pain at the injection site. It also has a slow onset of action. Its slow onset of action and the need for daily injections limit its use in children who respond to other biologics.

Although anakinra is effective, the ultimate place for this agent in the treatment of childhood arthritis is uncertain. It clearly is important in treating children with systemic-onset JA. In animal models, blocking IL-1 substantially reduced joint damage due to arthritis. It has also been shown that blocking IL-1 may be uniquely beneficial in children with systemic-onset JA. For some children with systemic-onset disease anakinra has been miraculous, but for others it is ineffective. There is a group of genetic conditions, w including NOMID and Muckle-Wells syndrome, that responds dramatically and almost immediately to anakinra. Familial Mediterranean fever also responds well.

Anakinra has all of the side effects associated with other biologics. Unfortunately, the combination of anakinra with etanercept increases the incidence of infections; as a result, physicians hesitate to combine anakinra with other biologics. There are children with psoriatic arthritis and with polyarticular JA who respond to kineret after failing with other biologics. Additional agents that block IL-1 but are given less frequently are under investigation and may ultimately replace anakinra.

Rituximab (Rituxan)

Rituximab was initially developed for the treatment of lymphomas. It is a monoclonal antibody directed against CD20, a surface marker present on "activated" B cells and perhaps other lymphocytes but not on mature plasma cells. When it was noted that some lymphoma patients who also had rheumatoid arthritis improved, studies of rituximab therapy for rheumatoid arthritis began.

It is now recognized the rituximab is effective in the treatment of rheumatoid arthritis, SLE, Wegener's granulomatosis, and juvenile dermatomyositis. It may prove effective in additional rheumatic diseases in the future. A number of studies are presently underway to determine the optimal regimen for rituximab in each of these conditions. In adults with rheumatoid arthritis, it is clear that rituximab may provide relief for severe cases that have not responded to TNF inhibitors. Rituximab has been very effective in children with RF-positive arthritis combined with cyclophosphamide or methotrexate. There is limited experience with this drug in other forms of JA, but it appears to be beneficial.

In adults with rheumatoid arthritis, repeated treatment seems necessary; this is likely to be true in children as well.

The combination of rituximab and cyclophosphamide often provides dramatic relief of symptoms in adults and children with SLE combined with normalization of serologic parameters for prolonged periods. While the therapy is aggressive, a number of children with SLE in my care have been able to wean themselves to minimal doses of prednisone and remained ANA-negative for several years. The long-term safety and efficacy of this regimen are being studied. The ability to cure SLE may be on the horizon.

One interesting aspect of rituximab therapy is that there is often an initial period of increased complaints lasting for one or two months after the rituximab is given. However, this is followed by steady improvement in most children. The current regimen is to give two doses of rituximab (600 mg/m^2 up to 1000 mg) two weeks apart (with or without cyclophosphamide) and repeat as necessary, but no more often than every four months.

Therapy with rituximab depletes CD20-positive B cells and is associated with an increased risk of infection. Infusion reactions also may occur, and rituximab should be administered in an experienced infusion center. Most often,corticosteroids and diphenhydramine are administered prior to the rituximab. The initial studies have shown substantial benefits from this drug. Many of my patients with SLE consider themselves to be cured.

Abatacept (Orencia)

Abatacept is a new agent that decreases the signaling between T cells and other cells in the immune system. Abatacept's mechanism of action is termed *costimulatory* blockade. In the presence of infection, cells in the immune system interact to alert the immune system to the need for an inflammatory response. To minimize inappropriate messages, cells communicating with each other need to interact at several different levels. They need to be HLA compatible, they need to be activated, and they need to interact with a costimulatory molecule (CD86). Abatacept blocks this costimulatory molecule and thus decreases the inflammatory response. I often explain abatacept's mechanism of action this way:

> Think of two Indians, strangers, who want to trade goods in the old West. They have to belong to the same tribe, they have to have something to trade, and they have to be friendly. Abatacept prevents them from shaking hands, so the trade isn't made.

There are studies of abatacept use in children with JA showing that it may be effective when TNF-blocking agents not useful. Whether it will prove to be most beneficial when used alone or in combination with other drugs is uncertain. The use of abatacept in other childhood rheumatic diseases has also been considered, but little information is available at the time of this writing.

Newer Biologic Agents

There are several agents under development that may be available soon, but the complex nature of the final stages of clinical testing and governmental approval make this uncertain. One is a different agent to block IL-1 that has a different site of action and needs to be given only every two weeks. Several other drugs undergoing testing block IL-6. This is a potent inflammatory mediator whose level rises and falls at the same time as the fever and rash come and go in children with severe systemic-onset arthritis. There are reports of excellent efficacy, but more information is needed regarding side effects. Many more agents are in the pipeline. Few people realize that hundreds of agents will undergo initial testing, of which only one or two will do well enough to go further. Of those few, only a small fraction will make it all the way to your drugstore

Older Immunosuppressive Agents

Cyclosporine (Neoral, Sandimmune) and Tacrolimus (Prograf)

Cyclosporine and tacrolimus are closely related immunosuppressive drugs that are primarily used to prevent organ transplant rejection. Cyclosporine was discovered first and is used more widely, but tacrolimus may be more potent and have fewer side effects. However, there is only limited experience with the use of tacrolimus for arthritis at present, and I restrict the rest of this discussion to cyclosporine.

Cyclosporine works primarily by blocking the synthesis of IL-2 (a messenger molecule) and preventing the recruitment of additional inflammatory cells to a site of inflammation. It also affects IL-3, IL-4, and interferon (IFN)-gamma, which are messenger molecules (cytokines) that promote inflammation. Since cyclosporine has an independent mechanism of action, in most cases it can be added to the other medications a child is taking.

Cyclosporine may be very beneficial in children with enthesitis-associated arthritis, systemic-onset arthritis, IBD-associated arthritis, dermatomyositis, and other vasculitic illnesses. It is also useful for the treatment of ocular inflammation (uveitis). However, a child's response to cyclosporine is unpredictable. Some children who have not responded to other medications have dramatically improved with the addition of cyclosporine. At the same time, I have used it in other children, in seemingly identical situations, without benefit.

Cyclosporine is associated with a variety of side effects. It interferes with the immune system and has essentially the same risks as the other immunosuppressive drugs. In addition, the larger doses used to prevent organ transplant rejection are often associated with kidney damage (renal toxicity). At the low dosages used for children with arthritis, these side effects are uncommon. However, children on cyclosporine should have all the normal monitoring tests (see above), especially to make sure that the urine and blood pressure are checked routinely. Changes in blood pressure or evidence of kidney irritation occasionally occur at low doses, but with proper monitoring the drug can be discontinued as soon as they appear. In children who are carefully monitored, side effects are infrequent and generally resolve quickly with discontinuation of the drug.

Cyclosporine has several peculiarities. One is that it promotes hair growth— not just on top of the head, but everywhere on the body. This may become unsightly, but if the cyclosporine is correcting the disease, it is acceptable. **Cyclosporine is also unusual in that it binds very strongly to glass.** This means that if you put the medicine in a glass of water, the cyclosporine will bind to the glass and none of it will be ingested by the child. Liquid cyclosporine is provided in a special container and must be administered directly to the child. You can't mix it in another container. Another peculiarity is that **children taking cyclosporine must avoid grapefruit juice.** There is a chemical in the juice that inactivates cyclosporine. Orange juice, grape juice, and other juices do not contain this chemical. If you are giving your child many juices or juice-flavored drinks, check the label carefully.

Leflunomide (Arava)

Leflunomide is another immunosuppressive drug that works by interfering with DNA synthesis. However, at the very low doses used by rheumatologists, it is suspected that leflunomide has other anti-inflammatory effects as well. In adult studies, leflunomide has proven effective for rheumatoid arthritis. Most physicians feel that leflunomide is appropriately used only after methotrexate and perhaps one of the biologics has been tried. However, this is a matter of individual judgment.

Leflunomide can be added to NSAIDs and other medications. It does not act at the same point as methotrexate, so the two drugs can be combined, but both may cause liver and blood cell abnormalities and their combined use requires careful monitoring. Like other immunosuppressive drugs, leflunomide has a slow onset of action but appears to be disease-modifying.

Leflunomide differs from most of the other immunosuppressive drugs by being highly concentrated in the enterohepatic circulation. This means that the drug is absorbed by the body, processed by the liver, and released from the liver into the intestine, but then reabsorbed into the body from the intestine. Instead of being removed from the body, like most drugs, the active part of leflunomide stays in the body for a long time.

To take advantage of the fact that leflunomide is very slowly removed from the body, patients are given a big dose the first few days and then a much smaller everyday dose. This is generally advantageous. However, if the drug must be removed from the system (e.g., because of a side effect), the child must be given cholestyramine. This is an agent that binds to the leflunomide products in the intestine and prevents them from being reabsorbed. Once bound to cholestyramine, the active compounds are carried out of the body quickly.

Leflunomide requires careful monitoring of the child, as with any other immunosuppressive drug. It may cause problems with the liver, the blood-forming cells, or elsewhere. It also may increase the risk of infection, as do the other immunosuppressive drugs. Diarrhea seems to be an occasional mild side effect. There was a lot of excitement when leflunomide first became available, but it seems less effective than methotrexate.

Mycophenolate Mofetil (Cellcept)

Mycophenolate mofetil is a newer immunosuppressive drug that inhibits DNA synthesis. It is primarily used for the treatment of organ transplant recipients but has been increasingly used in children with SLE and other vasculitic diseases. It has also been used in children with uveitis associated with JA and in adults with psoriatic arthritis. At present, the role of mycophenolate mofetil in the treatment of children with arthritis has not been defined. It is useful for some children with SLE and is seeing increasing usage. It has been reported to be as effective as cyclophosphamide in high doses, but most physicians have found that the necessary dose causes a significant incidence of stomach complaints that force patients to stop taking the medication. In addition, practical experience with the drug has not matched the success of the carefully selected patients in the published studies. A variety of investigations combining mycophenolate mofetil with other agents have been initiated. A lot of interesting information should be forthcoming.

Azathioprine (Imuran)

Azathioprine is one of the oldest immunosuppressive drugs. Like other drugs in its class, it works by inhibiting DNA synthesis.,. There is extensive experience with azathioprine in the treatment of children with arthritis and the vasculitic diseases. In the past, it was the primary immunosuppressive therapy used for children who failed to respond to NSAIDs and gold shots. With the widespread use of methotrexate, there has been much less need for azathioprine. It has all of the side effects of immunosuppressive drugs listed above. In addition, it is well known to sometimes cause liver irritation and problems with blood cell counts. It has also been associated with pancreatitis.

The proper role for azathioprine at present is unclear. It has been useful in children with severe polyarticular-onset and severe systemic-onset JA. Newer agents, such as leflunomide and mycophenolate mofetil, were developed with the intent that they would be more effective and have fewer side effects. At present, we do not have enough experience with the newer drugs to make a definite statement about their relative safety or effectiveness. However, many physicians will try leflunomide or mycophenolate mofetil before azathioprine.

The biologics etanercept, infliximab, and adalimumab may greatly reduce the need for drugs such as azathioprine. However, on a worldwide basis, many physicians continue to use azathioprine because they have extensive experience with it and because it is far less expensive. Azathioprine has been used extensively in the treatment of children with vasculitic diseases.

Cyclophosphamide (Cytoxan)

Cyclophosphamide is the most potent commonly used immunosuppressive agent. It is rarely used in the treatment of children with JA. Its use in the treatment of SLE is discussed in detail in Chapter 11. Cyclophosphamide can be given as daily pills or as intravenous injections. The injections are given on a variety of schedules, but the most common is monthly for a period of six months, followed by every three months until the course of therapy is completed. Except in special situations, daily pills should be avoided, as they have a much higher incidence of side effects than the intravenous injections.

Children receiving cyclophosphamide must be carefully monitored for evidence of bone marrow and bladder irritation. It is impractical to measure WBC counts and all other parameters daily. If the medication is being given intravenously at intervals, all necessary tests can be done before each dose is given. Daily use of cyclophosphamide pills is associated with an increased risk of infection and a greatly increased risk of bladder damage. The damage to the bladder can lead to persistent bleeding and has been associated with the later development of bladder cancer.

Periodic intravenous injections of cyclophosphamide not only allow more careful monitoring, but also permit the physicians to make sure that the child is well hydrated to prevent cyclophosphamide breakdown products from being allowed to remain in the bladder for a long period. In addition, most physicians administer MESNA intravenously after the cyclophosphamide. This compound binds to the cyclophosphamide breakdown products and neutralizes them, reducing the risk of bladder irritation.

Intravenous cyclophosphamide has been used for the treatment of children with systemic-onset JA who failed all other therapies. Although there are several small reports describing success, it is not generally utilized. The treatment is difficult for the child and the family, and at best some children improve. A number of years ago, I tested it on a group of eight children with severe disease. After one year, all elected to discontinue treatment. They did not think it made enough difference. With the current availability of many new therapies, the role of cyclophosphamide in the treatment of children with arthritis is extremely limited. However, it remains a mainstay of therapy for children with vasculitic diseases, including SLE, dermatomyositis, and scleroderma. The future of cyclophosphamide in the therapy of rheumatic diseases may well lie in combining its use with newer biologic agents to increase the efficacy of the biologics while significantly reducing the total amount of cyclophosphamide given.

Chlorambucil (Leukeran)

Chlorambucil is a very potent immunosuppressive agent that does not have the bladder-irritating properties of cyclophosphamide. It has been used for systemic-onset arthritis, vasculitic diseases, uveitis, and a variety of other life-threatening conditions. It is very effective. However, although chlorambucil does not irritate the bladder, it significantly impairs the body's ability to deal with infections.

Chlorambucil is not widely used because it has been associated with the development of leukemia, sterility, and other complications far more often than the other immunosuppressive drugs discussed here. It should be considered only in the most difficult situations and used only by physicians with experience. Nonetheless, there are situations in which its use is appropriate.

GLUCOCORTICOIDS: STEROIDS, CORTICOSTEROIDS, PREDNISONE, METHYLPREDNISONE, DEXAMETHASONE, CORTISONE, AND HYDROCORTISONE

The discovery of steroids was a major advance in the care of children and adults with rheumatic diseases. The beneficial effects of steroids result from their ability to block the effects of most inflammatory messengers (cytokines) and decrease the activity of the cells that promote inflammation. For children with severe diseases, the corticosteroids have vastly improved their quality of life. However, the excessive use of corticosteroids has many negative effects. These drugs should be used only when necessary. Excessive and unnecessary use may cause great harm.

Corticosteroids are simultaneously a blessing and a curse for children with JA. With a large enough dose, virtually all of the manifestations of JA will rapidly disappear. The discovery of these drugs at first was considered a miracle, but it quickly became obvious that their continued use caused an unacceptably high level of side effects. When considering the use of these drugs, it is important to remember that they may be absolutely necessary and lifesaving under certain circumstances but that prolonged use in a significant dosage is inevitably associated with complications.

For children with JA, corticosteroids should be thought of as a fire extinguisher next to the stove. If everything is going up in flames, the fire extinguisher is very handy. On the other hand, it makes a mess of your kitchen that takes some time to clean up. Further, if you have repeated need for the fire extinguisher, you're doing something wrong. With the ready availability of biologics, oral steroids should be necessary only in the treatment of systemic-onset JA, never pauciarticular-onset JA, and rarely polyarticular-onset JA. Corticosteroids are routinely used in the treatment of vasculitic diseases.

The adrenal gland in normally makes a certain amount of corticosteroids every day. If the adrenal gland fails, the result is a severe, life-threatening condition called **Addison's disease**. When the child takes extra corticosteroid every day, the body recognizes that there is no need for the adrenal gland to make more of it. If this process continues for a long period, the adrenal gland may not be able to produce an adequate amount of corticosteroids. This condition is termed *adrenal suppression*.

There are two important consequences of adrenal suppression. First, if corticosteroids have been given long enough to shut down the adrenal gland (weeks, not days), they cannot be stopped abruptly. Instead, they must be withdrawn slowly to give the adrenal gland time to resume its normal function. Second, if the child is taking corticosteroids and becomes ill with nausea and vomiting, or if for any other reason the child cannot take the normal daily dose, an injection is needed. This usually requires a visit to the doctor's office or the emergency department.

Even for children who have been able to discontinue corticosteroids, an extra dose should be given if they need surgery or are under any other form of significant physical stress, since their adrenal glands may not be able to produce the additional corticosteroids needed to deal with the stress. Be sure to inform any doctor caring for the child that he or she is taking or has taken corticosteroids if this is the case. The doctor will then know to take extra precautions, if necessary.

Side Effects of Corticosteroids

The side effects of corticosteroids are very common. They are not unusual; they are the normal effects of taking extra corticosteroids (see Box 23-1). In addition to the common side effects listed, corticosteroids may cause high blood pressure, mood changes, inflammation of the pancreas, and pseudotumor cerebrae, which is increased pressure in the brain associated with severe headaches and visual problems.

So why give corticosteroids? The answer is that most children with JA should not be given corticosteroids. However, children with diseases such as SLE and dermatomyositis often must take them. For children with arthritis, corticosteroids should be reserved for those who cannot carry out their normal activities

---

Box 23-1   Glucocorticoid side effects

Cushing's syndrome

Fluid retention

Increased appetite

Weight gain

Truncal obesity (thin arms and legs but increased fat on the back and stomach)

Moon facies (fat cheeks)

Stretch marks

Acne

Growth retardation

Bone-weakening calcium loss

Avascular necrosis

Muscle weakness

Poor sugar control (diabetes)

Cataracts

Increased intraocular pressure

Increased infections

Oral and vaginal thrush

Atherosclerosis

Hirsutism (extra hair growth)

Mood changes

---

of daily living despite an adequate trial of other medications. Preferably, children who are having trouble should be placed on a disease-modifying drug before they get to the point where they cannot function well.

In some cases, the disease is evolving rapidly or has a significant head start and the child requires corticosteroids. Even then, they should be used only for children with JA until one of the disease-modifying drugs can take over and the steroids can be withdrawn. In contrast, children with vasculitic illness often require chronic corticosteroid therapy. Most of the negative effects of corticosteroids are related to either the highest daily dose taken or the total amount taken over time, but side effects such as avascular necrosis of bone may occur after only the briefest exposure.

Many parents are very worried about the possible side effects of immunosuppressive drugs. It should be remembered that when these drugs are given by experienced physicians, their severe side effects are very rare. The negative effects of corticosteroids are very common. Before the widespread use of disease-modifying drugs, it was common to see a large number of obese children with weak hips sitting in wheelchairs waiting for the arthritis clinic to open. The obesity and hip weakness were side effects of excessive corticosteroid use. By avoiding such excess use, experienced pediatric rheumatologists have made these conditions rare.

Despite their negative side effects, there are times when corticosteroids are important. For children with life-threatening vasculitic diseases, they are often mandatory. Even so, the dosage should be minimized by the appropriate use of immunosuppressive drugs. This is discussed in greater detail in Chapters 10 to 16. For children with systemic-onset JA with macrophage activation syndrome or other severe manifestations, corticosteroids are also often mandatory. In the other forms of JA, corticosteroids can generally be avoided. However, if a child cannot attend school because of active arthritis, a short course of low-dose corticosteroids may be necessary.

A number of alternative corticosteroid regimens have been proposed. Many physicians have argued that, when given every other day, corticosteroids are less toxic. It is certainly true that 10 mg of prednisone every other day is less toxic than 10 mg every day. However, it is unclear that it is less toxic than 5 mg of prednisone every day, which may in fact be more effective. Some physicians claim that very high doses given every other day have few side effects. This is untrue.

In some situations, physicians use high doses of corticosteroids given intravenously. This is thought to have fewer side effects than high daily oral doses. On a one-time basis, this is probably true. However, it is not true when high intravenous doses are given routinely. Many physicians were very excited when deflazacort became available. It was thought to be a corticosteroid that would spare the bones. On an equal-dose basis that is true, but if the dose is adjusted to achieve an equal therapeutic effect, the bone loss is equal.

The widespread use of biologics, immunosuppressive drugs, and improved NSAIDs has significantly reduced the use of corticosteroids in the treatment of JA. As further methods of treating JA are developed, the number of children suffering from significant corticosteroid toxicity should continue to fall. However, until we have a suitable replacement, it is important to have corticosteroids available for those times when an immediate and dramatic effect is necessary.

Intra-articular Corticosteroids (Aristospan, Celestone, Depo-medral)

These corticosteroid preparations are often used for intra-articular injections. This means that the drug is injected directly into the inflamed joint. For many years, physicians were worried that this might weaken the joint. It is common to hear about athletes who received multiple joint injections and had badly damaged joints in the end.

In the 1990s, when MRI became widely available, a group of children who needed intra-articular steroid injections to treat arthritis in their knees were studied. This study took MRIs before injection, a few weeks after injection, and several months after injection. These serial MRIs demonstrated that the injections greatly reduced the inflammation and promoted healing of the cartilage. When athletes do badly, it is because they resume harmful activities after their knees are injected. Children with arthritis who receive intra-articular injections are instructed to rest.

With the increased use of intra-articular corticosteroid injections, it has become easier to control arthritis that is primarily affecting a single large joint. These injections should be considered for a child with a single swollen joint who is not responding well to NSAIDs. Studies even suggest that the liberal use of intra-articular injections has reduced the frequency of leg length discrepancy in children with true pauciarticular-onset arthritis. Since the therapy is generally safe and effective (see below), it should probably be done sooner rather than later.

A number of physicians believe it is appropriate to anesthetize a child with three or four swollen joints and then inject each joint. I believe that if there are more than two swollen joints, the disease is not under adequate control. These children should be given better systemic medication instead of multiple joint injections. The likelihood of achieving long-term benefit from multiple joint injections in this setting is small, but this issue remains controversial. The child will definitely feel much better for a period of days after several joints are injected because the corticosteroid slowly leaks out of the joints and has a systemic effect, just as it would if taken by mouth. This effect is minimal if only a single joint is injected.

I normally do not anesthetize children for joint injections. Anesthesia requires its own set of medications and carries its own risks. However, it can be done at the family's request. Since I rarely inject more than one joint, I find such injections to be a quick and easy procedure. The joint to be injected is cleaned with surgical soap (betadine). Numbing medicine can be injected around the area of the joint (this burns a little, and I give children the choice of skipping it).

Once the area is properly cleaned, the physician simply slips the needle into the joint and injects the corticosteroid. For an experienced physician, this is usually very easy. Although children up to age twelve years or so will need to be helped to hold still when it hurts, most children tolerate this very well with reassurance from parents and the doctor. Do not say that the injection will not hurt—that's not true. I always tell children that it will hurt for a minute and challenge them to say "Ouch" more loudly than I can. In the distraction of listening to me say "Ouch," many of them forget to say it.

It is very difficult to predict how long an intra-articular joint injection will provide relief. Sometimes only one knee is involved, and after it is injected the child never has trouble again. At other times, the knee is injected and there is no apparent improvement. Most often, joint injections provide two or three months of relief and allow other medications to take effect and control the disease. A frequent need for joint injections suggests that the disease is not being adequately controlled by the systemic medications.

There are very few risks associated with intra-articular joint injections. The greatest risk is that associated with anesthesia if it is used. Since I rarely inject multiple joints, I do not find anesthesia necessary except under unusual circumstances. Other risks associated with intra-articular joint injections include an infection as the result of being injected (I've never seen it), an unusual *crystal reaction* to the injected medication (I've never seen that, either), and damage to the skin around the injection site.

If corticosteroids leak into the skin and adjacent tissues during the injection, they cause loss of fat under the skin. This might seem to be a good thing, but it is not. Consider the hands of a person over the age of eighty. You can clearly see the veins and other tissues through the skin. This is due to the loss of all of the subcutaneous fat. A similar condition occurs if the corticosteroids leak under the skin. Often children come to me after being treated elsewhere who have pea-sized dimples at injection sites around their knees. These are not a big problem, but I have also seen larger areas of damaged skin that look like a bad scar. I can only assume that they are the result of poorly done joint injections.

Whenever a joint is injected, it is important for the physician to use a short-acting agent such as betamethasone if the area being injected is close to the surface (a tendon, a finger, or a wrist joint). Using a short-acting agent minimizes the risk of skin damage. Long-lasting agents such as triamcinolone hexacetonide should be reserved for large joints such as knees and hips.

There has been a lot of discussion about how much to limit activities after injecting a large joint. Our goal is to suppress the inflammation as long as possible. To accomplish this, we want the injected corticosteroids to remain in the joint as long as possible. Ideally, the child is not active for the first twenty-four hours after the injection. Some physicians even go so far as to place a temporary cast on the leg if the knee is injected, removing it the next day. Most of us settle for instructing the family to limit unnecessary activities for twenty-four hours.

It is also necessary to remember that the corticosteroids to be injected are typically mixed with lidocaine (the medicine used when the dentist numbs your teeth or when you need stitches in the emergency room). This has the advantage of immediately making the joint numb. **Be sure to find out if the patient is allergic to lidocaine.** Since the joint will be numb for several hours after the injection, everyone should be careful. Just as you could bite your lip and not know it after seeing the dentist, a child could injure the injected joint and not know it. This is one of the reasons why athletes who get joint injected and then go back in the game end up in so much trouble.

MISCELLANEOUS AGENTS

Thalidomide (Thalomid)

Thalidomide is a medication that was initially used as a sedative. It was rapidly withdrawn from the market because it causes significant birth defects if taken by pregnant women. It was subsequently discovered to have very potent anti-inflammatory effects. Although parents and physicians initially are concerned on learning that thalidomide is known to cause birth defects, **none of the immunosuppressive drugs can be given safely to pregnant women.** Fortunately, in pediatric rheumatology, pregnancy is rarely an immediate concern. There is no evidence that thalidomide has any lingering effects more than a month after it is discontinued. Thalidomide is very effective for some children with systemic-onset, psoriasis-associated, and polyarticular-onset arthritis who have not responded to other medications.

Thalidomide may cause abnormalities that show up on routine blood tests, including decreased WBC and elevated liver enzyme levels. Routine monitoring is required. Thalidomide is associated with nerve irritation that can produce pain and tingling, so this too should be monitored. Continued treatment with thalidomide could result in permanent nerve damage. However, in the dosage recommended for children with arthritis, this has not been a significant problem. Thalidomide also increases the risk of blood clotting. This has been a minor problem in adults receiving thalidomide for multiple myeloma, and physicians treating children with systemic-onset arthritis should be aware of the possibility.

The use of thalidomide currently requires extensive monitoring to make sure that the patient is not at risk of becoming pregnant. Although it seems improbable for small children, one can never be too careful. At present in the United States, only physicians who have registered with the company that provides the drug can prescribe thalidomide.

This drug may become more important in the future because it down-regulates the genes that are responsible for synthesis of many inflammatory molecules. (It tells the genes to make less of them.) In the United States, biologics are being used to attack these molecules, but the biologics are very expensive. When I teach in foreign countries, often the doctors are interested in hearing about the new biologic agents, but no one can afford them. Thalidomide may be similarly effective and is much less expensive.

Intravenous Gamma Globulin

Intravenous gamma globulin (IVIgG) received a lot of attention in the early 1990s. It is still used for many diseases by some physicians, but it is extremely expensive and it has largely been supplanted by the biologics. Intravenous gamma globulin always appeared to be helpful, but in controlled studies the benefits were always marginal. Some physicians still believe that this is an excellent medication for dermatomyositis. It is very effective for children with Kawasaki disease (KD) (see Chapter 17). The difference is that KD is an acute illness. Once you have treated a child for KD with IVIgG, in most cases the illness is cured.

The use of IVIgG seems to suffer from a phenomenon called *tachyphylaxis*. This means that the effect of treatment decreases with each successive dose. Children treated with IVIgG often seem much improved initially, but they require more and more IVIgG over time (usually, more frequent treatment) with less and less effect. As a result, the benefits of IVIgG for chronic conditions such as arthritis and dermatomyositis are less clear. It is a useful therapy for children with immune deficiency diseases who do not make enough of their own IgG, because in those cases it is simply a replacement therapy.

Many parents and physicians initially chose IVIgG because they felt that it was safer. With extensive experience, it has become clear that significant negative side effects may occur. Like infliximab, this therapy must be given as periodic intravenous infusions and may be associated with allergic reactions. In general, it should be restricted to specific conditions such as KD and some hematologic disorders.

Gold Sodium Thioglucose and Gold Sodium Thiomalate (Myochrysine, Solganol, "Gold Shots")

Gold shots were standard therapy for hard-to-control arthritis in adults and children when I began my career. For many children they were dramatically effective, bringing a slow but steady resolution of the arthritis. The major difficulty with gold shots is that they require painful intramuscular injections. The injections are given weekly until the arthritis is well under control and then are slowly spaced out over longer intervals.

Since gold shots can have a significant impact on the blood-forming cells, most physicians do routine blood tests before every dose. Frequent testing and doctors' visits are a major inconvenience. However, gold shots are effective for many children with arthritis. Side effects beyond the inconvenience of frequent physician visits are most often limited to minor changes shown on blood tests. Severe side effects do occur, but they are infrequent.

Over the past twenty years, most physicians have replaced the use of gold shots with methotrexate and now the new biologics. Methotrexate is usually given in oral form and is far more convenient. It is unclear where gold shots belong in the current approach to therapy. There are many children whose arthritis disappeared when they were treated with gold shots. However, some children ultimately relapsed after the shots were discontinued. The biologics, such as etanercept, clearly provide a quicker and greater level of relief with less apparent toxicity. I almost never use gold shots now, but there may still be a place for them.

Auranofin (Ridaura)

Auranofin is an oral version of gold salts given as daily pills. It was developed in an effort to eliminate the inconvenience associated with weekly gold shots. Unfortunately, auranofin does not seem to be as effective as gold shots. It has just as many side effects. It is rarely if ever used in children.

D-Penicillamine

D-Penicillamine is a chelating agent that was widely used for the treatment of children with JA, morphea, and scleroderma. It is clearly a disease-modifying agent but has a very slow onset of action and a high frequency of toxic reactions. Routine blood test abnormalities, skin rashes, kidney irritation, and neurologic abnormalities all occur. As a result of the slow onset of improvement and the high frequency of side effects, D-penicillamine was rapidly replaced by methotrexate for the treatment of children with arthritis. D-Penicillamine may still have a role for the treatment of children who have not responded to other medications, but it is rarely used for arthritis in childhood.

D-Denicillamine has long been the standard therapy for children with morphea and scleroderma (progressive systemic sclerosis). Although some physicians report good effects, most physicians with extensive experience find D-penicillamine to have a high frequency of toxicity and minimal efficacy. The right therapy for scleroderma remains controversial, but I prefer methotrexate. For most children with scleroderma or morphea, methotrexate has greater efficacy and less toxicity than D-penicillamine. Nevertheless, there are well-respected physicians who continue to use D-penicillamine for scleroderma.

Enzyme Replacement Therapies

For children who lack specific enzymes, such as children with MPS I, MPS VI, Gaucher's disease, Fabry disease, and a variety of other storage diseases, replacement enzyme therapy has made a major difference in the quality of life. Several pharmaceutical companies now make replacement enzymes such as laronidase for MPS I, galsulfase for MPS VI, imiglucerase for Gaucher's disease, and agalsidase beta for Fabry disease. These enzymes are infused intravenously to degrade the storage products that otherwise accumulate and cause damage. Infusion reactions are an occasional problem with all medications that are given intravenously and some children become allergic, but the benefits of these medications for affected children far outweigh the risks.

Other Modalities

Plasmapheresis (Apharesis)

At one point, plasmapheresis was considered a possible therapy for a wide variety of diseases. However, it was found to lack lasting beneficial effects. Today, plasmapheresis is not routinely used for the therapy of children with any rheumatic disease. However, it is occasionally beneficial for crisis management in children with SLE or antiphospholipid antibody syndrome. Controlled studies do not convincingly show any sustained benefit from plasmapheresis after the acute crisis. Over time, the toxic effects mount, while the therapeutic efficacy decreases.

COMBINATIONS OF MEDICINE

Suppose that you were given the job of reducing traffic in Manhattan. You would conclude that there are just too many cars! At first, you might simply close one of the bridges into the city. That would be effective when you first did it, but you would quickly notice that there are many bridges into Manhattan. Some people may have stopped going into the city, but others simply changed to a different bridge.

The next step would be to stop traffic on all the bridges. That would have a very good effect at first, but then you would realize that there are four tunnels. Tunnel traffic would quickly increase dramatically, and traffic into the city would begin to rise again. If you started blocking tunnel traffic, you would discover that people would start using the ferries more often.

To make matters worse, if you completely stopped traffic into Manhattan, the people living there would starve. Thus, there is no simple answer. You would need to adjust and test varying combinations of bridge and tunnel restrictions to find one that accomplished your goal of reducing traffic sufficiently without harming the people living in the city.

It is very frustrating for parents to have a child with active arthritis who is receiving multiple medications and is not getting better. When the physician recommends a new medication, parents inevitably ask, "Which one is this replacing?" Sometimes we add a new drug without discontinuing one of the others. This frustrates many parents. It is important to understand that the immune system is the body's defense against infection. Throughout history, infection has been a major cause of death in childhood. Thus, children who had strong immune systems were much more likely to survive.

As a physician prescribing medicine for a child with arthritis, I need to find the right combination with the best effect on the child and the fewest side effects. Often this means attacking the problem from several different directions. I try to stop one bridge and one tunnel to get the right balance of letting necessary traffic in and reducing the number of cars. There is no perfect solution for traffic or arthritis.

ROUTINE SUPPLEMENTS

Parents always want to make sure that they are doing everything possible for their children. In the United States, it is rare to find anyone whose diet is truly deficient. However, some children are fussy about eating meat, vegetables, and so on. The best way to deal with this problem is to make sure that the child takes a single multivitamin each day. It should be appropriate for the child's age.

Many children with chronic active disease are anemic. As a result of the chronic blood loss, some of them will become iron deficient. Other children don't utilize the iron in their bodies well. If a child has arthritis, be sure to give him or her a multivitamin with iron. However, remember that iron is toxic if the level is too high.

Calcium supplementation is also very popular at present. Calcium is included in our daily diet, but not all of us get enough every day. Most multivitamins don't contain a large amount of calcium. The reason is that calcium tends to cause upset stomachs and constipation. (People won't buy vitamins that cause these problems.) Calcium supplementation may be necessary for some children, but routinely recommending large amounts of calcium because a child has a chronic disease may not be beneficial. Many parents and physicians believe that children on corticosteroids should take extra calcium because of the effects of these drugs on bone. Careful studies have shown that calcium without vitamin D is of no benefit, and that the effect of corticosteroids is so dramatic that even with vitamin D the effect of adding calcium is minimal. The real effort should be directed at reducing the steroids.

Most of the other vitamins and minerals are adequately provided by a single multivitamin daily. There is always a lot of talk about extra supplementation. No one is quite sure when this is beneficial or not. However, it is clear that **too**

much vitamin A and too much vitamin D are harmful. In most cases, a daily multivitamin is more than enough.

> The best intentions don't always produce the expected results. One of my teenage patients had a strong family history of kidney stones. He had never had them, but some of his adult relatives had developed kidney stones in their forties. When my patient became ill, his mother wanted to do everything possible. She gave him extra calcium and extra vitamin C. As a result, she also gave him kidney stones.

IMMUNIZATIONS

The following are several important questions that I am repeatedly asked about immunizations:

- Do they cause JA or other rheumatic diseases?
- Are they safe for children with rheumatic diseases?
- Should a child with rheumatic disease be vaccinated?
- Should the siblings of a child with rheumatic disease be vaccinated?

Box 23-2   Recommendations for vaccinations in children with rheumatic disease

A child with arthritis off all medications and well for six months or more
All vaccines recommended may be given, but avoid rubella vaccination if the child has a positive titer, indicating immunity to rubella.

A child with arthritis on NSAIDs but well for six months
Most routine vaccinations are okay, but avoid rubella vaccination if the child has a positive titer.

No live vaccines should be given (e.g., chicken pox [herpes zoster] and smallpox). There is a risk of disease and Reye's syndrome.

A child with arthritis on immunosuppressive medications
(corticosteroids, biologics [e.g., etanercept, infliximab, anakinra, and adalimumab] and cytotoxics [e.g., methotrexate, mycophenolate mofetil, cyclophosphamide, and azathioprine])

No vaccinations should be given to the child (there are data indicating that pneumovax should be given if it hasn't already been given).

No live vaccinations should be given to siblings or household contacts.

Box 23-2 Continued

A child with active arthritis within the past six months (regardless of the medications)

No vaccinations should be given (not all doctors agree). This has to be reviewed on a case-by-case basis when issues such as college dormitory life, travel, or risk of epidemic exposure arise.

The most important thing to understand about immunizations is that they have saved millions of lives. Routine vaccination against smallpox eliminated a terrible and often fatal disease from the world (current bioterrorism issues are not relevant to this discussion; I discuss smallpox vaccination for children with rheumatic diseases below). Although it may take a full generation, routine immunization against hepatitis B will also save hundreds of thousands of lives. You will find it nearly impossible to locate a young American doctor with experience treating polio, measles, mumps, rubella, or their complications because routine vaccination has made these diseases very rare. This is a wonderful thing. At present, every American child is routinely vaccinated against polio, tetanus, measles, mumps, rubella, pertusis (whooping cough), and hepatitis B.

To meet the current recommendations of the American Academy of Pediatrics, children receive at least fifteen vaccinations during the first three years of life. Pauciarticular-onset JA frequently starts in children in this age group, so children often develop the disease within a few months of a vaccination. Since the injections cause fever and pain, it is natural for parents of a child with arthritis to suspect that the injection may have played a role.

A proper study would require evaluating the frequency of JA in a large group of children who were not properly vaccinated. However, it would be unethical to do this. I have been practicing for more than twenty-five years and have practiced in areas where routine vaccinations were not always done (because people did not go to the doctor). There does not appear to be an increase in the incidence of JA among properly vaccinated children. **We know that there are small risks associated with routine vaccination, but the risks of the diseases we are being protected against are far more severe.**

However, while I believe it is important that all normal children receive vaccinations, the situation for children who have arthritis is more complicated.

Here there is a diversity of opinion among doctors. In addition, the answer depends on what medications the child is taking. What I am stating here are only my own views.

Most often, the child has received polio, tetanus, measles, mumps, and rubella immunizations before developing arthritis. This will make life easier for everyone. Although several doses of vaccine are recommended, children get some protection from even a single dose. A child who has never been vaccinated against these diseases is a special case that will require careful consideration.

If a child has received the three routine vaccinations scheduled up to six months of age and the first measles, mumps, rubella vaccination, the child should not receive any further vaccines while the arthritis is active. For children who are off medications or taking only a routine NSAID, and in whom the arthritis has been fully controlled for six months, one can consider giving vaccinations that do not contain live virus.

Rubella is the only vaccine that routinely causes transient arthritis as a side effect. I would check to determine whether a child has a reasonable titer and would not revaccinate with rubella if the child is immune. I would avoid live vaccines (e.g., the chickenpox vaccine [herpes zoster] and potentially the smallpox vaccine) in any child who has active disease or is receiving immunosuppressive drugs. These recommendations are detailed in Box 23-2.

A major issue that is often overlooked is the possible spread of live virus vaccines among close contacts. If children are receiving medications that impede their ability to fight infection (including but not limited to corticosteroids, methotrexate, and biologics), not only should they **not** receive live vaccines but neither should their brothers and sisters. The altered virus contained in these vaccines can spread from one child to another and cause severe problems in an immunologically compromised child. Parents must also be warned about not letting their child come in close contact with other children who have been recently vaccinated with live virus vaccines.

Notes on Other Vaccines

Flu shots

The consensus opinion is that the benefits outweigh the risks. I let parents make their own decision.

Pneumovax

The American Academy of Pediatrics now recommends that young children receive the pneumovax vaccination early in life. Most older children have not gotten it. It should be given to children whom you think will be put on an immunosuppressive medication, but it must be given before you start the medication for it to be most effective. There is evidence that it has some benefit even if the children are on immunosuppressive medicine. It is safe because it is not a live vaccine.

Meningitis (meningococcal vaccine)

The meningococcal vaccine is increasingly being recommended for college freshmen and even for younger children.

Human papillomavirus (HPV)—Gardasil

The newly introduced HPV vaccine is being recommend for girls to reduce the risk of cervical cancer. There is some concern that it may stimulate the immune system enough to cause increased complaints in children with rheumatic disease, but preventing cervical cancer is an important goal that rheumatologists feel justifies any increased arthritis-related problems.

Bird flu

The reports in the media have become less frequent, but as I write this, bird flu is still a significant problem for birds and, rarely, for people. Should there be a new pandemic because bird flu does become an easily contagious human disease, the benefits of immunization with a satisfactory dead vaccine will outweigh the risks of increased arthritis.

Smallpox (vaccinia)

Smallpox was and still is a terrible disease that is often fatal. Worldwide vaccination programs have eliminated it except as a biowarfare threat. **This is a live virus and has a significant risk of causing trouble to anyone who is immunosuppressed**. It is also a member of the herpes family of viruses, which has been linked to Reye's syndrome.

Should the disease become a real threat, it will be necessary to immunize as many people as possible. For children on NSAIDs only, the risk would be acceptable under those circumstances. For children on immunosuppressive drugs, it would be necessary to stop these drugs at least fourteen days before vaccination and maintain the child off the drugs for a month after the vaccination (if the CDC makes official recommendations for this situation, we should all follow them. So far, they have not.) The risks of doing this will have to be considered for each child's situation.

24

Alternative Medicine: Vitamins and Supplements

Whenever I finish explaining a new medication and a parent asks, "Is there another choice?" I know that something is worrying the parent. One of the biggest problems in medicine is fear of side effects, and in talking to parents, I often make a comparison to flying. When you board the airplane and the flight attendant talks about the life jacket under the seat in front of you, you cannot help but think, "If there's a real chance we're going to land in the water, I'm getting off this plane." Surely, the flight attendant feels the same way. However, the government requires that passengers be informed about the life jacket and other safety precautions. Similarly, physicians are required to tell patients about the possible side effects of medications. If they thought there would be any serious ones, they would not prescribe the medicine. However, physicians and flight attendants are required to give patients and passengers this information, because no one knows for sure when something might go wrong.

No one can get to a faraway place without incurring the risks of driving, flying, taking a train, or taking a boat. And doctors cannot treat illness without the risk of side effects. **Whether patients take prescribed medications, buy over-the-counter medications, ignore the problem and believe it will go away, or buy health food "cures," there are risks associated with every choice. The only difference is whether or not those risks are clearly explained to patients.** The physician is required to do that, but parents have to read the warnings on over-the-counter medications.

A quick search of the Internet using the keywords *arthritis + alternative + cure* turned up over 120,000 Web pages. A search for *arthritis + diet* produced over 500,000 Web pages. Some recommend avoiding red meat, others rub-on creams, and still others dietary supplements. Can all of these sites really be wrong? Surely, some of them have useful information.

There are many things to remember when families consult you about using supplements and alternative medicines. First and foremost is that **none of these diets or creams or "supplements" is subject to any regulation regarding the truth of their claims, the purity of the product, or even the accuracy of the label.** Many supplements have been found to contain little if any of the ingredients highlighted on the label, and some have been found to be contaminated with heavy metals and other harmful substances. The harmful contaminants are not typically listed on the labels. (If you are curious, I found over 4000 Web pages discussing harmful contaminants in supplements. To check this, use the keywords *supplement + harmful + contaminant.*)

CAUTION PARENTS TO READ THE LABEL CAREFULLY AND NOT TO BELIEVE EVERYTHING THEY READ

There is no such thing as a pain-relieving medication or food with positive effects and no risk of side effects. It is with dismay that I see parents bring in all sorts of products found in health food stores, noted on the Internet, advertised on television, or seen in newspapers. They want me to say that it's all right to give these products to their children. But most would not be fooled for a moment if the item promised stock market riches or a new way to use their car without gasoline.

There are many unscrupulous individuals who will sell anything to get money. Health aids are a billion-dollar-a-year business. Most are harmless except for the expense, and may have a positive placebo effect. However, many others are potentially harmful, especially for people who have health problems. Moreover, their use may delay proper diagnosis and treatment. There are no rules restricting what salespeople can say in stores or what Web sites can claim. The small print always reads, "This item is sold as a food supplement, not a medication, and these claims have not been evaluated or validated by the FDA." Drugs approved by the FDA are made in factories that are carefully inspected. They are checked to be sure that they are as represented and that they contain no potentially harmful contaminants.

In the sections that follow, I discuss vitamin and mineral supplementation, alternative diets, dietary supplements, and herbal cures. You will find that I favor some types of supplementation and oppose others. Several key points need to be considered:

- Although the manufacturing, advertising, and distribution of medications are tightly regulated by the FDA, there is no regulation of recommendations for diets or dietary supplements.
- The manufacturers of supplements can claim whatever they wish without doing testing of any kind.
- There is no independent testing to determine whether the supplement actually contains what is listed on the label.
- There is no independent testing to make sure that the supplement does not contain harmful ingredients.

When you meet someone who is sure that a special diet or supplement improved his or her arthritis, remember that this person is probably well intentioned. Large-scale studies of adults with arthritis have clearly documented a substantial placebo effect associated with both diets and supplements. But I explain to my patients that there is no such thing as an active ingredient without possible side effects. **Anything that has real effects has the potential for side effects.** Physicians are prevented from owning pharmacies or selling medications in their offices. This is done to prevent them from having a financial gain in prescribing a medication. In contrast, the people selling vitamins and supplements have been trained to sell their products. Many are working on direct commission.

VITAMINS

Every child with a chronic disease should be taking a daily multivitamin that contains the appropriate amounts of vitamins A, B (all types), C, D, E, and K, folic acid, iron, and calcium. Children with iron deficiency may need additional iron supplementation. They should also be getting adequate daily calcium. However, iron-containing medications may cause an upset stomach. Overdosage of iron can be fatal.

Calcium in excess causes upset stomach and constipation. In severe excess, calcium can also contribute to the formation of kidney stones (especially if combined with a lot of vitamin C, which acidifies the urine). Beyond the recommended basic daily requirement, extra vitamins must be given with caution. Most vitamins have a tremendous safety range. However, vitamins A and D are stored in the body and may reach toxic levels.

SUPPLEMENTS

Supplements need to be divided between plant extracts and a large variety of chemicals. **We must remember that "all-natural" does not mean safe. The hemlock that poisoned Socrates was an all-natural product.** Sometimes parents or patients ask whether they can take the medicine in a more natural form. I find it is useful to consider the history of aspirin. The original form was derived from willow tree bark, clearly an all-natural product. When chemists looked at it carefully, they discovered that the active ingredient was salicin. However, while salicin was much more effective than the original bark extract, it caused severe upset stomach. Aspirin is chemically modified salicin that is much easier on the stomach than the all-natural form of the drug.

Box 24-1   Alternative therapies?

Remind parents who are considering supplements to consider the following: There is a large area containing many different remedies for coughs and colds in every health food and drug store. But if a patient has a documented streptococcal sore throat, every doctor recommends penicillin (unless the patient is allergic). **Why is only one drug recommended for streptococcal sore throat? Because it has been proven that penicillin works. Why are there so many different remedies for coughs and colds? Because none of them has ever been proven to work well.** If one had, we would all buy it and the other brands would be gone. **How many different products do you see in the health food or nutrition store claiming that they will cure arthritis?**

Glucosamine

One supplement that has been shown to be of benefit for people with **osteoarthritis** is glucosamine. Glucosamine is a raw ingredient used by the body in manufacturing cartilage. Several studies have shown that adults with osteoarthritis who were taking glucosamine felt better than those taking sugar pills. However, osteoarthritis is the breakdown of cartilage with age. This is not the cause of the problem in children with arthritis. Still, the side effects of glucosamine are usually mild. In contrast, chondroitin sulfate, which is often marketed with glucosamine, has failed to show benefit in studies and in fact has been shown to cause an increased frequency of stomach upset.

Fatty Acid Supplementation (Omega 3 and Similar Products)

Omega-3 fatty acids, oils found in large amounts in cold-water fish, have been recommended for people with arthritis since the 1980s. There was tremendous excitement when these compounds were initially described as helpful, and extensive studies were done. These fatty acids alter the synthesis of inflammatory mediators in the body. However, to achieve the claimed effect, it's necessary to take ten or more capsules every day.

Careful studies of patients taking omega-3 fatty acids showed that many of the adults with rheumatoid arthritis were much better in six to eight weeks. But by twelve weeks, the body had readjusted itself and began to make increased amounts of the inflammatory mediators again. All the benefits found in the early phase of the studies disappeared, and there were no long-term benefits. The major side effects of omega-3 fatty acids are increased bruising and prolonged bleeding. It also can be very expensive to take the amount necessary to produce a short-term effect.

Flaxseed oil is another source of essential fatty acids that is frequently recommended for the treatment of arthritis. There is no long list of negative side effects, but there is no convincing evidence that it helps, either. Other sources have suggested that by increasing omega-6 fatty acids, evening primrose, black currant, and borage oil may be beneficial. But all of these products have failed to demonstrate a positive effect when compared with identical-appearing fake capsules. In addition, they can cause side effects, especially if they are contaminated.

In the never-ending search for a better solution, a wide variety of additional agents are being screened and tested for use in patients with arthritis. Many new dietary supplements will appear claiming to help arthritis sufferers, and we hope that one of them will turn out to be beneficial. Yet, parents must be reminded that just as they would never accept a doctor's prescription for a new drug not yet approved by the FDA and on which no safety testing had been reported, and just because a friend told them it might help, they should not try new dietary supplements any more willingly. A number of them have been taken off the market after being proven unsafe. If something is proven safe and effective, everyone will know it very quickly. I'll be recommending it.

DIETS

I am a strong proponent of a healthy, balanced diet. Many different sources recommend that people with arthritis should avoid all sorts of foods. There are "no nightshade" diets, "no red meat" diets, "avoid fungus" diets, low-gluten diets, vegetarian diets, and many more. **Going on a special diet makes us feel that we have gained some control over our destiny**. Taking that important step to regain control makes us feel better.

I never argue with parents who tell me that they have adopted a special diet and that the child feels better (as long as it is a healthy diet). The truth is that large-scale testing has not shown any of these diets to be particularly beneficial for children with arthritis, with the exception of children with celiac disease. These children may develop arthritis as one manifestation of their disease and will do better on a low-gluten diet. If you are unsure, verify that the child has been checked for this disease; the initial screening is a simple blood test. Most children will not have celiac disease, but we need to find the few who do.

From time to time, I see children who have been placed on strict elimination diets because their parents believe that the arthritis is due to a food allergy. Although parents sometimes convince themselves that short-term benefits have been achieved, I've never seen improvement over the long term. These diets put the children through useless deprivation and damage to their growth and self-image. The only food intolerance truly associated with arthritis is gluten in celiac disease.

ALTERNATIVE MEDICAL SYSTEMS

We have all heard stories of people who got better after they prayed to a certain saint, went to Lourdes, had acupuncture, or took up Zen. Even after taking care of children for many years, I cannot always explain why their symptoms get better or worse on a given day. Diseases do wax and wane over time. Someone is going to get lucky and improve right after doing something unlikely to help.

There is no reason to argue with them that it is a coincidence. They will know they got better, and they will try to convince others of the same thing. Be very careful.

If anything worked consistently, we'd all recommend it. I'd be just as happy to recommend a certain acupuncturist, a church, or peanut butter as I am to prescribe medications. I have seen many parents who took their children to Lourdes, the Dead Sea, or the acupuncturist, or tried all the other things you hear about. If one of them worked more often than by random chance, I'd be telling you about it.

In this era of global travel and communication, there is no hidden cure being used in some remote part of the world that we do not know about. I frequently teach in Asia and Africa, and I am always asked whether I can help the people there get more American medicines. No one has ever come up to me and said, "Here, take this stuff home; it will cure everyone." In Vietnam, you will see vendors selling snake wine for rheumatism. The dead snake is still in the bottle. I wonder why the labels are in English and the prices are in dollars. Nothing on the bottles is written in Vietnamese.

CONCLUSIONS

All parents want to feel that they are doing everything possible for their children with arthritis. So, when they ask about a dietary supplement, I ask them the following questions:

- Would you accept a prescription for the same thing as a prescription from me?
- Have you ever heard of the manufacturer?
- Is any proof supplied for the claims made?
- Is there any certificate of approval of the plant where it was manufactured? Where is it?
- Who is recommending this product, and what is their training?
- Are they going to make a profit if you buy this product?
- If you are going to make your child take this, would you take it yourself?
- What do you know about the possible side effects or possible interference with the medicines your child is supposed to be taking?

The last thing we as physicians have to remember about supplements is that random studies suggest that at least half of the parents we deal with are giving their children supplements that they aren't telling us about. If things suddenly go wrong with the child or the blood tests show problems, be sure to ask if the parents have added a new vitamin, supplement, health food, and so on.

25

Understanding Laboratory and Diagnostic Tests

When I was a medical student first learning about diagnostic tests, I was present when a nervous mother asked the radiologist about the dangers of X-rays and whether it was really necessary to X-ray her child. The radiologist assured the mother that a single set of films would not cause problems, but she seemed only partially comforted. After she left, he smiled at me as I put the lead apron I had been wearing back on the rack with a questioning look. "That's what people don't understand," he said. "We do this all day, every day, for years at a time. That much exposure can add up and cause problem. I've never seen a patient with any problem that resulted from routine radiographs, but I've seen plenty of problems that became serious because people waited to long to do the appropriate tests."

X-RAYS

Each type of diagnostic test has its proper place in evaluating children with muscle, bone, or joint pain. If a bone is painful, it is appropriate to begin the evaluation (after a complete history is taken and a thorough physical examination is done) with a radiograph to eliminate the possibility of fracture or structural abnormality. X-rays are also useful in detecting malalignment or malformation. Radiographs may be sufficient to establish the diagnosis of a fracture, slipped capital femoral epiphysis, scoliosis, or many other orthopedic conditions (see Chapter 3). However, for children with JA, SLE, or many other rheumatic conditions, X-rays may be useful only to exclude orthopedic problems.

X-rays are almost always necessary when there is a history of trauma or a sudden change in the child's condition. However, the bones are not fully calcified in young children, and the use of X-rays to evaluate arthritis is of little value except in the most severe cases. Once the initial X-rays have been done, follow-up X-rays are necessary only if a fracture is suspected or if there is a structural abnormality that must be monitored. For children with rheumatic disease, periodic X-rays provide little information that cannot be gained from careful examination of the joints and their range of motion. However, X-rays are important if there is a sudden change or if the problem is not resolving in the expected manner.

MAGNETIC RESONANCE IMAGING

Magnetic resonance imaging (**MRI**) works on the principle of nuclear magnetic resonance. The MRI is excellent for imaging the soft tissues of the body. The bone marrow contains water and shows up well, as does the cartilage covering the ends of the bones. With special techniques, it is now possible to get excellent views of the bones themselves as well. Computed axial tomography (CAT) scans take less time than MRI, but both techniques give excellent pictures of the bone and the MRI can provide much more information about the surrounding tissue.

BONE SCANS

There are a number of other diagnostic tests that may be useful in dealing with bone and joint problems. One of the most common is the **bone scan**. Bone scanning is based on the uptake of the radioactive isotope technetium 99 (Tc-99) by active bone cells. Normal bone cells are not very active, but if there is an injury, arthritis, infection, or tumor, the bone cells become active in trying to repair the damage. When they become active, they take up more calcium and related substances. When Tc-99 is injected, active bone cells take it up. Because it is radioactive, its location in the body can be pictured using a gamma counter.

The bone scan may reveal abnormal areas that are too small to be obvious on regular X-rays or CAT scans. It can also find areas where the bone cells have been irritated but obvious changes have not taken place. As a result, this test is very good in finding conditions such as osteomyelitis and lesions such as osteoid osteomas before they become obvious on X-ray. Although the actual lesion may not be large, the irritated bone will show up quite brightly. One advantage of a bone scan is that it allows the physician to evaluate the entire body for areas of bone irritation with a single injection and a single visit to the hospital. Thus, it can help to find unsuspected problems.

GALLIUM SCANNING

Gallium scanning is another method of looking for areas of inflammation by injecting a radioactive substance (Ga-67). Areas of inflammation in soft tissues such as liver, spleen, lung, muscle, and other tissues take up the radioactive gallium to a greater degree than normal tissues do. Increased uptake of gallium can be used to find infections, tumors, and other problems. The machinery used is the same machinery used in the bone scan. Again, this has the advantage of allowing evaluation of the entire body. Nuclear medicine specialists have begun to recommend positron emission tomography (PET) scans, which detect areas of increased cellular activity due to increased sugar uptake. This is faster than gallium scanning and may ultimately replace it.

Although bone scans and gallium scans are done using the same machinery, they cannot be done simultaneously. Bone scans are completed the same day, and the Tc-99 is rapidly removed from the body. Gallium scans require three days because it takes the Ga-67 longer to reach the tissues. In addition, the Ga-67 takes a long time to leave the body. As a result, **if both tests are necessary, it is important to do the bone scan first**. The gallium scan can then be started the next day. It is necessary to wait more than a week after a gallium scan has been done (for the Ga-67 to clear the system) before a bone scan can be done.

DIAGNOSTIC ULTRASOUND (SONOGRAPHY)

Ultrasound is a relatively new technology that allows us to study muscles, bones, and joints at far less cost and without the risks associated with radiation and evaluate motion in real time. At present, the use of ultrasound to evaluate joint swelling and tendon inflammation is rapidly advancing. These tests may be available at your local diagnostic center and may be quite helpful in evaluating problems in the muscles and joints.

SYNOVIAL FLUID ASPIRATION

Synovial fluid aspiration is often done in the orthopedist's or rheumatologist's office. However, sometimes it is done in the radiology department with X-ray guidance (or ultrasound, as described above) to make sure that the needle is in the right place. The synovial fluid is then analyzed for evidence of infection, bleeding, or tumors. In children, the test is done most often to exclude the possibility of infection. Even children who are known to have arthritis can develop joint sepsis. If there is any question, an inflamed joint should be aspirated for testing. This testing should include a Gram stain, culture, cell count, protein, and sugar analyses. These tests are described in greater detail in the section on synovial fluid analysis later in this chapter.

Parents often wonder why the physicians do not simply remove all the fluid while they have a needle in the swollen joint. Unfortunately, the fluid will rapidly reappear. Medications are needed to stop the process. (Imagine that your kitchen faucet is stuck open and the sink is overflowing. If I come in with a bucket and empty the sink, the problem will stop for a short period. However, if I don't turn off the water or unplug the drain, the sink will fill up and start to overflow again.)

PULMONARY FUNCTION TESTING

Pulmonary function testing (PFT) consists of two parts. The first part measures the ability of the lungs to move air in and out. The second part measures the ability of the lungs to move oxygen from the air inhaled into the blood passing through the lungs. Both processes must work properly for a child to breathe easily.

Sometimes part of the test is repeated after a medication called a *bronchodilator* is given. The bronchodilator is used to reverse changes due to constriction of the airways by asthma or a similar illness. So, if the test results improve after the child uses a bronchodilator, this suggests that part of the problem is asthma or a similar disease. Difficulty with the forced expiratory volume (FEV1) indicates that the lungs are not moving well. There are two possible problems. In *obstructive lung disease*, something is impeding the air flow. This is rare in children with rheumatic disease. In *restrictive lung disease*, the lungs themselves are not moving well. This can be due to weakness, but more often it means that the lungs themselves are stiff. Most often, this happens when the lungs are involved by scleroderma, but it can happen with other rheumatic diseases.

The final part of PFTs is a test called a *diffusing capacity* (DL_{CO}). In this test, the child inhales a special sample containing a small amount of carbon monoxide. The child is instructed to hold his breath for ten seconds and then exhale. When the child exhales, the breath is analyzed to see how much of the carbon monoxide was exhaled. If most of it was exhaled, this means that it is hard for oxygen to enter the blood even though it is being moved in and out of the lungs properly.

OTHER TESTS

There are a number of other diagnostic tests that are specific to different diseases. Rather than discuss each of them here, I have included them in the sections related to those diseases where they are relevant.

LABORATORY TESTS

A few years ago, a child came to me complaining of hip pain on both sides. A physician had ordered an arthritis panel, and the report showed that she was both ANA- and RF-positive. Since these tests "confirmed" the diagnosis of arthritis, the child was begun on medications. She was sent to me to be evaluated for treatment with stronger medication for her arthritis because she had failed to improve with six months of treatment. X-rays revealed that the child had bilateral slipped capital femoral epiphyses. The original physician did not do X-rays or further testing once he had the positive ANA and RF results because those results had "confirmed" the diagnosis. Those tests were negative when repeated. The original laboratory's results were incorrect. **The most important findings on diagnostic testing are not the ones I expect to find. They just confirm what I already suspect. The most important findings are the ones I did not expect to find. They show that I need to do something different.**

Before I begin to discuss the details of various laboratory tests, it is important to understand that the results must be viewed as part of the total picture of the patient. **A set of laboratory tests is no replacement for a good history and physical examination. Abnormal laboratory tests can be a mistake; conversely, all laboratory tests can be normal and the child can still have severe arthritis.**

Children who complain of bone and joint pains but have "normal" laboratory test results often confuse parents and physicians. Many rheumatic diseases are associated with abnormal laboratory test results, but there are rheumatic and musculoskeletal diseases in which all test results are normal. **Normal laboratory test results do not mean that a child cannot have arthritis or another rheumatic disease. It is especially important to realize that JA is almost never associated with a positive test for RF.** Conversely, many children with mild laboratory abnormalities do not have rheumatic disease.

It is also important to remember that laboratory tests are not always accurate. In this day of cost saving, centralization, and rapid turnover, everyone should be very careful in interpreting laboratory values. Sometimes children are referred to me with abnormal laboratory test values that are normal when the test is repeated. At other times, children have been told that nothing was wrong because the test was normal, but a repeat test in my office is abnormal.

Over the years, many children have been referred to me because of laboratory tests that were incorrect. In addition, many children whom I care for (who repeatedly test positive for their disease) are occasionally reported to have negative tests. They are, of course, positive again when I repeat the test. Incorrect results may be a consequence of an improperly operating machine, mishandling of the blood en route to the laboratory, the wrong person's name on the sample, the wrong results being entered in the computer by a keyboard operator, and many other causes. **Always recheck a result that does not make sense, or a key result that would change the course of treatment, if it does not fit the clinical picture.**

Complete Blood Count and Mean Corpuscular Volume

A **complete blood count** (**CBC**) is one of the most routine blood tests, yet it provides a lot of useful information. The first values reported are the hemoglobin and hematocrit. If a child has a low hemoglobin level, the anemia should prompt further investigation. Many children with severe arthritis are anemic. However, a child may have normal results and still have arthritis or another condition. Anemia may be evidence of more severe disease, inadequate diet, bleeding (including bleeding from an irritated stomach lining), increased destruction of RBCs, or decreased production of blood cells. Each of these reasons for anemia has many possible causes. The hematocrit measures the same thing as the hemoglobin, although it is reported in different units. Most laboratories then report a group of tests called RBC, RDW, MCV, MCH, and MCHC. These tests indicate whether the RBCs are normal in size and help differentiate the causes of anemia. In general, only the **mean corpuscular volume** (**MCV**) is important in bone and joint conditions. This is just a fancy way of describing the size of the RBCs.

When the MCV is very low, it suggests that there is not enough hemoglobin in the cells. This is most often the result of iron deficiency but it can also be caused by genetic diseases like thalassemia (see below). In rheumatic diseases, the MCV is often low. In part this is because children with chronic disease often absorb iron poorly, and in part it may be due to irritation of the stomach lining by medications, which leads to chronic blood loss. Often anemia and a low MCV are due to a variety of factors acting together. A high MCV may indicate an increased number of reticulocytes. However, it can also be caused by folate deficiency. Sulfasalazine and methotrexate are two drugs used by rheumatologists that antagonize folate. Thus, a high MCV can be an early sign of problems due to these medicines. Children on methotrexate should receive supplemental folate to prevent this problem. If necessary, folate may also be given to children on sulfasalazine.

A normal MCV with a low hemoglobin level may be a *normochromic normo-cytic anemia*, which is the first phase of iron-deficiency anemia. It may also be a manifestation of hemolytic anemia. In hemolytic anemia, the body is rapidly destroying the RBCs. In an effort to compensate, the bone marrow starts releasing large numbers of reticulocytes. These are very large, so their MCV is high. However, the automated machine that performs the CBC typically produces an average reading. Thus, young cells that are large and old cells that are small may average out to a normal number despite low hemoglobin. (Some newer machines used to do CBCs will detect this situation.) This can be detected easily by ordering a reticulocyte count to identify the young cells. Often children with hemolytic anemia do need more iron. Hemolytic anemia may be an isolated problem, but it may also be caused by certain medicines and a number of rheumatic conditions, including SLE. Hemolytic anemia due to drugs occurs with increased frequency in children with **glucose-6-phosphate dehydrogenase (G6PD) deficiency** and is more common in children of African heritage. Hydroxychloroquine (Plaquenil) is a commonly used drug in pediatric rheumatology that may cause problems in children who are G6PD deficient. Any child with hemolytic anemia should be carefully investigated.

Genetic diseases in which hemoglobin is not properly made may cause bone pain because the bone marrow expands to make more RBCs. Diseases that produce bone pain include sickle cell disease and the carrier state for sickle cell disease. **Thalassemia** is another disease associated with abnormal hemoglobin production and very low MCV values that may cause bone pain. Mild thalassemia, or *thalassemia minor* (the carrier state), often has a low MCV but causes no symptoms. *Thalassemia major* is a severe disease associated with marked anemia. Because the bone marrow is overactive in children with thalassemia major, these children usually have bone pain and bones that appear very abnormal on X-ray. Abnormal hemoglobin production is best analyzed by hemoglobin electrophoresis.

Total Iron Binding Capacity and Iron

When a child is anemic, it is important to determine whether he or she is getting enough **iron** in the diet and absorbing it. If not, the iron level will be low, while the **total iron binding capacity (TIBC)** will be high. If these values are normal and the child is anemic, it suggests the possibility of thalassemia minor or a hemolytic anemia.

White Blood Cell Count

Very high or very low WBC counts are always cause for concern. With a very high WBC count, infection is always one of the possible causes. However, certain medications will also increase the count, particularly corticosteroids. Very high WBC counts can occur in diseases such as systemic-onset JA, severe infections, and leukemia. I have seen WBC counts as high as $95,000/mm^3$ in children with documented systemic-onset JA.

Very low WBC counts may also be the result of leukemia. More often, a low WBC count is the result of medications or viral infection. Many of the medications used in treating children with rheumatic diseases cause low WBC counts in some children. Whenever a child's WBC count is too low, careful attention should be given to all of the medicines the child is taking. This should not be limited to the medicines for rheumatic disease. The problem may be the result of another medicine or the interaction of two medicines. If a child you are caring for is having a problem, make sure that you know **all** the medicines and supplements the child is taking.

Certain diseases, such as SLE, may be associated with a low WBC count. Severe infections may also be responsible. Leukemia and some forms of cancer may make the WBC count too low or too high. A rare cause of very low

WBC counts is **aplastic anemia**. A sudden drop in the WBC count in a child with systemic-onset JRA may be a warning of MAS and is cause for immediate hospitalization, especially if accompanied by liver function abnormalities or significantly elevated D-dimer levels.

Certain uncommon rheumatic diseases (such as eosinophilic vasculitis, some cases of scleroderma, and Churg-Strauss syndrome) are associated with a significantly increased number of eosinophils. Significantly increased numbers of monocytes or basophils are very rare.

Platelet Count

Platelets are rapidly made in the bone marrow, and the number may fluctuate quickly. The platelet count is often very high in people who are under stress or chronically ill. Kawasaki disease and iron-deficiency anemia are often associated with platelet counts over 600,000, and the number may exceed 1,000,000 in KD, systemic-onset JRA, or, less frequently, iron deficiency. Low platelet counts may result from medications. In addition, the platelet count may go down because of increased destruction in children with idiopathic thrombocytopenic purpura (ITP), SLE, Felty's syndrome, MAS complicating systemic-onset JRA, thrombotic thrombocytopenic purpura (TTP), or an infection. It may also be low because of decreased production in a child with leukemia, lymphoma, or aplastic anemia. At times, there may be several different problems contributing to the low platelet count. If the platelet count is low with no obvious explanation, bone marrow aspiration may help determine the cause.

Erythrocyte Sedimentation Rate

There are several variations of the test for the **erythrocyte sedimentation rate (ESR)**, but all of them reflect the way the RBCs interact with each other in the blood and how fast they settle to the bottom of a test tube. Children with severe illness often have a high ESR. Often parents know that their referring physician became worried when he or she saw the high "sed rate," and they ask me what it means. It is important to understand and explain that the ESR is based on an observation and was not designed as a test. When blood collected from a patient is left to stand in the test tube, it will separate just like the oil and vinegar in salad dressing. The measurement of how far the RBCs settle to the bottom in one hour (in a specially designed tube) is the ESR.

Long ago, it was observed that the RBCs generally falls to the bottom of a test tube much faster in sick patients than in healthy ones. This is because of the electrostatic interaction between the RBCs, which is increased by acute phase reactants released by the liver when the body is under physiologic stress. But, of course, there are exceptions. Some people are sick and the ESR is normal, and in some people with abnormal ESRs there is no obvious explanation. The normal ESR value varies with the age and sex of the patient and from laboratory to laboratory, so it is important to know the normal value for the laboratory where your test was done. The problem is that *physiologic stress* is a very broad concept and elevated ESRs can result from many different conditions.

If the blood is left to sit for a long time or is not properly processed, the test result is unreliable. This is a problem with many large, centralized laboratories outside hospitals. The following warning is included with the results of every ESR specimen sent to a well-known national laboratory: "ESR specimens are stable for 4–6 hours at room temperature (12 hours if refrigerated). ESR results trend lower with increased specimen age." Unfortunately, doctors never are told the interval between the time the blood was drawn and the time the test was performed. Nor do they know whether the blood was refrigerated. Even if the specimen was drawn by the laboratory's own facility, the answers to these questions are unavailable. This is why I look at trends and never believe an isolated ESR value. C reactive protein is less subject to this problem, but it does not completely correlate with the ESR. Elevated C reactive protein values do occur in children with rheumatic disease and cannot be relied upon to distinguish infection from active rheumatic disease.

It is very hard to be comfortable when a child has an elevated ESR without an obvious explanation. The ESR is elevated in many children with rheumatic diseases and many other illnesses. In rare cases, children have abnormal ESRs with no apparent explanation. At the same time, children with pauciarticular JA or spondyloarthropathies may have all sorts of problems and their ESR may be normal (see Chapters 7 and 9).

C Reactive Protein

C reactive protein (CRP) is an acute phase reactant that is made in the liver. Levels of CRP rise and fall rapidly. Because the ESR measures a variety of acute phase reactants, the ESR and CRP generally move together. Some physicians prefer one test to the other, and many use both. The CRP may go up faster and come down sooner than the ESR. It is a common myth that CRP elevation indicates infection rather than another cause of inflammation, but many children who have rheumatic diseases have high CRP levels without infections. High CRP levels are common in children with systemic-onset JA who are not infected. The CRP is reported to be more stable after the blood is drawn and may have greater use for this reason, especially if there is a long delay between the time the blood is drawn and the time it is tested.

Chemistry Panel, Metabolic Panel, or a Serum Multichannel Automated Chemistry (SMAC)

Serum glucose is usually normal in children with orthopedic and rheumatic diseases. It may rise in children being treated with steroids. If the blood has been allowed to sit too long before being processed, the value will go down. The **blood urea nitrogen** (**BUN**) is elevated in children with impaired kidney function. It often rises to the top of normal or slightly above normal in children receiving NSAIDs because these drugs decrease the glomerular filtration rate (GFR). These slight elevations are normal and should not be a cause of concern. Unlike the BUN, the **creatinine** (**Cr**) level is not affected by mild changes in the GFR. Because children normally have lower Cr levels than adults, the BUN/Cr ratio may become very elevated. This is not something to be concerned about if the underlying values are normal. **One concern is that many laboratories do not report age-adjusted normal values. A Cr value of 1.2 mg/dl is normal for an older adult but very abnormal for a child under the age of ten years**. If the laboratory is not using age-adjusted normal values, the value of 1.2 mg/dl will not be flagged as abnormal in the child's results.

Abnormal levels of the electrolytes **sodium, potassium, chloride, and carbon dioxide** may indicate abnormal kidney function, dietary problems, or other metabolic abnormalities. Their levels should be normal in children with orthopedic and rheumatic conditions unless there is significant internal organ involvement. **It is important to recognize that the electrolytes, like the glucose and the ESR, are very sensitive to proper handling**. If the specimen is mishandled (too warm, too cold, or sits too long before being processed), the reported values become very unreliable.

A low **sodium level** may be the result of fluid retention, brain injury, or medications. Children with very low sodium levels may have problems including weakness and muscle cramps, but values above 130 are rarely troublesome. High levels of sodium suggest excessive salt intake, dehydration, or kidney disease. Like the sodium level, the **potassium level** is normally regulated by the kidneys. Low levels of potassium may cause weakness and muscle cramps. High levels may interfere with heart rhythm, and very high levels are dangerous. Don't give extra electrolytes to a patient unless you know that the kidneys are working properly. **A number of the sport drinks and body builder supplements can cause serious problems in children with borderline kidney function**. Low sodium levels with high potassium levels can occur in diabetics and in children with compromised adrenal function.

Serum **calcium** may be abnormal in children with parathyroid diseases. Sarcoid is the rheumatic disease most often associated with elevated calcium levels. The level may also be abnormal in children with renal disease, vitamin D intoxication, or other metabolic abnormalities. These problems may result in bone and joint abnormalities or pain if they persist for an extended period. Low calcium may be associated with severe muscle cramps. **Vitamin D–dependent rickets** may cause joint problems in children and is associated with a low calcium level and joint pains. However, rickets is extremely rare in the United States because most dairy products contain supplemental vitamin D. Rickets is typically diagnosed by a characteristic abnormal appearance of the bones on X-rays. It is important to take a careful dietary history in small children who may be subjected to stringent diets by their parents that do not offer adequate intake of calories, vitamins, or essential amino acids (in some cases, it is the child's unusual food preferences that cause problems).

Most often the serum **chloride** level is normal. A very low chloride level can occur in someone who is sick and vomiting frequently. **If you are dealing with a teenager who chronically has a low chloride level, you should consider the possibility of bulimia.** Teenagers won't always admit having this condition unless confronted with the evidence. If an increased amylase level accompanies the low chloride level, it strongly suggests the possibility of bulimia. The amylase comes from irritation of the salivary glands caused by the persistent vomiting.

Carbon dioxide (CO_2) levels in the blood go up and down as part of the mechanism that controls the acid-base balance. If the CO_2 level is significantly off, a thorough metabolic workup should be done by the physician. Note that the CO_2 level is another test that often is abnormal because the blood specimen was allowed to sit too long before it was processed.

Phosphorus is another electrolyte that is often measured. The phosphorus level is closely related to calcium metabolism. Children with kidney problems or calcium metabolism problems may have too high or too low a phosphorus level. Otherwise, the phosphorus level is rarely abnormal. Note that children who are using too much antacid may develop low phosphorus levels (hypophosphatemia). Antacids contain chemicals that bind the phosphorus in the intestines and prevent it from being absorbed.

Albumin is a serum protein manufactured by the liver that serves as both a building block and a carrier molecule. A low level may be the result of decreased production or increased loss. Decreased production may be due to liver disease or poor nutritional intake. Increased loss may result from loss through either the gastrointestinal system or the kidney. In either case, it needs to be investigated. Systemic lupus erythematosus and amyloidosis are among the many diseases that may cause increased loss of albumin through the kidney. This is easily detected by urine tests for protein.

Whenever the serum albumin level is low, the body must compensate by increasing the levels of other elements in the blood to maintain an appropriate osmotic balance. Most often the body increases the level of cholesterol in the blood to accomplish this. High cholesterol and low albumin are commonly found in children with renal disease, often nephrotic syndrome. Changes in diet are not likely to have any effect on these problems if the underlying conditions are not corrected. If the body is unable to maintain an appropriate osmotic balance, water will leak out of the blood vessels, producing edema. Painful, swollen feet in children may be a sign of kidney malfunction and low albumin levels. Sometimes the first clue is that socks are leaving deep marks on the feet or calves.

In addition to measuring the albumin level, the comprehensive metabolic panel includes the **total protein, the total globulin, and the albumin/globulin ratio**. These are obtained by measuring the total protein and the albumin. The globulin is then determined by subtracting the albumin from the total protein, and the albumin/globulin ratio is determined by dividing the albumin level by the globulin level. Globulins are larger proteins in the blood that include a number of acute phase reactants as well as immunoglobulin molecules. The level of acute phase reactants rises in people who are ill, so the globulin level goes up in these people as well. At the same time, the albumin level often goes down when people are sick. The combination of factors often leads to a decreased albumin/globulin ratio. Low globulin levels also may be an indication of low immunoglobulin levels.

Bilirubin is commonly included in the comprehensive metabolic panel. Most often it is reported as *total* and *direct* bilirubin. Direct bilirubin has been completely processed by the liver, while indirect bilirubin has not. Liver disease is the most common cause of a significantly elevated bilirubin level. If the bilirubin level is too high, the child will look jaundiced.. In children with rheumatic or musculoskeletal disease, the most common cause of a significantly increased bilirubin level is hemolysis. This can occur after internal bleeding or in children with hemolytic anemia. Hemolytic anemia is often seen in children with SLE. Because RBCs also contain aspartate transaminase (AST), physicians may initially be confused, thinking that children with elevated bilirubin and AST levels have hepatic disease, when in fact the liver is fine and the problem is excessive hemolysis.

Serum glutamic-oxaloacetic transaminase/AST (**SGOT/AST**) is contained in muscle cells, liver cells, and RBCs. Damage to any of these can result in increased amounts of AST being present in the blood. If the AST is elevated with no obvious explanation, it is important to be sure that muscle enzyme testing (CK and aldolase) is done to look for muscle diseases, as well as a reticulocyte count to look for hemolytic anemia. Normal CBC and chemistry panels do not include the proper tests for these problems, and an elevated AST level may be the only hint. In a child with hemolysis the bilirubin level will also be elevated. This does not happen with muscle disease. If the elevated AST is the result of problems with the liver, there should be a significant elevation of the alanine aminotransferase (ALT) as well. However some children with muscle disease do show elevated ALT as well as AST.

Serum glutamate pyruvate transaminase/ALT (**SGPT/ALT**) is another enzyme that is primarily found in the liver. Thus, if the AST level is elevated but the ALT level is not, it suggests that the source of the AST is outside the liver. Mild elevations of the ALT level can occur from disease outside the liver if the AST level is also elevated. There are many different liver diseases that may result in an elevation of the ALT level. The ALT level may also rise if the liver is being irritated by medications, supplements, or environmental toxins. Methotrexate is known to irritate the liver in some children, but the NSAIDs and many other drugs may also cause liver irritation in some children. This is why it is important to monitor these tests routinely in children on medication.

It should always be remembered that some rheumatic diseases may cause damage to the liver, and some liver diseases may cause bone and joint discomfort. This is especially true in patients with infectious hepatitis. All children with significantly elevated liver enzyme levels need careful evaluation.

Lactic dehydrogenase (**LDH**) increases with damage to RBCs, muscles, hepatocytes, or other types of cells. When there is increased cell turnover, the LDH level can be very high. Many physicians believe that an LDH level over 1000 units means that the child must have a tumor, but children with rheumatic diseases such as systemic-onset JRA or dermatomyositis and other systemically ill children may have very high LDH levels (well over 1000 units). Know that if a child is thought to have pauciarticular JRA and the LDH is very high, something is wrong. These children should be carefully evaluated for leukemia or bone tumors.

Like children with an elevated AST or ALT level, children with an elevated LDH level must be investigated carefully. The problem may be located in any of many different organ systems. Damage to many tissues—including the brain, heart, lungs, liver, blood cells, muscle, or spleen—all may result in elevated LDH levels.

Alkaline phosphatase is an enzyme associated with bone turnover. Because children have actively growing bones, the normal alkaline phosphatase value for children is much higher than the normal value for adults. If the laboratory is not reporting age-adjusted values, a normal value in a child may be reported as abnormal. Alkaline phosphatase is also found in the gallbladder. In an adult, an elevated alkaline phosphatase level may indicate gallbladder disease, but this is a rare problem in children. (Note: Children with sickle cell disease can develop gallbladder problems.) Occasionally, children have alkaline phosphatase values many times the expected normal value with no apparent illness. Bone tumors with increased cell turnover (e.g., osteogenic sarcoma) may be associated with bone pain and elevated alkaline phosphatase levels.

The level of **uric acid** is another laboratory value frequently reported in the comprehensive metabolic panel. Uric acid is a breakdown product of DNA. Thus, increased uric acid means either that there is increased breakdown of cells, or that the kidneys are not properly clearing the uric acid, or both. Children with hemolytic uremic syndrome have high uric acid levels. So do children with leukemia. Sometimes children with elevated uric acid levels and joint pain are referred for possible gout. These children should be carefully evaluated for other problems. Gout is essentially unheard of in childhood except in the setting of kidney disease or cancer chemotherapy, where the drugs are causing many tumor cells to die very quickly and the kidneys cannot handle the load. For all intents and purposes, children do not develop gout.

Muscle Enzymes: Creatinine Kinase and Aldolase

Creatine kinase (CK) is produced by a variety of cells in the body. It can be released from both skeletal and heart muscle and from the brain. Although it may be elevated in adults with myocardial infarctions, the most frequent cause of elevations in childhood is muscle inflammation. This may occur in children with dermatomyositis, scleroderma, or MCTD. Sometimes CK is elevated with extensive exercise. A number of children have been referred to me over the years because of elevated CK levels after working out with weights or practicing for the football team. They often had CK levels many times the upper limit of normal. After two weeks of rest, the results were back to normal.

The level of CK is also elevated after some viral infections. One winter there was a viral epidemic (most likely influenza B) in which many children began to complain of pain in their calves. Their CK levels were in the thousands, and many physicians became concerned. All of these children had normal test values a few weeks later when their viral infection had resolved. There are children with elevated CK levels that persist despite rest and for which no explanation can be found. This situation is discussed in Chapter 6. Fractionation of the CK may be helpful to exclude cardiac or brain tissue as the origin of the elevation.

Aldolase may be elevated in children with muscle damage. In general, the aldolase level is less sensitive to muscle inflammation than the CK level, but there are children with dermatomyositis who have elevated aldolase levels and a normal CK level. Aldolase can also be increased in children with liver inflammation secondary to infectious mononucleosis or viral hepatitis.

One of the biggest problems with our current system of ordering laboratory tests is that many useful tests have been eliminated from the standard panels. As a result, the test results may all be "normal" because the right test to diagnose the disease was not included. Lactic dehydrogenase and CK are well-known examples of this. Children with dermatomyositis are tired all the time and want to be carried because their muscles are painful and weak. Early in the course of the disease, the LDH, CK, and aldolase levels may be elevated before there are any other indications of muscle disease. However, LDH and CK are no longer included in the normal metabolic panel, and aldolase was never part of the panel. Thus, it is not uncommon for me to see a child because the parents keep insisting that something is wrong, but the pediatrician cannot find anything and "the lab tests are all normal." The answer may be obvious when the proper tests are done.

Quantitative Immunoglobulins (IgG, IgA, and IgM)

Immunoglobulin levels are reflected by the measurement of the total protein, but they can be measured more precisely by specific testing. In a normal immune response, the body recognizes and processes a foreign antigen and begins making antibodies against it by making IgM. As the immune response matures, the body begins to make IgG. IgA is also made in the secondary stage. There are additional antibody classes—IgE and IgD—that play a role in specific diseases.

Children who cannot make any antibodies have **agammaglobulinemia**. These children usually die of infections unless they receive a bone marrow transplant or repeated infusions of IVIgG. Less severe forms of partial IgG deficiency are more common. There are several subclasses of IgG. If only one is missing, the child may have frequent infections but otherwise do well. Children may also have a generalized low level of IgG. Children with a generalized low IgG level may have trouble handling viral infections, and have an increased frequency of joint pains and limping episodes when viral infections develop. Defining these low IgG levels is difficult. Large studies have shown that the normal levels of immunoglobulins in young children are highly variable. I have seen a number of young children (four to six years of age) with low levels that are still "normal" who limp whenever they develop viral infections. Thorough investigation has not found any additional abnormalities. As the children get older and their immune system matures, this limp stops.

IgA deficiency is an important special case of immunoglobulin deficiency. IgA is the body's defense at mucosal surfaces. Thus, IgA is found in the gut, the saliva, and the upper airways. Children with IgA deficiency have an increased incidence of colds and ear infections but in general do well. However, IgA deficiency is much more common in children with rheumatic disease than it would be if the two conditions were unrelated. It is important to identify children with IgA deficiency not only because they have an increased incidence of infections and rheumatic diseases, but also because they can have major problems with transfusion reactions. There are many stories of these children getting into trouble when they need a transfusion because all of the tests for RBC compatibility are done correctly, but the children have a transfusion reaction due to the IgA in the donor's blood.

IgE is primarily associated with allergic reactions. High levels of IgE usually indicate a very allergic individual. These high levels can also be found in children with eosinophilic vasculitis (see Chapter 15). IgD levels are almost never measured. There is a very rare syndrome called *hyper-IgD syndrome* that causes children to have recurrent fevers and abdominal pain.

Specialized Tests

In trying to understand all of the specialized laboratory tests, it is necessary to understand how these tests come about. Imagine that I have asked you to develop a quick, rapid test to detect the presence of fire engines. Since we need fire engines to conduct the test, I have sent you to the scene of several fires to start your work. You quickly come back and report that you have found a very useful test to detect a fire engine. It is almost invariably a big red truck at the scene of a fire. You and I go to a few fires, and the test looks extremely useful.

Then we stand on the corner of the highway and pull over all of the big red trucks that go by. Few, if any, are fire engines. What went wrong? All tests have important two characteristics called *sensitivity* and *specificity*. Sensitivity means no false negatives (everybody with the disease is found by the test). Specificity means no false positives (everybody who has a positive test has the disease). No test has perfect sensitivity and specificity. Further, the results depend on where the test is done. At the scene of a fire, the red truck test is useful—it has both high sensitivity and high specificity—but not on the highway. A positive test should always be considered in light of the setting (i.e., why it was done).

Antinuclear antibody testing

Antinuclear antibody testing used to be very significant in diagnosing children with rheumatic disease. When it was originally developed, a positive test in a child who did not have rheumatic disease was rare. The main problem with the test was that the results were difficult to compare between different laboratories. Each lab used its own materials and did its own validation. In the early 1980s, it was decided that a standardized test would be better. This requires that every laboratory use the same substrate.

A uniform cultured human cell line, called Hep2, was agreed on for the standard. But there are so many variables in performing ANA testing that it is still not safe to compare results between different laboratories. Furthermore, this cell line gives low-titer (see below) positive results much more frequently than the old method did. As a result, positive tests that do not mean that the child has a rheumatic disease have become very common. In one reported study, one-third of children who were admitted to the hospital for tonsillectomy had low-titer positive tests for ANA. None of these children had rheumatic disease. Higher-titer positive tests are more meaningful. However, having only a low-titer ANA does not guarantee that the child does not have disease.

The ANA titer refers to how much the patient's sera can be diluted and still give a positive reading. Sera are initially screened after being diluted forty times (1:40). If the screen is positive, then further tests are done at 1:80, 1:160, 1:320, and so on, until there is no detectable fluorescence. The last dilution at which the fluorescence can be seen is the ANA titer.

Positive tests for ANA are found in a wide variety of conditions. They are certainly found in children with SLE, but they are also found in children with many other rheumatic diseases, including JA. They may briefly appear after a wide variety of infections (especially viral infections where the virus has damaged the nuclei of the cells it infected). Positive tests for ANA have been seen in many children with no identifiable disease and in some children with many different diseases. A positive ANA should prompt consideration of a rheumatic disease, but it may be a false lead.

A positive test for ANA is also important in children with arthritis. In children with any of the various forms of JA, the complication of eye disease occurs more frequently in children who have a positive ANA test than in children who have a negative test (see Chapters 7 and 8). Despite extensive investigation, the explanation for this association is unknown.

The most common ANA pattern is called *homogeneous*. Some children have a speckled ANA, and others have a shaggy or **rim pattern ANA**. A **homogeneous ANA pattern** occurs in many different people and is not disease-specific. A **speckled pattern** is also common at low titer, but at higher titer it may be associated with MCTD or scleroderma. **A rim pattern is almost always a sign of active SLE.**

Determining whether the different ANA patterns were associated with antibodies to different parts of the nucleus was very difficult in the 1970s. Researchers did not have all the advanced techniques that are available now.

At that time, scientists tried dipping the cells in different chemicals to see whether they changed the ANA test. In doing this, it was discovered that the test results for one group of patients went from positive to negative, and whatever the antibodies were reacting to could be "extracted" by the chemical solution. This led to the term **extractable nuclear antigen** (**ENA**).

After many years of research, we now understand that ENA consists of many different pieces: Ro, La, Sm, and RNP (Ro comes from Robert, the name of the patient in whom the antibody was first found; La from Lane; Sm from Smith; and RNP stands for ribonucleoprotein). Different patterns in the way antibodies react to these pieces tend to correlate with different patterns of disease. The interpretation of these various patterns is found in Chapters 11 and 12.

Another early finding was that some of the antibodies detected by the ANA test were directed against DNA and that people with high titers of anti-DNA antibodies were often sicker. At first, the tests for antibodies to DNA were fairly crude, but they have improved over time. These tests were formerly separated into tests for single-stranded DNA (ssDNA) and tests for double-stranded DNA (dsDNA). Tests for ssDNA have mostly disappeared, as they were very nonspecific and occurred in a wide variety of situations. Most anti-DNA tests today measure dsDNA. High titers of anti-dsDNA are much more specific for SLE than a positive ANA. However, there are children with anti-DNA antibodies who have other diseases. Sometimes a child is very sick with a viral infection and anti-DNA antibodies appear as part of the immune response to the virus. These antibodies usually disappear within a few months. When you are looking at anti-DNA antibody tests, the lab may have run a *Crithidia lucilliae* assay. Many sources of DNA contain DNA in chains, and these chains may have damaged ends. The damaged ends often cause positive test results that are not meaningful. *Crithidia* is a microorganism that has circular DNA. There are no loose ends. Thus, the *Crithidia* test avoids this problem. A positive test for anti-DNA antibodies using *Crithidia* is more meaningful. However, even this test is occasionally positive in children who don't have SLE. Nonetheless, any child with a positive test result for anti-DNA antibodies should be thoroughly evaluated.

Antineutrophil cytoplasmic antibodies

Unlike antinuclear antibodies, which react with materials in the nucleus of the cell, antineutrophil cytoplasmic antibodies (ANCAs) react with elements in the cytoplasm of neutrophils. There are two major variations: cANCA reacts with proteinase 3, a substance found in granules that are spread diffusely throughout the cytoplasm of neutrophils, and pANCA reacts with myeloperoxidase. This is also a component of neutrophil granules, but because of its electrostatic charge, when the cell is fixed for staining, myeloperoxidase tends to move toward the nucleus. The resultant staining pattern is perinuclear. With continued investigation, it has become clear that pANCA may also represent antibodies to lactoferrin and other substances.

How and why pANCA and cANCA occur is unclear. Their importance lies in their association with Wegener's granulomatosis, pauci-immune glomerulonephritis, Churg-Strauss syndrome, other systemic vasculitis syndromes, and IBD. If the antibodies are present, more extensive testing is indicated. For example, if a child with arthritis is complaining of stomach pains, it may be due to medications. If the child has pANCA, I will be quicker to investigate by endoscopy the possibility of IBD. Unfortunately, the association of the antibodies with these diseases is incomplete. Some patients with the diseases do not have the antibodies, and some patients with the antibodies do not have the diseases. As with so many other tests in rheumatic disease, we recognize the association but do not yet fully understand the how and why.

Anti–*Saccharomyces cerevisiae* antibodies

Saccharomyces cerevisiae is a fungus that commonly occurs in the large intestine. Antibodies to this fungus (**anti-*Saccharomyces cerevisiae* antibodies, or ASCA**) occur more often in children with IBD than in normal children. These antibodies are not routinely measured by rheumatologists, but they are increasingly being used by gastroenterologists in the evaluation of children who may have IBD. Studies have shown ASCA to be common in children with Crohn's disease, which is one type of IBD. However, they are also common in children with spondyloarthropathies whether or not they have IBD.

Serum complement levels

Complement levelsare most commonly measured in children with possible SLE. Although the complement system consists of many separate components, only C3 and C4 are routinely measured. **C3** is typically depressed in children with active SLE and may be a warning of more active disease to come. However, the predictive value of a change in C3 level is the subject of much debate. Few diseases other than SLE cause a low C3 level.

C4 is also frequently low in children with SLE. However, the significance of a low C4 level is less clear. This is discussed in much more detail in Chapter 11. Many laboratories will also report the result of **CH50**, but this is not a complement component. CH50 is a test that measures the function of the entire complement system. If any one of the components of the system is low, the CH50 will be low.

C1q and **C2** are two other complement components that can be measured, but these are not tested routinely. Genetic deficiency of C1q is associated with an increased risk of developing SLE. The risk of developing SLE is also increased in children who are deficient in C2 or C4. Deficiency of C4 does not cause any obvious illness, but deficiency of either C2 or C3 is associated with increased infections. Children with complete genetic deficiency of C3 often die of infections. Children genetically deficient in C2 have an increased incidence of infections and of rheumatic diseases but may live a normal life if they are recognized and given antibiotic prophylaxis. Most physicians think that C2 deficiency is extremely rare, but I have seen several children with C2 deficiency in my practice. You have to look for it to find it.

Anticentromere and anti-Scl-70 antibodies

These antibodies are associated with forms of scleroderma. Anticentromere antibodies are often present in children with CREST syndrome, and anti-Scl-70 antibodies may be present in children with systemic scleroderma. These antibodies are very significant if they are present. Most children who test positive for them will turn out to have the disease. However, I have seen false-positive results and low-titer positive results that have turned out to mean nothing. In addition, I have followed several children with worrisome levels of these antibodies who have not developed obvious disease over several years. However, they still may.

Like all diagnostic tests, tests for anticentromere and anti-Scl-70 antibodies are useful when they are done in children whom you suspect have the disease, but you must be very careful in interpreting the results if they do not fit the clinical picture. Not every laboratory does these tests well. Before you become concerned about a positive test result that does not make sense, make sure that the test has been repeated in one of the nationally recognized laboratories (see the Appendix). Unfortunately, the absence of these antibodies does not guarantee that your patient does not have one of these diseases. The antibodies are found in less than half of affected patients and less often in children than in adults.

Anti-Jo-1 antibody

This is one of a variety of antibodies (anti-synthetase antibodies) that have been described in adults with muscle disease. It is very uncommon in childhood. Adults with this antibody tend to have a more difficult disease course. There is a growing belief that patients who test positive for this antibody have a completely different disease from that of other patients with myositis.

Factor VIII

Factor VIII, or Von Willebrand's factor, is one of the blood clotting factors. In children with inflammatory disease, the factor VIII level will rise and fall as an acute phase reactant. Some physicians like to follow this level in children with muscle disease or other diseases in which the blood vessels tend to be involved. A rising level suggests more disease activity.

Antigliadin antibodies, antitissue transglutaminase, and antiendomyseal antibodies

These antibodies are part of a celiac disease panel. It is important to detect them in children with celiac disease (gluten-sensitive enteropathy). Children with celiac disease develop arthritis and other autoimmune diseases more often than would be expected. Antigliadin antibodies can be of either the IgG or the IgA type. IgG-type antigliadin antibodies are very common and probably are not meaningful. IgA-type antigliadin antibodies should raise the suspicion of celiac disease. Antitissue transglutaminase and antiendomyseal antibodies are much more specific for celiac disease. Unfortunately, not all patients who test positive have the disease, and a negative test does not guarantee that they do not. However, these tests are helpful in determining which children with abdominal complaints should be evaluated further. The diagnosis of celiac disease depends on a biopsy of the small bowel that demonstrates the classic findings.

Rheumatoid factor

The most important thing to know about RF is that children with arthritis are most often negative. The test is positive only in one small subgroup of children and should not be used to make the diagnosis of JA.

The RF test measures the presence of IgM antibodies directed against IgG. This test is very useful in diagnosing an adult with rheumatoid arthritis and must be positive for the patient to be seropositive. However, most children with JA are negative. Why these antibodies are present in adults with rheumatoid arthritis remains unclear. It is thought to mean that the IgG in these patients is altered in some way. Rheumatoid factor is found in some normal people, in people with a variety of rheumatic diseases, and in people with various infections, especially subacute bacterial endocarditis (SBE).

Positive tests for RF in children with bone or joint pain occur in a few specific situations. Adult-onset rheumatoid arthritis by definition occurs after sixteen years of age. However, since the disease does not always proceed as described in the literature, it occasionally starts earlier. There are children with true adult-type rheumatoid arthritis that starts in the early teenage years or even younger. This is not common. Children with certain infections, including SBE, also can have a positive RF test, as can children with other rheumatic diseases. A child with joint pains, a positive RF, and a positive ANA should be carefully evaluated for the possibility of scleroderma or MCTD. These conditions are often associated with a positive ANA and a positive RF.

You may hear about "hidden" RF. This is a very confusing subject. Typical RF is IgM directed against IgG. Because IgM has a unique structure that is very large, it is easy to detect these antibodies. Using special techniques, one can measure IgG and IgA antibodies against IgG, which are smaller and not are detected by the normal RF test. These hidden RFs are found in some children with JA. However, these tests are not commonly done, and their proper interpretation remains unclear. There are many false-positive tests for IgG RF.

Lyme disease testing

This is a key element in the evaluation of any child with arthritis in areas where the disease is endemic. Many laboratories do Lyme disease testing, and a variety of techniques are used. It is very important to understand the difference between a screening test and a meaningful positive test. If you have a very good test for a disease that is expensive to perform, you do not want to do it on every child who might have the disease. This is especially true if there is an easier test that will identify children who do not need the costly test. This is the situation with Lyme disease. The easy test is an ELISA that identifies antibodies in the blood against spirochetal antigens. *Borrelia burgdorferi* is the agent that causes Lyme disease. It is a spirochete and has spirochetal antigens. However, there are many spirochetes, all of which have spirochetal antigens. Some of these spirochetes are normally found in saliva. If a child has Lyme disease, he or she will have a positive ELISA for antibodies to spirochetes, but so will many children who have been exposed to spirochetes other than those of Lyme disease. All children with a positive ELISA should then be tested on a Western blot. The Western blot determines exactly which spirochetal antigens the antibodies in the child's blood are reacting with. Since it separately tests many different spirochetal antigens, the Western blot can distinguish between antibodies found only in people with Lyme disease and antibodies found in people exposed to other spirochetes. **Thus, a positive Lyme ELISA identifies only the people who need to be tested further. A positive Western blot indicates definite exposure to *B. burgdorferi*, the spirochete that causes Lyme disease.** The Western blot isn't done on everyone because it is a much more expensive test.

There are several points to remember. A child with a positive Western blot has definitely been exposed to *B. burgdorferi* and needs to be treated for Lyme disease. However, this does not prove that Lyme disease is the cause of the child's symptoms. Lyme disease and exposure to *B. burgdorferi* are very common in many parts of the United States. Thus, people with other conditions may also have a positive test for Lyme disease even though Lyme disease may have nothing to do with their symptoms. In one study, people who lived in an endemic area for Lyme disease, who felt well and were shopping in a local shopping center, were asked to give blood specimens for testing. Over 10 percent were positive for Lyme disease. If more than 10 percent of the random population tests positive for Lyme disease, this means that over 10 percent of the people with other conditions will test positive for Lyme disease even though that disease is not the cause of their problem. **If a child tests positive for Lyme disease, he or she certainly should be treated. But if the symptoms continue, retreatment may not be the right answer. There may well be another problem.** Conversely, some people worry about having Lyme disease but test negative. This is unlikely unless the laboratory makes a mistake. It is always a good idea to repeat the test if you are concerned. Treatment and repeated treatment in the absence of a positive test may lead to a delay in the diagnosis of the real problem.

> I have seen and treated many children with real Lyme disease, but the child who stands out was sent to me from an area where many children develop this disease. His test was negative, but he had a very painful hip. Over a period of six months he was treated with antibiotics repeatedly for Lyme disease, without improvement. Then he was referred to me for treatment of difficult Lyme disease. I did further testing and found that he had a tumor irritating his hip. Only when we removed the tumor did he get better. The problem was never Lyme disease.

Thyroid function tests

These tests are often done in children with joint problems because both **hyper-thyroidism** and **hypothyroidism** are often associated with diffuse aches and pains. Both of these conditions also may be associated with fatigue and muscle weakness. In addition, autoimmune diseases such as SLE may be associated with antibodies that interfere with thyroid function.

The main thyroid function tests are **T3 (triiodothyronine), T4 (thyroxine), and TSH (thyroid-stimulating hormone)**. The first two hormones regulate the body's metabolism. Thyroid-stimulating hormone is secreted by the pituitary gland and influences the function of the thyroid. In children with rheumatic disease, we occasionally see TSH abnormalities without T3 or T4 abnormalities. This can be a warning of problems to come. The best way to think of this is as if you were evaluating a car. If the car is going at normal speed and the driver is pushing normally on the gas pedal, everything is fine. However, if the car is going too fast and the driver is not touching the gas pedal (high T3 and T4 but normal TSH), something is wrong. If the car is going at normal speed but the driver has depressed the gas pedal all the way, that also suggests problems (normal T3 and T4 but high TSH). Children with SLE and related conditions often develop autoimmune thyroid disease. Normal T3 and T4 with a high TSH may be the first sign.

Some children with autoimmune diseases have high titers of **antithyroid antibodies** long before they actually develop thyroid disease. These may be **antithyroid peroxidase antibodies** or **antithyroglobulin antibodies**. Often children with antithyroid peroxidase antibodies have a family history of Hashimoto's thyroiditis. These children should be monitored carefully for the possibility that they, too, may ultimately develop Hashimoto's thyroiditis. Thyroid antibodies are also seen in some children with SLE and occasionally in children with celiac disease and other autoimmune diseases.

Serum protein electrophoresis

Serum protein electrophoresis (SPEP) measures the pattern of the proteins in the blood. It is a useful test for multiple myeloma. In multiple myeloma, one particular line of cells is causing the problem, resulting in a *monoclonal spike* (a single sharp peak) that can be easily seen on the SPEP. This virtually never occurs in children. In children with rheumatic diseases, the SPEP usually shows a polyclonal (a broad peak) increase. However, the SPEP may detect IgA deficiency or low levels of other immunoglobulins.

Anticardiolipin and antiphospholipid antibodies

These antibodies were first recognized in patients with SLE who had bleeding problems. Doctors noted an association between patients with SLE who bled too much because of what was called the *lupus anticoagulant* and false-positive tests for a venereal disease (syphilis). When this was examined, it was found that many patients with SLE had an antibody that reacted with the cardiolipin backbone of the spirochete that causes syphilis. Further testing led to the description of anticardiolipin and antiphospholipid antibodies.

Anticardiolipin and antiphospholipid antibodies are not identical, but the same information applies to both. These antibodies were first noted in SLE patients with excessive bleeding, but it was discovered that they were also present in SLE patients who had clotting problems (deep vein thrombosis, strokes, etc.). These antibodies are also present in some adults and children with a variety of rheumatic diseases, as well as in people who do not have any other identified autoimmune disease.

The anticardiolipin and antiphospholipid antibodies can interact with varying components of the clotting system (see Chapter 11). These antibodies are not all the same. Some have no effect on clotting. Others get in the way and slow down clotting. Still others make the molecules stickier and promote clotting. One source of confusion is the presence of these antibodies in children who have no clotting problems. No one is sure what to do. In children who have blood clots with no other explanation, most turn out to have anticardiolipin antibodies. However, it is risky to give anticoagulants. It appears that most people with anticardiolipin antibodies are at very little risk. Therefore, if the child has never had clotting problems, most rheumatologists either do nothing or just give a baby aspirin daily. However, a child who has demonstrated clotting problems should be treated with an anticoagulant.

Anticardiolipin or antiphospholipid antibodies can also affect pregnant women. Women known to have anticardiolipin antibodies should be carefully monitored when they become pregnant. Women who have had an excessive number of spontaneous abortions (miscarriages) in middle or late pregnancy often turn out to be anticardiolipin antibody–positive.

Clotting studies: prothrombin time and partial thromboplastin time
Routine clotting studies consist of two tests: the **prothrombin time (PT)** and
the **partial thromboplastin time (PTT)**. The PT measures the ability of blood
to clot once it is exposed to thromboplastin (a substance that starts clotting).
The values are usually ten to fourteen seconds. The PTT measures the ability
of blood to clot without being exposed to a stimulus to start clotting. The two
tests measure different parts of the clotting system—the intrinsic and extrinsic
clotting systems.

Anticardiolipin antibodies can prolong clotting, as can many drugs. Some
children have prolonged clotting times because they either do not make or do
not make enough of the clotting factors. These are variants of hemophilia. Low
levels of clotting factors may be a genetic defect or the result of liver disease.
Vitamin K is important for the synthesis of clotting factors, and children with
prolonged bleeding should be given a vitamin K injection. It is unsafe to operate
on children with a significantly prolonged bleeding time without explanation.

HLA B27
HLA B27 is a genetic marker. Our knowledge of HLA B27 demonstrates both
how much and how little we understand about the role of genetics in rheumatic
diseases. HLA B27 is inherited, and, like other markers, it is common in some
populations and rare in others. HLA B27 seems to have arisen in Asia. It is
common among Northern Europeans (e.g., Scandinavians) but also among the
Chinese and some North American Indians.

Eight percent of the Caucasian population is HLA B27–positive, but over
90 percent of adults with ankylosing spondylitis are positive. The vast majority
of people who are HLA B27–positive do not have arthritis. However, if a child is
being evaluated for arthritis, the finding of HLA B27 positivity increases the risk
of his or her having chronic complaints and possibly progressing to ankylosing
spondylitis.

The easiest way to conceptualize this situation is to view HLA B27 as a
multiplier, That is, if the child has no other genetic predisposition to arthritis,
being HLA B27–positive is not significant. However, if he or she has any genetic
predisposition to arthritis, HLA B27 doubles that predisposition. Thus, the very
worst cases are HLA B27–positive, and children who are HLA B27–positive are
at increased risk of developing problems. They may have problems because of

their genetic predisposition and still be HLA B27–negative, and they may be HLA B27–positive and have no problems because they have no other genetic predisposition. (Note: While this is a helpful way to think about the role of HLA B27, we do not know how HLA B27 actually works.)

HLA B27 is strongly associated with ankylosing spondylitis. It is less strongly associated with Reiter's syndrome, the arthritis of IBD, psoriatic arthritis, and other forms of spondyloarthropathies (see Chapter 9). As with all genetic factors that seem to increase the risk of having arthritis, it is logical to ask why the gene has not disappeared from the population. Although all the details are not conclusively proven, it is hypothesized that being HLA B27–positive may protect against certain infections. Thus, it is beneficial to keep HLA B27 in the population even though it has a negative effect on individuals who have additional genetic factors that predispose them to having arthritis.

Urinalysis

Urinalysis is the easiest way to evaluate kidneys damage or inflammation. Hematuria and proteinuria both suggest renal irritation. The urinalysis report will describe the **specific gravity**, which reflects how well the kidney is concentrating the urine. This must be evaluated with reference to whether the person has been drinking a lot or is dehydrated. If the person is dehydrated, the urine should be concentrated and have a high specific gravity. If he or she has too much fluid in the body, the urine should be dilute.

Sugar in the urine is called **glycosuria**. Children being treated with high doses of corticosteroids sometimes begin to lose sugar in their urine. If they do, this is an indication that they are moving toward diabetes, and efforts should be made to reduce the dose of corticosteroid. **Ketones** are also reported if they are present. Normally, there are no ketones in the urine. Ketones are an indication that the body is metabolizing fat instead of carbohydrates. In someone who is sick or has not eaten well for a significant period, this is a normal finding. In a diabetic patient it may be a sign of ketoacidosis. There may be ketones in the urine because the person has not been eating, but there shouldn't be glucose, too. Anyone with ketones and glucose in the urine needs immediate further evaluation.

Protein in the urine needs to be monitored carefully. Some people have **orthostatic proteinuria**, which means that their kidneys leak protein when they are standing for a prolonged period. This is a common and unimportant condition. It can be determined by checking a morning specimen. Since the person has been lying down all night, there should be no protein in the urine. Other people have protein in their urine after a lot of physical activity, especially running. This, too, is not significant, but persistent proteinuria is a symptom of other problems. Excessive protein loss results in **nephrotic syndrome**. This is determined by measuring the twenty-four-hour urine protein excretion (discovered later in the chapter) or by determining the protein/creatinine ratio. Children with SLE may develop nephrotic syndrome as a result of kidney damage. Children with amyloidosis, a rare complication of JA, often have protein in their urine and also may develop nephrotic syndrome. Many children have idiopathic nephrotic syndrome that is not associated with other diseases.

Small amounts of protein in the urine may be an indication that drugs or other chemicals are irritating the kidney. If protein appears in the urine after a new drug has been started, it needs to be monitored carefully. One problem is that some of the NSAIDs are excreted in the urine and cause a false-positive test for protein on the dipstick. This situation can be clarified by having the laboratory perform a more sophisticated test for protein in the urine.

Urobilinogen indicates the presence of bilirubin in the urine. This occurs only in the setting of liver damage or disease that results in an elevated bilirubin level in the blood (discussed above). It may occur in children with **hemolytic anemia** because all the broken-down blood cells are metabolized into bilirubin. Another cause of a positive test for urobilinogen is the NSAID etodolac (Lodine). When etodolac is excreted in the urine, it will react with the test strip and give a false-positive test for urobilinogen.

Occult blood in the urine indicates the presence of hemoglobin from broken RBCs. It suggests that there is bleeding somewhere in the urinary tract. This bleeding may be occurring in the kidney or further down the urinary tract. Most often it is associated with the presence of RBCs. However, mild bleeding in which all of the cells are broken before leaving the body may show up only as occult blood. Another cause of a positive test for occult blood is myoglobin. Myoglobin is a muscle breakdown product that is detected by the dipstick test for occult blood. It can show up in the urine after muscle damage from crush injuries or even vigorous tackle football games. It may also be seen in newborn babies who had a difficult delivery. It is rarely present in children with dermatomyositis.

Red blood cells in the urine are reported as RBCs/hpf. This is a simple count of the number of RBCs per high-power field when the urine is examined under the microscope. Zero to five is a normal finding. Small amounts of blood can be present after vigorous exercise, but these should disappear quickly. While five to ten RBCs/hpf may not be significant, investigation is necessary if it is consistently present. The RBCs in the urine may come from the kidney, the bladder, or anywhere else in the urinary tract. Many different diseases, renal stones, or drugs may cause RBCs to be present in the urine. This condition can also be caused by injuries if a child is struck hard in the stomach or on the back and the kidneys are injured. Some children with JA occasionally have blood in their urine without an obvious cause. Blood may also show up in the urine of girls during menstruation. Sometimes a specimen is contaminated with blood before a girl realizes that her period has started. This is not a cause for concern; the test simply needs to be repeated after menstruation is over.

White blood cells in the urine are reported as WBCs/hpf. Most often, a few WBCs in the urine result from a specimen collected without proper cleaning. However, large numbers of WBCs or clumps should be considered an indication of infection, and a urine culture should be performed. White blood cells in the urine may also result from irritation of the kidney. Leukocyte esterase in the urine helps to differentiate between WBCs from infection and other causes.

Casts are clumps of RBCs or WBCs in the urine. They are called casts because they are clumps of cells that are held together in the shape of the urine tubules. The presence of RBC or WBC casts is considered an indication of ongoing significant kidney damage. This is most often seen in SLE but can also occur in other diseases that damage the kidneys. Hyaline casts are not significant.

Bacteria in the urine suggest that either the specimen was not collected in a clean manner or that there is a urinary tract infection. If there is a urinary tract infection, it is usually due to a single bacterium, though a poorly collected specimen may contain many different types of bacteria. A leukocyte esterase test may help detect a urine infection, as the level of leukocyte esterase increases when the WBCs (leukocytes) are trying to fight an infection. This is not always a reliable finding.

Some compounds that are excreted into the urine may condense into **crystals**. Uric acid crystals and calcium apatite crystals are very common. If there are many of these crystals, one must consider the possibility of kidney stones. These types of crystals are not normally associated with any of the rheumatic diseases.

Twenty-four-hour urine studies are done to determine exactly how much protein and calcium are being lost in the urine. "Spot" protein/Cr ratios done on a voided sample are becoming more accurate and may fully replace the twenty-four-hour test. In the past, the twenty-four-hour test was the best way to quantify the amounts. The dipstick test for protein in the urine is relatively inaccurate and may vary from specimen to specimen during the day. However, the twenty-four-hour tests are accurate only if the child collects **all** of the urine. This is best done by collecting the specimen over the weekend. The proper procedure is to have the child get up in the morning and discard the first urine specimen. Then everything is collected, including the first specimen the next morning. If the laboratory collects on Sunday, the specimen can be taken there for analysis on Monday. If the laboratory collects on Saturday, they will have to keep the specimen refrigerated on Sunday.

Testing Cerebrospinal Fluid

The only time it is unsafe to do a lumbar puncture is if there is increased pressure in the brain. This can be detected by examining the patient's eyes for evidence of increased pressure (papilladema). A CAT scan or MRI of the brain may also detect increased pressure.

Cerebrospinal fluid can be analyzed for evidence of infection, irritation of the brain, bleeding, or other disease. The most important thing is to make sure that there is no infection. In diseases such as SLE that may affect the brain, the child may start acting strangely. Often there is confusion as to whether the strange behavior is due to the drugs being used to treat the SLE, the child's upset about being ill, the illness itself, or an infection. Examining the spinal fluid is the only way to be sure that there is no infection.

The report on the CSF will describe its color, which may be reddish or yellow if there has been bleeding. If the tap is bloody, it may indicate that a blood vessel was nicked during the procedure. Fresh bleeding does not discolor the CSF after the RBCs are spun out, and there will be no damaged or "crenated" RBCs in the specimen. If there is a lot of fresh blood in the specimen, the number of WBCs must be adjusted.

In the absence of infection or irritation, there should be fewer than ten WBCs per milliliter in the CSF. Larger numbers suggest infection. In addition to the cell count and Gram stain, the CSF is analyzed for the amount of sugar and protein present. The amount of sugar will decrease if there are bacteria in the specimen. A low sugar level and a high protein level suggest infection, but a high protein level with a normal sugar level suggests irritation. Oligoclonal bands are another finding that suggests irritation of the central nervous system. They are sometimes found in SLE and sometimes in multiple sclerosis, but there may be other causes.

Testing Synovial Fluid

Synovial fluid is the normal lubricating fluid secreted by the cells that line joints (synovium). Synovial fluid testing is very similar to CSF analysis except that the normal values are different. Again, the most important reason to do this test is to eliminate the possibility of infection. Just as someone with a rheumatic disease that affects the brain could still get an infection, children with known JA can still get infections in their joints.

Whenever you see a child with a hot, swollen joint, it is important to be sure that there is no infection. An experienced physician may be confident that he or she can distinguish a joint that is not infected, but whenever there is doubt the joint must be aspirated. All the tests done on the synovial fluid are the same as those done on the CSF. However, in the synovial fluid there may be up to 100,000 cells without infection. A count of less than 5000 cells is considered normal. Cells numbering 5000 to 50,000 are consistent with arthritis but can also be seen with Lyme disease and irritation of the joint. Cells numbering 50,000 to 100,000 may indicate arthritis, Lyme disease, or an infection. More than 100,000 cells indicates probable infection.

A Gram stain to test for bacteria is always done, no matter what the cell count is, and some of the fluid should be sent for culture by the bacteriology laboratory. If tuberculosis is a possibility, special stains should be done on the fluid (it won't show up on the Gram stain). Special culture techniques are also required if the bacteriology laboratory is required to detect tuberculosis. Protein and sugar are measured just as in the CSF.

The laboratory will typically look for crystals in the synovial fluid. In adults, this is useful in detecting gout, in which there are uric acid crystals in the joint, or pseudo-gout, in which there are calcium hydroxyapatite crystals in the joint. However, neither of these diseases occurs in children under normal circumstances. If the synovial fluid is bloody, it may indicate that a vessel was nicked during the procedure. However, there is an infrequent disease called **pigmented villonodular synovitis** that causes bleeding into the joint. Usually, this is suspected when there is evidence of old blood in the joint. Old blood in the synovial fluid may also come from an injury.

One important source of error in evaluating synovial fluid may occur when the end of the bone near the joint is infected. In this situation the child may complain of knee pain, but the synovial fluid does not reveal evidence of an infection. This is correct in that the joint is not infected, but there is an infection in the end of the adjacent bone. This can be suspected after careful physical examination. A bone scan or MRI will reveal the infection in the bone. During the first few days after they start, infections in bone may not be apparent on X-rays.

26

Reconstructive Surgery

Rebecca's parents were very nervous. Rebecca had severe arthritis that had affected her hips. Despite taking multiple medications from a variety of physicians, things had slowly gotten worse over the past year. Now Rebecca was in my office. She and her parents had hoped that I would have a medication to reverse all of her problems and allow her to walk normally again. Unfortunately, it wasn't so. Rebecca's hip pain was so bad that she rarely ventured out of the house except to go to school. She had begun to use a wheelchair to get from class to class. Careful review of her X-rays made it clear that medications would cause no improvement. Rebecca needed hip replacements.

Her parents were very resistant to the suggestion that Rebecca's hips be replaced. I explained that she would have much less pain and much better function. When I had Rebecca walk down the hall, she had an abnormal gait because of the hip pain. Her parents told me that other children had picked on Rebecca because they thought she walked oddly. They were afraid of what would happen if her hips were replaced. I had one of my volunteers bring in a pamphlet on total hip replacement. The volunteer, a young lady, walked in, smiled, gave me the pamphlet, and walked out. I asked Rebecca's parents whether they had noticed anything. They replied that I was lucky to have such an attractive volunteer working in my office. They were stunned to learn that she was one of my patients who had had her hips replaced a year earlier. No one could tell that she had had this surgery. The only ones who knew were her friends, who saw how much better and how much happier she was after her recovery.

The goal of every pediatric rheumatologist is to maintain and restore the fullest possible level of function. In an ideal world, every child would receive proper medical attention early in the disease course and respond dramatically to therapy. Unfortunately, in the real world, children do not always receive proper medical attention early in the course of their disease. In addition, some of those who do receive proper medical attention fail to respond well.

Many parents are afraid of reconstructive surgery. However, the ability to replace severely damaged joints is one of the most dramatic improvements in the long-term prognosis for children with arthritis. I discuss a number of surgical joint replacements in this chapter. With all the modern medications available, these are rarely necessary for my patients. Moreover, there are very few institutions that have the experienced surgeons and necessary facilities to perform joint replacements on children and adolescents with rheumatic diseases.

At present, we have useful replacements for hips, knees, and shoulders. We can also do useful reconstructive surgery on wrists, elbows, ankles, and feet. These surgeries often dramatically relieve pain and improve function. If a child's activities are being significantly limited by the damage to a joint and medications have failed, it should be replaced if possible.

ANESTHESIA

Most joint replacement surgery was formerly done under general anesthesia. For children with severe arthritis, this was always a major problem. They frequently have neck involvement, and it is difficult (and sometimes dangerous) to intubate them. In the past, if a child had severe neck involvement, it might have been necessary to perform a tracheotomy. Now, almost all joint replacement surgery can be done using regional anesthesia. This eliminates the risk of injury to the neck that in the past made it so complicated to do joint replacement surgery for children with severe arthritis.

TOTAL HIP REPLACEMENT

Total hip replacement (THR) surgery is one of the most significant advances in the care of children with severe arthritis. Prior to the widespread availability of THR for children, any child with severe arthritis in the hip was simply placed in a wheelchair when the pain became too great. Few of these children were ever able to resume walking. Now we are able to replace the hips of children with severe pain, and wheelchairs have become far less common.

Total hip replacement surgery is not performed by a pediatric orthopedist. Instead, it is necessary to find an adult orthopedist who does THR surgery and who is experienced in working with children. Those with sufficient experience are primarily found only in large academic centers with extensive experience in pediatric rheumatology. In addition, there are relatively few centers that have the sophisticated resources required to manufacture custom hip replacements for young children. The normal outcome of THR surgery is excellent. I care for a number of children and young adults who have had this surgery. They could walk right past you on the street unnoticed.

Many parents are concerned about the timing of THR surgery. The appropriate time is as soon as the child's arthritis begins to limit significantly his or her ability to walk around outside the house. If a child's hip pain is so severe that you are considering a wheelchair, it is time to arrange THR surgery instead. For all of us, it is far easier to be pushed than to walk; for a child with arthritis, this is even more true. As soon as the child starts to use a wheelchair, he or she begins to lose strength in the legs and begins to develop flexion contractures in the knees. Both of these complications make it much more difficult to recover the ability to walk after surgery. The best outcome is obtained when the use of a wheelchair has been minimized or avoided completely.

Parents sometimes hesitate because they are concerned that the child will stop growing if the hip is replaced. However, if the hip is so damaged and painful that the child cannot walk, it is not going to grow. Two-thirds of the growth in length of the femur occurs at the distal end. That growth is not affected by THR.

Other parents are concerned because they do not know how long the THR will last. It is true that the prosthesis may ultimately need to be replaced, but confinement to a wheelchair is not a better option. In experienced hands, hip replacements that become loose or otherwise need revision can be fixed repeatedly. The key is to have an experienced surgeon who is familiar with working with children. I have seen children who were denied hip replacement because "hip replacements are not made small enough." At centers such as the Hospital for Special Surgery, we have a custom fabrication unit that can make a prosthesis of any size we need. We have done surgery on children as young as nine years of age and as small as 60 pounds with excellent long-term results.

ARTHROSCOPIC KNEE SURGERY AND KNEE REPLACEMENT

Total knee replacement (TKR) surgery has been very successful in maintaining the ability of children to carry out the activities of daily living. With improved medications and the ability to suppress arthritis in the knees using intra-articular corticosteroids, TKR in response to arthritis has become rare in children. Continuing active synovitis in a knee that has not responded to routine medications or intra-articular corticosteroid injection may be treated by an arthroscopic synovectomy. This therapy often provides significant relief but may have to be repeated.

Some children develop avascular necrosis in their knees as the result of corticosteroid usage. This is best treated with TKR. Usually, this does not need to be done in small children and does not result in significant loss of growth. Like hip replacements, knee replacements may need revision over time. However, surgeons at experienced centers can do this when necessary.

ANKLES

The ankle joint is difficult. At the time of this writing, it is generally better to fuse the ankle than to replace it. Fused ankles force children to walk without bending their ankles (it's clumsy, but it works). Because the joints of the ankle have been fused, they do not move—but they do not hurt, either. The mechanics of the ankle joint are relatively complex and to date, the mechanical replacements are not satisfactory.

FOOT SURGERY (TARSAL FUSION)

One of the more difficult problems for children with arthritis is involvement of the joints between the tarsal bones of the feet. These joints are important when you walk over an irregular surface or bend your feet. If they become significantly involved by arthritis, there may be a lot of pain when walking. A surgical procedure called a *triple arthrodesis* will fuse these bones. This results in a stiff foot and will cause difficulty when the child walks over an uneven surface, but it will relieve most of the pain.

WRIST SURGERY

The wrist is often significantly involved in children with psoriatic arthritis and some related spondyloarthropathies. It may also be involved in polyarticular-onset JA. There are two major problems. One is a wrist that hurts whenever it is bent. In some children, the symptoms are relieved by wearing a splint. If there is active arthritis, the splint may even result in fusion of the wrist.

If the splint does not provide adequate relief, it may be necessary to fuse the wrist surgically. This is not a major surgery. If the wrist is not splinted or fused, there is a risk of progressive subluxation and deformity. When this happens, the wrist may become permanently flexed, with permanent loss of function.

With progressive active arthritis, children may develop marked wrist subluxation. This subluxation causes the extensor tendons of the fingers to rub against the ulnar styloid process. If this continues, the tendons may rupture, with loss of ability to extend the fingers. Surgery to remove the ulnar styloid process is minor and may relieve the problem.

SHOULDER SURGERY

In some children with severe arthritis the glenoid can be damaged, limiting the ability to raise the arms over the head and perform other activities. This interferes with dressing and other activities of daily living. Surgical replacement of the glenoid head is easily done in an advanced center.

27

Family Issues

In one of my families there were three children; the oldest was a twelve-year-old boy with severe arthritis. It was decided that he would have a hip replacement after the end of the school year. Both parents were very concerned, and everyone knew that Johnny was expected to be in the hospital for five days after the surgery. All of us would have the same initial response: Ask a sitter or a relative to care for Sally and Timmy (eight and ten years old) so that Mom and Dad can be at Johnny's bedside for the five days. Summer travel plans are off, because Johnny will need a lot of physical therapy to recover and will not be able to travel. **This all sounds reasonable, but it's the wrong answer.**

Instead, Grandma came to take care of Sally and Timmy for the first two days. After it was clear that Johnny was recovering as expected, Dad took off with Sally and Timmy on a trip to one of their favorite places. Mom and Grandma relieved each other in the hospital. At the end of the week, everyone was back home feeling that they had gotten a lot of attention. Further, it was agreed that if Johnny made good progress in physical therapy, the whole family would go to an amusement park at the end of the summer. Otherwise, Sally, Timmy, and Mom would go, and Dad would stay home with Johnny. Everyone got attention. Everyone had a shared goal. No one felt deprived or held back.

Physicians must be a major resource for the families of children who have a serious chronic condition. In addition to the medical care necessary, these families are in need of psychosocial support. **Often if a child has a significant disability, his or her medical care starts to take over everyone's life.**

If you have lived with a child with a chronic condition for a period of time, you know that it places a strain on everyone in the family. **A chronic childhood illness is not the child's problem; it is the family's problem. No one in the family is spared the impact of the child's disease. If they try to pretend**

otherwise, everyone suffers. Everyone will feel the impact of the attention diverted to take care of the ill child, everyone will feel the impact of the financial burden, and everyone will feel the impact of missed vacations. Divorce and psychiatric disease are much more common in families of children with chronic illness than in the general population.

IS THERE ANY ESCAPE?

There is no single answer that works for everyone. Families are different. Children are different. The degree to which a child's illness interferes with the family will be different. **Still, there are important points of which everyone should be aware.** First, parents have more control over the situation than they think, but they may need your help in recognizing the need to confront the situation. Second, ignoring the problem does not make it go away; it makes it worse. I deal with families every day. The successful ones allow everyone in the family personal time and space. If all family members are recognized as having important needs, everyone can work together for the good of the whole family. **Do not allow families to neglect their healthy children (or spouse) for the sake of the child who is ill. In the end, everyone will be unhealthy because of the psychological problems this causes.**

None of this advice means that you should neglect the child who is ill. None of this advice is easy. Caring for children is hard work. Caring for a child with a chronic disease is much harder. The key to success is encouraging family members to communicate their feelings. Often you will hear quiet comments in the office or you (or your receptionist) will notice things in the waiting room that indicate that family members are under stress. In many families, Mom is in charge of taking care of the children, including all the doctors' appointments and so forth. She often starts to feel overburdened. The other children may start to feel neglected because of the time it takes for Mom to deal with the needs of the ill child. Dad can start to feel neglected as well. This situation will not work if there is a chronic problem.

Remind your patients that the families that cope most successfully do so by having everyone pitch in. Sometimes Dad brings the child to the appointment and Mom stays home with the other children. Everyone must enjoy special activities. There will be times when the family makes a sacrifice for the child with disease. Equally, there should be times when everyone gets to go somewhere special as a reward for pitching in. Life is not fair, but it can be balanced. Encourage parents who have several children to make sure that each one gets the attention he or she needs. **Don't forget to tell parents to include themselves on the list of people who need attention and special activities.**

WHOSE FAULT IS IT? THE BLAME GAME

Imagine that you and your spouse are going to the movies on Saturday night. Your spouse gets home late from visiting with friends, and both of you have to rush to get ready. By the time you reach the theater, they've turned down the lights and are showing the previews. The easy-to-reach seats are full, and you have to squeeze past many people to reach two seats together on the side.

As you squeeze past one gentleman, you hear a plop and your foot gets cold. You have just knocked over the large container of soda that he'd set on the floor. "Oh, my goodness—I'm so sorry!" You struggle into your seat, feeling guilty and wondering whether you should get up and offer to buy him another soda or give him the money for it. Now you are angry at yourself for knocking it over.

In a few minutes, as you think about it, you are angry at your spouse for making you late in getting to the theater. If you'd been on time, you would have arrived while the lights were still on and found better seats. Then you are angry at the man who set his soda down on the floor. He should have known better than to put it there and forget to pick it up when he saw you moving into his row. The rows of seats shouldn't be so close together in this theater anyway. Who designed this place? Maybe we shouldn't come back here!

It's the blame game! These are all minor issues. It is unfortunate that all of them are true. Nonetheless, no one of these problems is the explanation for what happened. In reality, no one is to blame and everyone is to blame. Trying to assign blame to any individual won't solve anything. It's just a normal process of rationalization that we all go through. **If you said out loud any of the things you were thinking to yourself, it would just make the situation worse.** Swallow hard and concentrate on moving on so that everyone can enjoy the movie.

It is not someone's fault that the child has an illness. No one should feel that he or she is being deprived or punished as a result. Parents must devote time to the child with disease, but they should also give time to the other children and to their spouse as well. They must always look for a way to make things special and balanced for everyone. It's hard work—but it's well worth it. If you feel that a family under your care is off to a bad start, sit down with everyone and talk about it. Not every pediatrician has the time or the rapport with families to approach them directly with specific suggestions. However, every physician is a counselor to the families he or she cares for and should be able to suggest a psychologist or another mental health care professional to help the family cope with the inevitable strains of chronic disease. There are psychologists, psychiatrists, and social workers who are trained specifically in dealing with the families of children who are chronically ill. **There are many stories of mothers who selflessly devoted their lives to a child with serious disease. Most of these stories include divorce, unhappy brothers and sisters who did not do well, and a child with chronic illness burdened by guilt over the disruption of the family.**

GROWING UP IS HARD TO DO

Another difficult situation for families of children with chronic disease is allowing the young adult to accept increasing responsibility and ultimately total responsibility for his or her care. Some hospitals have special adolescent clinics, while others sponsor specialized transition clinics for older children with chronic disease. In most situations, this type of clinic is unnecessary. If the physicians and family have done a good job of preparing them, as they get older these children will make the transition naturally.

When my patients obtain driver's licenses and begin to come alone to their appointments, they quickly recognize their responsibility. Getting the driver's license is the only transitioning experience they need. Just as they can drive themselves to their appointments, they realize that they are responsible for being sure that their blood tests are done in a timely fashion, their prescriptions are obtained or renewed, and their medications are purchased. It's amazing how much more responsible they suddenly become when they can travel independently.

There are physicians who feel that all patients need to be transferred to an internal medicine specialist once they reach a certain age. It is certainly true that patients need to be cared for by a physician who treats them in a manner that is appropriate for their age. If a physician is unable to adapt to patients' changing needs as they grow older, the patients should move on. However, many physicians are quite comfortable caring for patients of diverse ages. Every physician must make this decision personally and be comfortable with it.

If the physician and patient have been working well together and trust each other, it is not necessarily in the patient's best interest to be forced to move on. I have learned a lot about how to deal with younger patients from my patients who have grown up and feel comfortable talking about how they used to feel. If you treat children as responsible participants in their own care from the beginning, nothing necessarily needs to change when they get older. In each case the parents, the patient, and the physician must come to a mutually agreeable arrangement. I have had other patients who clearly felt the need to move on.

Some children with debilitating disease are forced to remain dependent on their parents even when they are clearly no longer children. This is always a difficult situation. Some continue to rely on their parents for all types of support, while others recognize that they qualify for appropriate aid for the disabled (Social Security disability benefits, etc.) and assume responsibility for their own care. If the individual physician is uncomfortable providing the appropriate resources to deal with these issues, it may be best for the patient to be helped through the process by a multidisciplinary team in a transition clinic. Ask your local foundations what resources are available so that you can help the family choose the course that best meets their needs. Do not be afraid to suggest that there are social workers who can help families deal with the system. These people are there to help.

DEPRESSION (PATIENT FATIGUE)

Katherine was a young lady who had suffered from chronic recurrences of dermatomyositis since the age of six. Although she was always the official patient of one of the senior physicians, many of us took care of her during our training. By the time she reached her late teens, she had experienced more hospitalizations and setbacks than anyone could count. However, when I last saw her, she was doing well. Her medications had been reduced to acceptable levels, and she was preparing to go to college. I left and moved on to another institution.

Two years later, she came to the hospital between scheduled visits complaining of symptoms similar to those she had had during a very difficult period. When she asked whether the symptoms might mean that her disease was flaring, she was told that this was possible. She drove her car into a freeway pillar at high speed that afternoon. There were no skid marks. Maybe she just lost control?

I have been discussing how hard it is to be the parent of a child with arthritis. What I have not talked about is how hard it is to be the **child** in this situation. When children are young, their problems are the responsibility of their parents. They expect their parents to help them get better. For most children with arthritis and related conditions, this is possible. The vast majority of the children I care for go on to live productive lives. However, the adolescent years of increasing self-awareness and increasing self-responsibility are difficult for everyone. They are even more difficult for children with chronic disease and require heightened awareness on the part of their physicians.

During the course of a chronic illness, there will be times when a child or young adult becomes depressed. **He or she would be abnormal if this never happened**. Parents and physicians need to pay attention. While a certain amount of depression can affect anyone, it is well known that some adolescents with chronic disease become suicidal. They feel that they have lost control over their lives and cannot see the light at the end of the tunnel. This feeling may take the form of overt actions or simply failure to take their medications. Everyone should be listening for comments such as "It doesn't make any difference," "I don't care anymore," and "Why do I have to come to the doctor?" It's important that parents and physicians know whether the medications are being refilled at appropriate intervals.

No one should try to tell adolescents with chronic disease not to complain. It isn't helpful to tell them that things could be worse. **What adolescents need is someone with whom to discuss their concerns honestly.** It is important to acknowledge their problems while pointing out the positives. It is also important to be proactive. If you are the physician and you must give a child depressing news in the office, talk about it. Don't leave the child to "stew alone." If you think the child is significantly depressed, try to make sure that he or she gets help.

There are psychologists and psychiatrists who specialize in dealing with adolescents and children with chronic illness and their families. Some children can be helped simply by having an honest conversation with their doctor. Others need an outsider to talk to. Some need medication. **It is important to remember that there is no direct correlation between the doctor's view of how well or how badly an adolescent is doing and the adolescent's view.** Parents and physicians must be vigilant.

28

Getting the Best Results

After I get a family settled down and the child's care on the right track, someone frequently asks, "Why do I have to come back so often?" I always compare this to making soup. Anyone can take down a cookbook, read the soup recipe, and get two pounds of beef, a large onion, a carrot, noodles, assorted seasonings, a good-sized pot, and a stove. However, there is a lot of room for interpretation when the instructions say, "Cut up the beef and slice the carrot and onion thinly. Add the ingredients to a large pot with water just to cover. Heat over medium heat for two hours, adjust the seasonings, and serve."

To someone with a lot of experience making soup, those are adequate instructions. If you make soup every day, you know exactly how to do it to get the result you want. But compare two cooks. One cook reads the book, finds the ingredients called for, puts them in a pot of water, sets it on medium heat, and walks away for two hours. The cook who makes soup all the time has picked exactly the beef, onion, and carrot he or she wants and knows how to prepare them for the soup. After the pot is on the stove, the experienced cook checks the soup every ten to fifteen minutes, adjusts the heat, tastes the seasonings, and makes all the other small adjustments that come from experience. Which cook do you think is likely to make the better soup? Similarly, children with rheumatic diseases require continual monitoring, reevaluation, and adjustments for the best outcome. As the primary physician, you have an important role to play in their care. You must help them choose their specialists and interpret what the specialists recommend. If they appear not to be following the specialist's recommendations or keeping appointments, you need to notice and discuss the reasons with them.

Many primary care physicians view their relationship with the specialist as a one-way street. They send the patient to the specialist, and the problem becomes the specialist's. Optimal care requires that both the primary care physician and the specialist view their relationship as a two-way street. The specialist should be communicating with the primary care physician, and when questions or concerns arise, the primary care physician should share his or her concerns, or the family's concerns that have been voiced to him or her, with the specialist. Communication has to be two-way to get the best outcome.

This is the most important chapter in this book. Everyone wants the best results for the children they care for, but not everyone understands that you have to go out and get them. Reading this book means that you are off to a good start. You are reading this book because you want more information. If you were planning a vacation to Hawaii, it would not be a good idea simply to call the first travel agency you found in the phone book or walk into the first one you saw on the street. Most of us would begin by asking our friends if they or someone they knew had been there. Were they pleased with the trip? What airline did they use? Where did they stay? What did they see? Who made the arrangements? Similarly, you should invest as much time as possible in picking the specialist to care for the children you care for.

MAJOR DETERMINANTS OF THE PROJECT OUTCOME

There are three major determinants of the outcome of any project:

- Your level of effort and knowledge
- The level of effort and knowledge of the people who work with you
- Luck

No one can control luck, so it is very important to maximize your efforts and choose carefully the people with whom to work.

CHOOSING A SPECIALIST

You should be looking for the best doctor for the child's problems. It may be the one in your health plan, the one in the same building, the one in the same group, or the one in the same hospital. Or it may not. No one doctor is the right one for everyone.

Children with muscle, bone, joint, or arthritis pain often are sent to an orthopedist for a possible injury. If there is no history of an injury, be suspicious. Some orthopedists have little or no experience with childhood arthritis.

I often see children with arthritis who were originally told that they must have a hairline fracture that did not show up on the X-ray. If the problem is promptly resolved, there is no cause for concern. **If the problem keeps coming back or if there are repeated problems in many joints, a more detailed investigation is needed.** Finding a specialist on your own is not difficult. In every large urban center, there are organizations such as the Arthritis Foundation, the Lupus Foundation, and the American Academy of Pediatrics (see the Appendix). These organizations can direct you to the certified doctors in your area, but they may not be willing to choose among them. See which doctors are associated with the better hospitals in your area. In major cities, there are often newspaper or magazine articles identifying the top doctors. You can even find books listing the top doctors in America. The doctors on these lists are not all the same, but they should be well trained and well regarded in their specialty.

Unless you live in a very small town far away from any large academic center, you want a physician who fulfills the following criteria:

- Is board certified in the specialty
- Preferably is certified in the pediatric specialty (many specialists trained in internal medicine rarely see children)
- Answers your questions and the family's questions in a way you can understand
- Takes time to explain what is happening
- Treats everyone in a way that makes both of you comfortable

AGGRESSIVE VERSUS CONSERVATIVE APPROACHES

Some physicians are very active in their fields They attend the annual scientific meetings of their medical specialties each year, teach at universities, and publish their own work describing advances in the field. Other doctors take care of children the same way they were taught to do during their training many years ago. Fortunately, medicine has been making rapid advances, and there are many new and exciting therapies. You want a specialist who will make sure that the children you refer get the best possible care. They may not be teaching or publishing, but they should be up-to-date.

There are both aggressive and conservative physicians. **What you want is a specialist who is conservative when appropriate and aggressive when appropriate, not one who is always aggressive or always conservative.** Some muscle, bone, and joint diseases tend to resolve over time. These are best treated conservatively. Others get steadily worse, and the longer you wait before you stop them, the more damage accumulates. You need a physician who can tell which is which and respond appropriately.

Second Opinions

One of the most difficult issues for primary care physicians is when the child they referred to a specialist is not getting better. First, be sure that the family is doing what the specialist recommended. If they are, let the specialist know your concerns. Parents are always worried about getting a second opinion. A good doctor knows that the child's health is the most important thing. If a family wants a second opinion, a good specialist will not act insulted. Instead, he or she will encourage the family. However, make sure that the family goes to a well-qualified physician for the second opinion. Ask the family's specialist if they are afraid to do so. If the specialist is confident, he or she will give you the name of someone believed to be a valuable source of further information. If the specialist is not confident or acts insulted, that may be all the more reason to suggest that the family get a second opinion.

CONFLICTING ADVICE

Suppose that you wanted to buy a really good chocolate cake. If you asked your neighbors to recommend a bakery, they might all agree. More likely, they would recommend several different bakeries. If they all agree, it's easy. But suppose you went to the different bakeries and asked each baker how he made his chocolate cake. They probably would not agree on all the ingredients. However, it's unlikely that any of them would stay in business very long if their cakes did not turn out well.

Conflicting advice is one of the hazards of getting a second opinion. What should you do when you get conflicting advice from two different doctors?

Sometimes some of the advice is just plain wrong. However, far more often, it reflects different points of view.

If you get widely differing opinions, discuss them with the physician you trust. Often there are varied approaches. Is the specialist flexible? Can he or she explain the choices? But remember, while either of two different ways to bake a cake may work, a combination of the two often will not.

Frequently, when I am evaluating children for a second opinion, the parents are quite confused if I give advice different from that of the original physician. Rheumatology is not a textbook science. If there were one correct answer, everyone in the field would agree and life would be simple. Parents are confronted by the need to make the right choice for their child. Yet, every physician brings a different level of training and experience to the examining room. As a physician, I can only make sure that I explain the plan well, discuss the options, and explain why I prefer the option I recommend.

In some situations, I recommend a course of treatment that is not in the books. If all the answers were in the books, experience wouldn't count. Since I see children from all over the world with difficult conditions, it is my job to offer the benefit of my experience and to test new ideas. These children were sent to me because the answers in the books didn't work. New therapies that work ultimately make it into the books, but there are often delays of several years between the time when a new therapy is tested and found to work and when it is described in the books.

Some physicians feel that it is up to the parents to decide which treatment plan to follow. They lay out all the options and say, "You choose." If the physicians, with all of their training, cannot agree, how can the parents choose? **Physicians must not take away the parents' ability to choose for their child, but they should certainly accept the responsibility of recommending what they think is the best course.** The primary care physician has an important role in this process. Often he or she is the person the family turns to and asks for help.

There is no easy answer to the problem of conflicting advice. You need to know the doctors' backgrounds and level of training. Is one specialist widely respected in his or her field? Is the specialist someone who is teaching new physicians in the field? Ask these questions. Sometimes the advice that is most difficult to accept is what really needs to done.

FOLLOWING ADVICE AND KEEPING APPOINTMENTS

Mrs. Smith could never understand why Jennie didn't do well. Jennie always seemed to have some type of joint complaint, but every time Mrs. Smith took her to see a doctor, the doctor wanted to do all sorts of blood tests and make Jennie take medicine. Frequently, she'd fill the prescription because Jennie was complaining a lot. But when Jennie wasn't better in two weeks or complained of a stomachache, Mrs. Smith would stop giving her the medicine and cancel the follow-up appointment. After all, there was no sense in going back to have the doctor see how Jennie was doing on the new medicine; she wasn't taking it. After a few months or a year, Jennie's complaints would increase and Mrs. Smith would go back to the doctor and try another medicine for a few weeks, but none of them ever controlled Jennie's arthritis. Mrs. Smith even tried a couple of different doctors. She couldn't understand why Jennie didn't do well in the long run. **You'd think this story couldn't be true, but I've seen and heard it over and over again.**

It may seem obvious, but encouraging your patients to follow the specialist's advice and keep their appointments are the most important things you can do. All of us are a bit lazy. All of us want to believe that the problem will just go away if we ignore it. But if you smelled smoke in your house, would you just ignore it?

All too often, I see children who were supposed to come back in two weeks but who return in six months. They still have the problem. The parents say that the child took a few of the pills and then had a stomachache, so he or she stopped. Instead of calling the doctor to discuss the problem, the parents did nothing until the situation got worse again. The more damage they let accumulate, the harder it is to undo. If parents tell you that they did not like the specialist's advice, encourage them to discuss it with the specialist or find another specialist. Prescriptions left in pockets or purses and pills sitting in bottles in the medicine cabinet will not solve the problem.

Every parent is concerned about giving his or her child medication. Every parent is worried about side effects. These are valid concerns. Medicines do have possible side effects. You need to be sure that your patients are following up with the specialist and that the specialist is monitoring appropriately (see Chapter 23).

However, imagine how silly it would be to let your house burn down because you were afraid of water damage. I have seen many children do poorly because their parents were afraid of the medications and wouldn't give them. If the doctor thought the medicine was a greater risk than the disease, he or she would not recommend it. Primary care physicians have an important role in convincing families to follow through.

PROPER MONITORING

Careful monitoring is the way physicians minimize problems. The reason for periodic blood tests is to detect problems before they become obvious. Encourage families not to skip appointments because the child looks fine. Doing so robs the child of the chance to have a problem detected before it becomes serious. Of course, most children don't experience side effects, but no one knows who will and who will not. By the time a child looks ill, the problem may have progressed to a serious stage that is not easily reversed.

It's easy to skip the periodic monitoring appointments when the child is off medication. However, the same principle applies. We can never be sure that a rheumatic disease is gone forever. If the family did not notice the child's problems at the beginning, will they immediately notice that they have come back? The specialist is trained to detect the earliest signs of disease activity. Do you want to take advantage of his or her skills? The families most likely to skip appointments are the ones in denial, and they are the ones most likely to overlook early symptoms of disease recurrence.

DEALING WITH SCHOOLS

Many children with relatively minor problems have no significant problems at school. But if a child has a chronic condition that is obvious to everyone or even a mild condition that prevents full participation in physical education, the school will need to know. Some schools are extremely obliging, and a note saying that the student should be allowed to "self-limit" in physical education is sufficient. Other schools follow stricter guidelines.

There are a number of things to know when dealing with schools. The most important one is that the Americans with Disabilities Act gave all the power to the family. If a few notes and an occasional phone call are all that is needed, it's great. However, if the school is being difficult, the child may need an individual education plan (IEP), as described below.

For most children with mild to moderate disease, everything can be handled easily. Often these children need some leeway in physical education and perhaps a second set of books so that they do not have to carry a heavy load of books back and forth to school. A note from the doctor's office is often sufficient. If many classes will be missed, or if a child needs extra time to get from class to class or extra time on exams because of difficulty writing, he or she will probably need an IEP. In most districts, this is not a major problem, but IEPs take time and effort and often cost the school district money. If the school administration discourages a family from asking for an IEP because "you do not want to label your child," make sure that the student is getting what he or she needs. If the student's needs are being met, great! Otherwise, push for the IEP.

Remind parents that they are entitled to have a parent advocate present at the IEP meeting. The teachers, the administration, and the counselors will also be there to help devise a good plan. The school district is supposed to supply whatever is necessary to facilitate the child's education. Some parents go too far, but some school districts resist senselessly. A child's basic needs should be met. The IEP should be designed with the child's best interests in mind. Moreover, the rules are slanted in the child's favor. But some school districts "forget" to tell families what they are entitled to. Wise parents speak with their physician and their local specialty society before the meeting. If necessary, lawyers who specialize in representing parents can be present at IEP meetings. Fortunately, they are rarely necessary.

LOCAL HELP ORGANIZATIONS

There are local help organizations for parents of children with a wide variety of conditions. See the Appendix for a listing. These organizations can be very helpful in directing you to other parents who have had similar experiences. They can provide useful information regarding the nature of your child's condition, experienced doctors, and other resources. They can also help you to find experts for dealing with the many problems of insurance, school, and so on. Many of the national help organizations now have Web sites as well.

Appendix: Resources

There are thousands of organizations, Internet sites, books, and similar resources for families of children with musculoskeletal diseases and other problems. It is impossible to list all of them here. I have listed the major organizations and others with which I have worked. I'm sure that this list is incomplete. Many of these organizations have a Web page that may direct you to many others. I have also listed some Internet-based groups that provide support for children with chronic illness and their parents. But be careful: some of the information on the Internet is excellent, but much of it is not reliable.

My own Web page is the pediatric rheumatology home page: http://www.goldscout.com.

There is more information in this book than I can post there, but I regularly update that site with the latest information.

Organizations Dedicated to Helping Children with Musculoskeletal Diseases

Organizations without a Specific Disease Focus

National Institute of Arthritis and Musculoskeletal and Skin Diseases

> (301) 495-4484 or (877) 22-NIAMS (toll free)
> Information Clearinghouse
> National Institutes of Health
> 1 AMS Circle
> Bethesda, MD 20892-3675
> http://www.niams.nih.gov

The Food and Drug Administration (FDA)

> (888) INFO-FDA (1-888-463-6332)
> U.S. Food and Drug Administration
> 5600 Fishers Lane

Rockville, MD 20857-0001

http://www.fda.gov

The American Academy of Pediatrics

(847) 434-4000

National Headquarters:

The American Academy of Pediatrics

141 Northwest Point Boulevard

Elk Grove Village, IL 60007-1098

http://www.aap.org

The American College of Rheumatology

(404) 633-3777

1800 Century Place, Suite 250

Atlanta, GA 30345

http://www.rheumatology.org/index.asp

The American Academy of Orthopedic Surgeons

(847) 823-7186 or (800) 346-AAOS (toll free)

6300 North River Road

Rosemont, IL 60018-4262

http://orthoinfo.aaos.org

Organizations Dedicated Primarily to Arthritic Conditions
(JRA, spondyloarthropathy, ankylosing spondylitis, psoriatic arthritis; information on other conditions may be found at some of these sites, as well.)

The Arthritis Foundation

(800) 283-7800

Arthritis Foundation

P.O. Box 7669

Atlanta, GA 30357-0669

http://www.arthritis.org

The American Juvenile Arthritis Organization (AJAO)

> http://www.arthritis.org/events/ajao_programs_services.asp
>
> The AJAO is now part of the Arthritis Foundation and may be accessed via its contact numbers.

The Arthritis Society of Canada

> (416) 979-7228
>
> The Arthritis Society (National Office)
>
> 393 University Avenue, Suite 1700
>
> Toronto, Ontario M5G 1E6
>
> Canada
>
> http://www.arthritis.ca

Arthritis Insight

> http://www.arthritisinsight.com
>
> This is a Web-based question-and-answer site with information for children and adults.
>
> The children's information is at http://jraworld.arthritisinsight.com.

Creaky Joints

> http://www.creakyjoints.com
>
> This is a site where children, teenagers, and young adults can share ideas, complaints, and the knowledge that they aren't the only ones in the world with arthritis.

The Spondylitis Association of America

> (800) 777-8189
>
> 14827 Ventura Boulevard, #222
>
> Sherman Oaks, CA 91403
>
> http://www.spondylitis.org
>
> This group works with persons with ankylosing spondylitis and spondyloarthropathies.

National Psoriasis Foundation

(503) 244-7404 or (800) 723-9166 (toll free)
6600 SW 92nd Avenue, Suite 300
Portland, OR 97223-7195
http://www.psoriasis.org

Organizations Dedicated Primarily to Vasculitic Diseases
(SLE, scleroderma, KD, dermatomyositis)

The Lupus Foundation of America, Inc.

(301) 670-9292
1300 Piccard Drive, Suite 200
Rockville, MD 20850-4303
http://www.lupus.org

Juvenile Scleroderma Network, Inc.

(310) 519-9511 (phone or fax)
24-hour helpline: (888) 881-2848
1204 West 13th Street
San Pedro, CA 90731
http://www.jsdn.org

The Scleroderma Foundation

(978) 463-5843 or (800) 722-HOPE (4673) (toll free)
12 Kent Way, Suite 101
Byfield, MA 01922
http://www.scleroderma.org

Raynaud's Association

(914) 682-8341; fax (914) 946-4685
94 Mercer Avenue
Hartsdale, NY 10530
http://www.raynauds.org

Kawasaki Disease Foundation

(978) 887-9357

6 Beechwood Circle

Boxford, MA 01921

http://www.kdfoundation.org

The American Behçet's Disease Association

(800)-7behcets

P.O. Box 19952

Amarillo, TX 79114

http://www.behcets.com/home.ivnu

Sjögren's Syndrome Association

(800) 475-6473

8120 Woodmont Avenue, Suite 530

Bethesda, MD 20814

http://www.sjogrens.org/

The Myositis Association

(202) 887-0082

1233 20th Street NW, Suite 402

Washington, DC 20036

http://www.myositis.org

Organizations Dedicated to Other Diseases

Genzyme Corporation

(617) 252-7500

500 Kendal Street

Cambridge, MA 02142

http://www.genzyme.com/patient/patient_home.asp

Although this is a corporate Web site, it provides a wealth of information for patients with rare genetic syndromes that may be mistaken for rheumatic diseases (fibromyalgia, chronic fatigue syndrome, etc.).

The Chronic Fatigue and Immune Dysfunction Syndrome Association

(800) 442-3437

The CFIDS Association of America, Inc.

P.O. Box 220398

Charlotte, NC 28222-0398

http://www.cfids.org/

The American Fibromyalgia Syndrome Association

(520) 733-1570

AFSA, Inc.

6380 East Tanque Verde, Suite D

Tucson, AZ 85715

http://www.afsafund.org

The National Fibromyalgia Association

(714) 921-0150

2238 N. Glassell Street, Suite D

Orange, CA 92865

http://fmaware.org/index.html

The Pediatric Network

http://www.pediatricnetwork.org/index.htm

This site is intended for children with fibromyalgia, chronic fatigue syndrome, and related conditions and their families.

Specialized Laboratories for Rheumatic Disease Testing (Selected List)

Rheumatology Diagnostics Laboratory

(310) 253-5466 or (800) 338-1918 (toll free)

RDL, Inc.

10755 Venice Boulevard

Los Angeles, CA 90034

http://www.rdlinc.com

Specialty Laboratories

(800) 421-7110

2211 Michigan Avenue

Santa Monica, CA 90404-3900

http://www.specialtylabs.com/contact_us.asp

Prometheus Laboratories, Inc.

(888) 423-5227

5739 Pacific Center Boulevard

San Diego, CA 92121-4203

http://www.prometheuslabs.com

Mayo Medical Laboratories

Multiple sites and phone numbers.

See the Web page for details for your area.

http://www.mayoreferenceservices.org/mml/index.asp

Miscellaneous Resources

Individual Education Plans (504)
(There are many organizations discussing IEPs found on the Web, but I have no recommendation for a particular one.)

"A Guide to the Individualized Education Program by the Office of Special Education and Rehabilitation Services U.S. Department of Education" (July 2000)
http://www.ed.gov/offices/OSERS/OSEP/Products/IEP_Guide

Parent Advocacy Coalition for Educational Rights

(952) 838-9000

8161 Normandale Boulevard

Minneapolis, MN 55437

http://www.pacer.org

Other School-Related Issues

"Bandaids and Blackboards"
Joan Fleitas, Ed.D., R.N, Associate Professor of Nursing
Fairfield University
Fairfield, CT 06430
http://www.lehman.cuny.edu/faculty/jfleitas/bandaides/
This site is dedicated to helping children with chronic disease and their
parents deal with school-related issues.

Information for Patients on Various Medical Procedures

The virtual hospital total hip replacement page:
http://www.vh.org/adult/patient/orthopaedics/hipreplace/index.html
The virtual hospital total knee replacement page:
http://www.vh.org/adult/patient/orthopaedics/kneereplacement/index.html
The virtual hospital has a variety of other useful pages found at
http://www.vh.org

Textbooks for Physicians

Anderson, Steven J., and J. Andy Sullivan, eds. *Care of the Young Athlete.*
Rosemont, IL: American Academy of Pediatrics and American Academy of
Orthopedic Surgeons, 2000.

Cassidy, J., and R. Petty. *Textbook of Pediatric Rheumatology*, 4th ed. Philadel-
phia: W.B. Saunders, 2001. This is the standard textbook. All of the
rheumatic diseases discussed here are covered, with many references.

Greene, Walter B., M.D., ed. *Essentials of Musculoskeletal Care*, 2nd ed. Rosemont, IL: American Academy of Pediatrics and American Academy of
Orthopedic Surgeons, 2001.

Isenberg, David A., Patricia Woo, and P. J. Maddison, eds. *Oxford Textbook of
Rheumatology*, 2nd ed. New York: Oxford University Press, 1998.

Books for Parents

Aldape, Virginia Tortorica, and Lillian S. Kossacoff. *Nicole's Story: A Book About a Girl with Juvenile Rheumatoid Arthritis.* Minneapolis: Lerner Publications, 1996.

Horstman, Judith, William J. Arnold, Brian Berman, J. Roger Hollister, and Matthew H. Liang, eds. *The Arthritis Foundation's Guide to Alternative Therapies.* Atlanta: Arthritis Foundation and Longstreet Press, 1999.

Lane, Nancy E., ed. *The Osteoporosis Book.* New York: Oxford University Press, 1998.

Lockshin, Michael. *Guarded Prognosis: A Doctor and His Patients Talk About Chronic Disease and How to Cope with It.* New York: Hill & Wang, 1998.

Wallace, Daniel J. *The Lupus Book: A Guide for Patients and Their Families.* New York: Oxford University Press, 2000.

Wallace, Daniel J., and Janice Brock Wallace. *All About Fibromyalgia.* New York: Oxford University Press, 2002.

Index

reactive or infection-associated arthritis, 94,
110–111, 136–139, 145, 153
Reiter's syndrome, 138–139
shoulder pain as symptom of, 59
temporomandibular joint pain (jaw pain), 99
uveitis with, 131
Spondyloepipheseal dysplasia tarda, 33
Spondylolisthesis, 42–43, 75–76
Spontaneous abortions, 356
Sports drinks, 341
Sports injuries. *See* Athletic-related injuries
"Spot" protein/Cr ratios, 361
Sprains, 48, 61
ssDNA (single-stranded DNA), 349
Staphylococcal bacteria, 33, 44, 45
Sterility, 189, 192, 289
Sternocleidomastoid muscle. *See* Necks
Stiff neck, 98
Stomachs. *See* Gastrointestinal conditions
Storage diseases, 67
Strains, 48, 61, 73–75
Streptococcal infections, 33, 149–150
Stress fractures, 72–73, 82, 261, 262
Stress ulcers, 178
Stretch marks, 190
Strokes, 174
Subacute bacterial endocarditis (SBE), 174, 353
Subcutaneous or intramuscular calcifications,
230–231, 234
Submandibular gland, 200
Subtalar joints, 54–55
Sucralfate (carafate), 286
Suicide, 374–375
Sulfa drugs, 285, 286
Sulfasalazine (azulfidine), 286–287
for infection-associated arthritis, 138
for psoriatic arthritis, 141, 142–143
for resistant JA, 119
side effects, 132, 286–287
for spondyloarthropathy, 131–132, 286
Sun exposure, 162, 288, 291
Supplements. *See also* Vitamins (multi), 322–329
accuracy of labels, 323–324
body builder supplements, 341
disclosure to physicians, 329
fatty acid supplementation, 326
food supplements, 224
glucosamine, 325–326

herbal supplements, 12, 224
overview of, 316–317
risk of side effects, 276
sports drinks, 341
Surgical treatment. *See also* Reconstructive surgery
for infection-associated arthritis, 138
for pauciarticular-onset juvenile
arthritis, 100–101
polyarticular-onset juvenile arthritis, 107–108
for psoriatic arthritis, 143
for systemic-onset juvenile arthritis, 116
Sympathetic effusion, 27
Synechiae (see also uveitis), 98
Synovectomies, 26, 101, 133
Synovial fluid, 22, 332–333, 362–363
Synovitis in the hip, 148–149
Synovium. *See also* Uveitis, 123
Syphilis, 156–157, 356
Systemic lupus erythematosus (SLE), 160–194
adjunctive therapies, 191–192
albumin loss, 342
anti-Ro antibodies, 193
cardiac involvement, 173–174
central nervous system abnormalities, 170–173
clotting system: antiphospholipid syndrome,
177–178
complications in childhood, 184–185
described, 160–162
diagnosis, 154, 162–166
drug-induced SLE, 183–184, 288
eye complications, 124
gastrointestinal system involvement, 178–180
as genetic condition, 161, 165–166
in girls, 177
hematologic involvement, 176–177
IBD associated with, 145
joint replacements, 180–181
laboratory tests and typical patterns of disease,
181–183
liver involvement with, 179, 191
MCTD mistakenly associated with, 195, 196
neonatal systemic lupus erythematosus,
193–194
prognosis, 192–193
PSS associated with, 220
pulmonary involvement, 175–176
Raynaud's syndrome associated with, 205